Library of Congress Cataloging-in-Publication Data

Bonci, Leslie.
 Sport nutrition for coaches / Leslie Bonci.
   p. cm.
 Includes bibliographical references and index.
 ISBN-13: 978-0-7360-6917-5 (soft cover)
 ISBN-10: 0-7360-6917-8 (soft cover)
 1. Athletes--Nutrition. 2. High school athletes--Nutrition. I. Title.
 TX361.A8B66 2009
 613.7'11--dc22

                                                    2008043483

ISBN-10: 0-7360-6917-8 (print)   ISBN-10: 0-7360-8610-2 (Adobe PDF)
ISBN-13: 978-0-7360-6917-5 (print)   ISBN-13: 978-0-7360-8610-3 (Adobe PDF)

The Web addresses cited in this text were current as of October 2008, unless otherwise noted.

Acquisitions Editors: Patricia Sammann and Nate Bell; **Managing Editors:** Pamela Mazurak and Carla Zych; **Copyeditor:** Julie Anderson; **Proofreader:** Anne Meyer Byler; **Indexer:** Nan N. Badgett; **Permission Manager:** Martha Gullo; **Graphic Designer:** Robert Reuther; **Graphic Artist:** Julie L. Denzer; **Cover Designer:** Keith Blomberg; **Photographer (cover):** © Human Kinetics; **Photographer (interior):** © Human Kinetics unless otherwise noted; **Photo Asset Manager:** Laura Fitch; **Visual Production Assistant:** Joyce Brumfield; **Photo Production Manager:** Jason Allen; **Art Manager:** Kelly Hendren; **Illustrators:** Alan L. Wilborn unless otherwise noted; F 2.1 (page 11) Alan L. Wilborn and Denise Lowry; **Printer:** Versa Press

Copies of this book are available at special discounts for bulk purchase for sales promotions, premiums, fund-raising, or educational use. Special editions or book excerpts can also be created to specifications. For details, contact the Special Sales Manager at Human Kinetics.

Printed in the United States of America   10 9 8 7 6 5 4 3 2 1
The paper in this book is certified under a sustainable forestry program.

Human Kinetics
Web site: www.HumanKinetics.com

United States: Human Kinetics
P.O. Box 5076
Champaign, IL 61825-5076
800-747-4457
e-mail: humank@hkusa.com

Canada: Human Kinetics
475 Devonshire Road Unit 100
Windsor, ON N8Y 2L5
800-465-7301 (in Canada only)
e-mail: info@hkcanada.com

Europe: Human Kinetics
107 Bradford Road
Stanningley
Leeds LS28 6AT, United Kingdom
+44 (0) 113 255 5665
e-mail: hk@hkeurope.com

Australia: Human Kinetics
57A Price Avenue
Lower Mitcham, South Australia 5062
08 8372 0999
e-mail: info@hkaustralia.com

New Zealand: Human Kinetics
Division of Sports Distributors NZ Ltd.
P.O. Box 300 226 Albany
North Shore City
Auckland
0064 9 448 1207
e-mail: info@humankinetics.co.nz

Sport Nutrition for Coaches

Lesli   **LDN**

*I dedicate this book to all the athletes, coaches, and athletic directors who have had
a profound influence on my sport nutrition career. You have made me a better professional.*

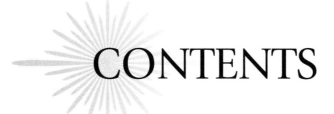

CONTENTS

ASEP Gold Level Series Preface vii
Preface ix
Acknowledgments xi
Creating a Coach's Notebook xii

PART I   Essential Concepts   1

Chapter 1   Sport Performance and Energy Systems 3
Getting Energy for Exercise   4
Matching Energy Systems to Sports   6

Chapter 2   Foods That Fuel 9
Carbohydrate   11
Fat (Lipids)   17
Protein   21
Striking a Nutrient Balance   25

Chapter 3   Eating Timed for Top Performance 35
Pre-Exercise Eating   36
Pre-Event Eating   39
Postexercise Eating   42
Getting Athletes to Eat   44

Chapter 4   Hydrating for Top Performance 47
Why Do Athletes Become Dehydrated?   48
What Should Athletes Drink?   49
How Much Should Athletes Drink?   50
What Are Salty Sweaters?   52
What About Caffeine and Alcohol?   53
How Can You Get Athletes to Hydrate?   53

Chapter 5   Reducing Body Fat 55
Assess Where the Athlete Is   57
Consider Diet Options   69
Create an Action Plan   74
Seek Referrals   77

Chapter 6   Increasing Muscle Mass..................**81**

How Can Athletes Add Muscle Mass?   82
Determine a Starting Point   83
Set Up an Exercise Regimen   86
Implement an Action Plan   87
Decide What and When Your Athlete Should Eat   89

Chapter 7   Sizing Up Supplements **99**

Vitamins and Minerals   101
Other Common Supplements   105
Supplement Safety   109
Anabolic Steroids   109
Supplement Legality   112
Supplement Education   113

PART II   Special Situations   117

Chapter 8   Preventing Common Complaints **119**

Muscle Cramps   120
Gastrointestinal Distress   122
Hitting the Wall or Bonking   126

Chapter 9   Coping With Special Diets **129**

Vegetarian and Vegan Diets   130
Diets for Athletes With Diabetes or Hypoglycemia   136
Food Allergies and Food Intolerances   143
Religious Diets and Fasts   144

Chapter 10   Dealing With Disordered Eating............**147**

Eating Disorders   149
Female Athlete Triad   152
Fostering a Positive Eating Environment   155
Getting Help for Your Athletes With Eating Disorders   157
Including Parents in Treatment   158

Chapter 11   Dealing With Alcohol Use **163**

What Alcohol Does in the Short Term   165
What Alcohol Does in the Long Term   166
Talking to Your Athletes About Alcohol   167
Setting Team Policies on Alcohol   169

PART III   Planning Tools   173

Chapter 12   Facing Logistic Challenges **175**

Off-Season Nutrition   176
Athletes' Busy Schedules   177
Institutional Food   178
Nutrition on the Road   180

Chapter 13   Budgeting Good Nutrition **185**

Packing Food for Contests   186
Getting Help from Families and the Booster Club   187
Choosing Affordable (and Healthy) Chain Restaurants   188
Negotiating Food Budgets   188

Chapter 14   Implementing a Sport Nutrition Plan **191**

Creating a Sport Nutrition Game Plan   192
Getting Athletes and Parents to Buy In   195
Presenting Nutrition Information   195
Providing Incentives for Good Nutrition   198
A Final Word   198

Appendix A: Restaurant Dining Guidelines 201
Appendix B: Performance Eating Handouts 204
Appendix C: Nutrition Screening Form 236
Appendix D: Answers to Game Plan Questions 241
Glossary 246
Bibliography 249
Index 251
About the Author 256

ASEP GOLD LEVEL SERIES PREFACE

The American Sport Education Program (ASEP) Gold Level curriculum is a series of practical upper-level texts that provide coaches and students with an applied approach to sport performance. The curriculum is designed for coaches and for college upper-level undergraduates and graduate students pursuing professions as coaches, physical education teachers, and sport fitness practitioners.

For instructors of college courses, the ASEP Gold Level curriculum provides an excellent alternative to other formal texts. Most undergraduate students complete basic courses in exercise physiology, mechanics, motor learning, and sport psychology—courses that are focused on research and theory. As students move into more complex areas of study, many want to know how to apply what they learn in the classroom to what they can teach or coach on the court or playing field. ASEP's Gold Level series addresses this need by making some of the higher levels of sport science easier to understand and apply to enhance sport performance. The Gold Level series is specifically designed to introduce these topics to students in an applied manner. Students will find the information and examples user-friendly and easy to apply in the sport setting.

The ASEP Gold Level sport science curriculum includes the following:

Sport Nutrition for Coaches—This text not only covers the fundamentals of sport nutrition but also describes practical ways to use this information to improve athletes' performance and health.

Social Issues for Coaches—In this book, the findings of sociology related to common coaching issues are described and then translated into guidelines that coaches can use when working with athletes, their parents, and the school or sport organization.

Risk Management for Coaches—A coach's legal and ethical responsibilities to control risk to athletes are explained, followed by practical steps coaches can take to ensure players' safety.

In addition, sport-specific books providing advanced knowledge of conditioning and instructional methods will be part of the Gold Level.

A variety of educational elements make these texts student- and instructor-friendly:

- Learning objectives introduce each chapter.
- Sidebars illustrate sport-specific applications of key concepts and principles.
- Coach's Notebook actions appear throughout the text, where they are marked with a special icon. By writing the results of these actions in a notebook, coaches will create a personalized handbook for working with their team.
- Coach's To Do Lists provide steps that coaches can take to apply the content of the chapter to their coaching.
- Chapter summaries review the key points covered in the chapter and are linked to the chapter objectives by content and sequence.
- Key terms at the end of most chapters list the terms introduced in that chapter and remind coaches and students that these are important words to know. The first occurrence of the word in the chapter is boldfaced, and the words also appear in the glossary.

- Game Plan Questions at the end of each chapter allow coaches and students to check their comprehension of the chapter's contents. Answers to questions appear at the back of the book.
- A glossary defines all of the key terms covered in the book.
- Appendixes provide useful tools, such as guidelines to healthy eating in restaurants.

- A general index lists subjects covered in the book.

These texts are also the basis for a series of Gold Level online courses to be developed by Human Kinetics. These courses will be offered through ASEP's Online Education Center for coaches and students who wish to increase their knowledge through practical and applied study of the sport sciences.

PREFACE

Everyone knows that food is essential to survival, but few of your athletes realize that what, when, and how much they eat and drink may be the difference between optimal and subpar performance. *Sport Nutrition for Coaches* is designed to help you provide practical, concise, realistic, and positive nutrition strategies for your athletes. As a high school or college coach, you assume the roles of educator, enforcer, counselor, and role model. Your ability to provide your athletes with sound, practical, and safe sport nutrition information can enhance their health, growth, and sport performance.

Many obstacles prevent athletes from eating an optimal diet. These obstacles include misinformation about fluid and food requirements. Many athletes place a negative focus on eating—what not to do, rather than what *to* do—and want the outcome (increased muscle mass) without going through the process (eating more and strength training).

Many athletes focus more on what to eat than on the timing and quantity of intake. Another concern involves abnormal or harmful eating behaviors and weight issues: These can destroy team dynamics, carry serious health consequences, and impair performance. Other variables that affect performance include supplement use and alcohol use and abuse.

You may have athletes on your team who are not in the best physical condition. A summer spent indoors can be a recipe for disaster on the first day of practice, especially under hot and humid conditions. Some athletes have pre-existing medical issues, including asthma, diabetes, and food allergies. Some athletes may be latchkey kids who are responsible for their own meals, and some athletes may be vegans whose diets do not meet their nutritional needs.

You may have athletes on your teams whose parents follow special diets that are not appropriate for your athletes.

To effectively educate athletes on the benefits of sport nutrition, you need to have your own house in order. This doesn't mean eating perfectly, but do you walk the talk? Do you eat small, frequent meals? Do you eat something before and after practice? Do you take supplements? Do you review any supplements that athletes want to take *before* they take them? Do you weigh your athletes or give weight recommendations? Do you encourage fluid breaks during practice and insist that your athletes come to practice hydrated and fueled?

Because most of you travel with your athletes, you need to think about eating on the road. Do you travel with snacks or tell your athletes to bring snacks? Do you get your booster clubs involved with pregame meals and snacks? Do you educate your athletes about eating on the road, including how to make healthy choices in restaurants?

This book addresses all aspects of sport nutrition by providing answers to the questions you hear from your athletes most often. It also address some of the most common nutrition mistakes that athletes make and gives you guidelines on how to advise your athletes. I work with and speak to coaches daily, and I've included information on select sport nutrition topics that coaches often ask about. I've also included examples from real-life consultations with athletes to show you how what you learn can be applied to your players. The goal is not to make you a sport dietitian. But because you spend a lot of time with your athletes and they value what you say, you owe it to them to be their nutrition coach.

Most coaches and athletes are looking for information on gaining the performance edge. Oftentimes, this involves tweaking the diet rather than totally overhauling it. No one has the time or desire to spend all day thinking about what and when to eat, but if eating is always an afterthought, the effects on sport performance may include a decrease in strength, speed, stamina, and recovery and an increase in injuries—not a recipe for success.

Sport Nutrition for Coaches can help your athletes reach their potential. Eating and hydrating before practice improves mental and physical performance and decreases the risk of injury. Your athletes' well-being is a priority to you and your institution, so you must ensure that your athletes' nutritional needs are met.

This book is divided into three sections:

Part I: Essential Concepts—This section covers fueling essential for your athletes. Topics include energy needs for exercise, fuel sources for sport, timing of eating to optimize performance, and hydration needs. This section also addresses weight management and supplements.

Part II: Special Situations—This section addresses common complaints such as muscle cramps and gastrointestinal distress and provides guidance on how to address nutrition needs in athletes who are vegetarian, have diabetes, are hypoglycemic, have food allergies, or need to fast for religious reasons. This section also addresses eating disorders and alcohol use.

Part III: Planning Tools—The final section covers day-to-day issues such as eating on the road, food budgets, and program implementation. Strategies are presented for teaching parents and athletes about the importance of fueling appropriately for sport.

Throughout each chapter are suggestions for using what you've learned in real-life activities to help your team succeed. These are marked with this special icon:

If you combine the results of these activities into a Coach's Notebook, you'll have a resource that will help you promote good nutrition for your athletes year-round.

At the beginning of each chapter is a list of learning objectives. A summary is provided at the end of each chapter, followed by a list of key terms (introduced in the chapter in boldfaced type) that are commonly used in sport nutrition instruction. Also included are a number of Game Plan Questions you can use to check your comprehension of the chapter's content and your ability to apply it in your teaching. At the end of the book you will find appendixes, a glossary that contains all the terms introduced in the chapters, references, and an index. Throughout the book you will find additional resources such as Web sites, articles, and books of interest.

Finally, keep this in mind:

If you resist, don't expect your athletes to make nutrition a priority.

If you insist, your athletes will listen.

If you persist, proper fueling and hydration will become a regular part of training.

ACKNOWLEDGMENTS

I would like to thank all the coaches in my life:

My life coaches—my husband Fred, sons Gregory and Cary, parents Annabelle and Jay Joseph, and brother Louis Joseph—for your love, support, patience, humor, and understanding.

My writing coaches—Pat Samman, Pam Mazurak, and Carla Zych at Human Kinetics—for your guidance, suggestions, and commitment to bringing this book to fruition.

My professional coaches—Nancy DiMarco, sports dietitian and professor of nutrition and food sciences, Texas Women's University; Dr. Freddie Fu, chairman, department of orthopedic surgery, University of Pittsburgh Medical Center; and Christine Bonci, co-director, division on athletic training and sports medicine, University of Texas—for your encouragement, enthusiasm, insight, and feedback.

My real-world coaches—
from the university of Pittsburgh: Coach Buddy Morris, Coach Dave Wannstedt, Coach Marian Clark, Coach Chuck Knoles, Coach Alonzo Webb, Coach Joe Jordano, Coach Jamie Dixon, Coach Agnus Berenato, Coach Joe Luxbacher, Coach George Dieffenbach, and Coach Debbie Yohman;
from the University of Texas: Coach Jeff Madden;
from the University of Florida: Coach Mickey Marotti;
from the Pittsburgh Pirates: Coach Frank Velasquez and Coach Chris Dunaway;
from the Milwaukee Brewers: Coach Chris Joyner;
from the Pittsburgh Steelers: Coach Mike Tomlin, Coach Dick LeBeau, Coach John Mitchell, (former head) Coach Bill Cowher, and (former strength) Coach Chet Fuhrman;
and all the collegiate, club, and high school coaches who trusted me with their athletes—for the real-life experiences you've shared with me and the value you place on the role of sport nutrition in helping your athletes to succeed.

Thank you all for being part of my team.

CREATING A COACH'S NOTEBOOK

Throughout this book we've noted ways that you can work good nutrition into your sport program using what you've learned in each chapter. Each activity is marked with an icon:

If you do each of these activities, write up the results, and keep them in a notebook, you'll build your own individualized manual to guide you in working with your current team (and future ones as well).

To create your notebook, set up the following tabs:

- Start-Up Activities
- Off-Season Activities
- Preseason Activities
- Beginning-of-Season Activities
- Season-Long Activities
- Activities for Athletes Who Want to Lose Fat
- Activities for Athletes Who Want to Gain Mass

Each activity will state the tab under which the completed activity should be filed. For example, the following activity would be filed under Beginning-of-Season Activities:

> *Explain the importance of hydration to your athletes. Educate them on appropriate fluid choices. (Beginning-of-Season Activities)*

You may want to order the results even further within each tabbed section. Here's a suggested table of contents for your notebook:

Start-Up Activities

- Identify which energy systems are most used in your sport and what nutrients fuel them. (chapter 1)
- Become familiar with your sport's list of banned substances. (chapter 7)
- Identify which common complaints are most widely seen in your sport. (chapter 8)
- If your school or organization does not have a written policy banning steroid use, consider developing one in conjunction with your school's or organization's administrators, the athletic staff, and student and parent representatives. (chapter 7)
- Learn about your school's or organization's policy on student-athlete alcohol use. If no policy exists or you believe the existing policy should be changed, meet with administrators to develop a more appropriate policy. (chapter 11)
- Create a sport nutrition game plan. Describe that game plan to parents and athletes during the preseason meeting. (chapter 14)
- Design an incentive program to encourage athletes to eat and drink properly. (chapter 14)
- Develop a list of dietitians and other health professionals in your area to whom you could refer your athletes. (chapter 5)

Off-Season Activities

- Develop and provide your athletes with guidelines for off-season nutrition. (chapter 2)

- Encourage athletes who want to lose body fat or gain muscle mass to work on their goals in the off-season under the supervision of a health professional. (chapters 5 and 6)

- Send out a letter to all athletes one week before the start of preseason reminding them to eat and drink before practice and to bring snacks and fluids to practice. (chapter 3)

- Have returning athletes calculate their sweat rate for a few days prior to the start of preseason so that they know how much fluid they are going to need during practice. (chapter 4)

Preseason Activities

- Arrange for students to be able to eat in the period before practice during the school year. (chapter 3)

- Brainstorm ideas on how to supply and prepare the necessary food. Consider resources such as parents, the booster club, local grocery stores, and restaurants. (chapter 13)

- Before the season begins, sit down with your coaching staff and determine your food budget. Be sure to include snacks for both practices and competitions, along with meals while on the road. (chapter 13)

- Before the season begins, have your athletes fill out a preseason nutrition screening form. In addition, ask your athletes to complete a three-day food diary. Review the results and discuss any food issues with the athletes individually. (chapter 10)

- Identify any athletes on your team who need special diets. (chapter 9)

- During the preseason parent meeting, describe the school's or organization's alcohol policy. Have students and their parents sign a contract stating that they understand and will follow the policy. (chapter 11)

- At the beginning of the season, provide athletes and their parents a written policy banning steroid use and have every athlete fill out a supplement and medication form. Follow up with athletes as necessary. (chapter 7)

- Create a nutrition plan for a typical road trip using the food guidelines in this chapter. For example, select what types of food to bring in the vehicle, determine what restaurants are available on the road, and decide how to handle any anticipated logistic issues. (chapter 12)

Beginning-of-Season Activities

- Have players fill out the food frequency form. Also give them the handouts on proper fueling for male and female athletes. Ask the players to compare their food frequency form results to the handouts. (chapter 2)

- Post or hand out the ratings for food choices table so that your players can make proper food and beverage choices. (chapter 2)

- Explain the importance of hydration to your athletes. Educate them on appropriate fluid choices. (chapter 4)

- Have athletes weigh themselves before and after exercise to determine their sweat rate. (chapter 4)

- Identify athletes who are salty sweaters and teach them how to take in more salt. (chapter 8)

- Educate athletes on ways to prevent food-borne illness. (chapter 8)

- Have athletes identify when and what to eat before and during exercise. (chapter 8)

- Make 30-gram carbohydrate snacks available to athletes during exercise or encourage athletes to bring their own snacks. Another option is to designate one player, each practice, to provide a snack for the rest of the team. (chapter 8)

- Assign someone on your staff to do blood glucose checks on diabetic athletes. (chapter 9)

- Ask diabetic athletes to track their eating and exercise using the blood glucose monitoring form. (chapter 9)

- Have 15-gram carbohydrate foods available at all times to treat hypoglycemia. Have a glucagon injection and someone who knows how to administer it on hand. (chapter 9)

- Make a list of all your athletes' food allergies and food intolerances. Keep these in mind when providing food before, during, or after practice and on the road. (chapter 9)

- Meet with food service staff and a team member to plan what healthy foods to offer and how to present them. (chapter 12)

Season-Long Activities

- Implement a firm policy of "No eat, no play." (chapter 3)

- Give players multiple fluid breaks during practice. (chapter 4)

- Make sure that players rehydrate after exercise. (chapter 4)
- Remind your athletes with diabetes to take in carbohydrate and fluid during exercise. (chapter 9)
- Encourage salty sweaters to consume salty foods or drinks following exercise. (chapter 4)
- Discuss supplement and steroid use with athletes during the season and encourage them to talk with you about supplements before beginning to use them. (chapter 7)
- Have athletes compare the cost of supplements with the cost of foods with similar nutrients. (chapter 7)
- Educate athletes about how supplements can contribute to digestive distress. (chapter 8)
- Encourage athletes to bring familiar foods and a good gut travel kit on road trips. (chapter 8)
- Educate vegetarian athletes about nonmeat sources of protein and vitamins. (chapter 9)
- Locate a sports dietitian in your area and have her discuss with your team the role of food in sport performance. (chapter 10)
- Post signs and posters reminding athletes to eat and drink for performance. Allow your athletes to decide which phrases or messages to use. (chapter 14)
- Select a few easy-to-prepare, healthy food recipes. You or a parent, chef, or dietitian can teach athletes how to prepare the recipes. (chapter 12)
- Have your athletes complete the alcohol questionnaire from the DISCUS tool kit. Following a review of the answers, invite a guest speaker to address the performance and health consequences of alcohol use. (chapter 11)
- If you suspect any of your athletes have an eating disorder, talk with them individually. Make it clear that they will retain their place on the team, but that their health comes before participation in sports. Form a treatment team for each athlete, and include parents in the treatment. (chapter 10)

- Plan a recognition event for parents during the season or at the end of the season to show your appreciation for their role on the sport nutrition team. (chapter 14)

Activities for athletes who want to lose fat (chapter 5)

- Have a health professional assess the athletes' weight and body composition.
- Assess your athletes' caloric expenditure by having them keep an activity log.
- Have the athletes keep a food diary for one week. Also, ask them to fill out a food pattern form and the eating style questionnaire. Review the results with the athletes.
- Set up individual meetings with athletes to discuss their reasons for wanting to lose weight.
- Select and form a weight-loss team to monitor and support your athletes.
- Talk with athletes about how to decrease their number of calories eaten daily.

Activities for athletes who want to gain mass (chapter 6)

- Have a health professional assess the athletes' weight and body composition.
- Assess the athletes' caloric expenditure by having them keep an activity log.
- Develop a strength training plan for athletes who want to increase mass.
- Select and form a weight-gain team to monitor and support your athletes.
- Have the athletes keep a food diary for one week.
- Encourage athletes to gradually increase the number of times a day they eat.
- Set up individual meetings with athletes to discuss how to increase the number of calories eaten daily.

Use the Coach's Notebook you create to help present sport nutrition concepts to your team so your players can eat right, stay hydrated, and perform at their very best.

PART I

Essential Concepts

As a coach, you need to know the basics of nutrition and how it affects your athletes' performance. In this section you'll learn how to use nutrition to get your team working optimally. Chapter 1, Sport Performance and Energy Systems, begins with an explanation of how the body gets the energy needed during exercise and which energy systems are most used in each sport. In chapter 2, Foods That Fuel, you are introduced to the three major food components—carbohydrate, protein, and fat—and learn how much and what types of each component are needed for good health and sport performance. Another important aspect of eating for performance is selecting when and what to eat before, during, and after exercise; this topic is covered in chapter 3, Eating Timed for Top Performance. An often overlooked part of nutrition is hydration. In chapter 4, Hydrating for Top Performance, you find out what causes athletes to become dehydrated and what types of liquids athletes should drink when they exercise, as well as when and how much. It even includes information on salt, caffeine, and alcohol intake.

Often when athletes report for the new season you find that they've gained too much weight or need to build more muscle. That's where chapters 5, Reducing Body Fat, and 6, Increasing Muscle Mass, come in. Both chapters lay out, step-by-step, how to work with health professionals to help your athletes meet their weight goals for play. An issue frequently related to building muscle mass is the use of supplements, and in chapter 7, Sizing Up Supplements, you find out which supplements are and aren't effective. You also get information on the safety and legality of supplement use, as well as ideas for educating your athletes about supplement use and prohibiting the use of steroids.

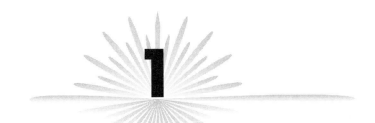

Sport Performance and Energy Systems

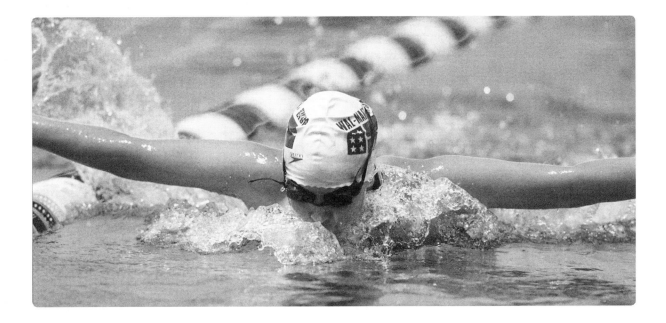

Marty is a freshman on his high school swim team. In the eighth grade he was a standout in school as well as on his club team, and his coach told him he had a chance to make varsity. Marty started to show up early to morning practices and swim laps for 30 minutes before practice began. He also swam extra after evening practices and on the weekends. As his time spent in the water increased, his performance decreased. His times were slower, he didn't sleep well, his appetite was almost nonexistent, and he complained of a rapid heartbeat when he woke up.

His parents and the coach were very concerned, and the athletic trainer at school suggested that Marty see a sports medicine physician. Marty was diagnosed with overtraining. His body was working overtime without sufficient rest or fuel. He was told to cut back on his time in the water and fuel his body better. As a result, his times improved, he felt better, and he ended up making varsity!

When you finish reading this chapter, you should be able to explain

- the nutrients that athletes need to fuel exercise,
- the energy systems involved in exercise, and
- which energy systems are used in which sports.

It takes more than talent, practice, and perseverance to create a good athlete—it also takes good nutrition. The amount and type of food and drink that your athletes consume, as well as when they consume these items, affect the output of the energy systems that athletes need for exercise. When a baseball pitcher throws, the efficacy of his pitch isn't determined just by the number of hours he spent perfecting his technique or the amount of weight he lifted; his pitch is also influenced by how fast his muscles contract and how many muscle fibers contract, and these factors depend on the amount of fuel available in those muscles. Nutrition plays a large part in how well energy is stored and transferred during sport performance.

Most sport activity is fueled by a combination of aerobic and anaerobic energy systems, which require different types and amounts of energy (or fuel). In addition, the body's ability to digest, absorb, and use nutrients affects performance. Athletes need to realize what types and amounts of energy their sports require for optimum performance over the course of the season. You may have athletes who feel great and perform well in the preseason, or early season, only to take a nosedive halfway through. The energy that they need is not going to come from a bar, a can, or a pill but rather from consistent fueling of the body with appropriate food as well as adequate rest and recovery.

Getting Energy for Exercise

When athletes move, chemical reactions occur in the body at the cellular level whereby energy is stored and released so that the muscles can continue to work. These reactions are called **metabolism.** They break down nutrients to release energy (**catabolism**) or to synthesize fuel or build body tissues (**anabolism**). Both of these processes are important components

of exercise, and they can occur together. For example, strength training is catabolic, making fuel available to the muscles so they can move, as well as anabolic, making muscles grow in size in response to lifting and to the intake of adequate protein and calories. Eating also can be anabolic; the carbohydrate in a granola bar eaten after exercise can help resynthesize fuel that will be available to the muscles for the next practice session. Food consumed before or during exercise is broken down into smaller components, or nutrients, and stored by the cells so that energy can be released to fuel the physically active body.

The major fuel source for the cell is the molecule called **adenosine triphosphate (ATP).** When the bonds of this molecule are broken, it releases large amounts of energy. ATP provides the energy that allows the muscles to contract and relax; in addition, it is used in the synthesis and repair of muscle tissues and in the transport of nutrients to the cells of the body. Although the body has very limited stores of ATP, it is constantly being formed, broken down to be used as an energy source, and then reformed. A very efficient mechanism indeed!

Three energy systems in your body are able to generate ATP: the phosphagen system, the anaerobic system, and the aerobic system. The type of activity and the length of time the athlete performs the activity determine which energy system the body uses.

Phosphagen System

Short spurts of intense activity, such as a six-second sprint or a tennis serve, are fueled through the **phosphagen system.** The basis of this system is the **creatine phosphate (CP)** molecule, which is stored in the muscles. Creatine is found in foods such as meat, poultry, and fish and is also produced in small amounts in the liver, kidneys, and pancreas. CP can use its energy to create ATP very rapidly during muscle contraction, but the ATP is quickly used up and then

replenished during rest periods. This system does not need oxygen to work, unlike the aerobic system, which comes into play later.

Anaerobic System

When the muscles run low on CP, short bursts of activity (one to three minutes) are supported by the **anaerobic system** (also known as the glycolytic or lactate system). *Anaerobic* means "without oxygen"; this system, like the phosphagen system, does not require oxygen to generate energy.

In the anaerobic system, the body generates ATP from glucose. **Glucose,** which comes from carbohydrate, is stored in the active muscles and in the liver as **glycogen,** a large molecule that can break down quickly into glucose as needed for muscle movement. The glycogen stored within a given muscle can be used only within that muscle; it can't be moved from one part of the body to another.

The anaerobic system is very efficient, quickly producing energy for the body to use when energy needs increase rapidly, such as when an athlete goes from standing still to a burst of activity in soccer, football, basketball, or hockey. The anaerobic system is the one called into action until enough oxygen is available to the body so that the next system, the aerobic system, can kick in.

A limitation of the anaerobic system is that during high-intensity exercise, the process of **glycolysis** breaks down glucose to ATP, pyruvate, and hydrogen. As high-intensity activity continues, the hydrogen combines with pyruvate to form lactic acid, or **lactate.** The liver will try to eliminate lactic acid from the body, and if lactate production by the muscles and lactate clearance by the liver are equal, exercise can continue. However, if an athlete reaches his or her **lactate threshold** and lactate production exceeds lactate clearance, excess lactate can accumulate in the blood. This is why carbohydrate intake is so critical. The athlete who shortchanges his or her carbohydrate intake is not going to have adequate glycogen stores to produce enough ATP in this system; therefore, he or she will not perform at optimal levels. However, as athletes adapt to training, their bodies are better able to handle lactate clearance and they can exercise at higher levels of intensity and output.

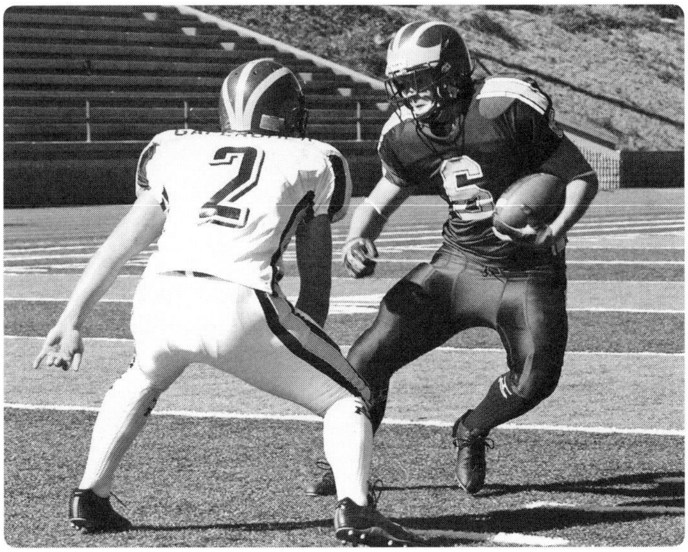

The anaerobic energy system provides energy to fuel sudden, short bursts of activity.

Aerobic System

Because not all sports finish in less than three minutes, a system is needed to generate energy for longer-duration activity. That is the **aerobic system,** which requires oxygen. This system primarily uses two fuel sources:

- Carbohydrate, stored as glycogen and broken down to glucose
- Fat, stored as triglycerides and broken down to fatty acids

These are the major energy sources, or substrates, for exercise.

The amount of ATP derived from the breakdown of carbohydrate when combined with oxygen in the aerobic system is much higher than that generated with the anaerobic system. The body can also break down fat and use the fatty acids as an energy source in this system, but adequate oxygen and carbohydrate must be present for this to occur, as would be the case during an activity performed at a low intensity such as a run instead of a sprint. On the plus side, more fat is stored in the body, within adipose (fat) tissue and muscle, than glycogen. And, over time, those who engage in endurance training develop the ability to use fat for energy more efficiently, sparing glucose and extending endurance. In fact, for stop-and-go as well as endurance sports, a better-trained athlete relies less on glycogen and more on fatty acids, thus sparing muscle glycogen so exercise can be prolonged.

If the muscles run out of glycogen, they will take up glucose from the blood. The hormone glucagon signals the liver to break down the glycogen stored there to glucose and to release it into the blood.

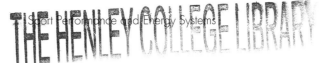

If glucose levels in the blood become low, as when endurance exercise lasts several hours, this system can use muscle protein, broken down into amino acids and converted by the liver into glucose, as an energy source. However, protein is not the most efficient source of energy for the exercising muscles, and using it as fuel depletes the supply of muscle protein available to the body for other purposes.

Even though it may seem that the phosphagen system would be used first, followed by the anaerobic and then the aerobic system, all three systems can operate at the same time. However, one will predominate, depending on the nature, duration, and intensity of the exercise. For example, a soccer player would use a combination of the anaerobic system for sprinting and the aerobic system for running at a slower pace up and down the field.

Matching Energy Systems to Sports

For your athletes to excel in their sports, they must have enough fuel to produce the energy needed to get them through practices and competition. For example, sprint athletes and powerlifters rely on the phosphagen and anaerobic systems for energy production; therefore, these athletes must consume adequate amounts of carbohydrate to make sure they store enough glycogen in the liver and muscles.

Endurance athletes, such as distance runners and Nordic skiers, as well as athletes involved in stop-and-go sports such as soccer, lacrosse, basketball, hockey, and football rely on both the anaerobic and aerobic systems to fuel their muscles. These athletes need to eat a varied diet, consuming carbohydrate, protein, and fat sources at every meal, so that they can tap into these fuel sources during activity. Table 1.1 lists various sports and the primary energy systems that are used to fuel that activity.

There is a delicate balance between training and intake. The goal is to increase the efficiency of the body for the demands of the sport, but this can only be accomplished if energy needs are met. The body can produce energy from stored fuel but relies on the energy derived from food sources to allow for sustained physical activity and improvements in performance. Therefore, if you want your athletes to get the most out of their bodies, remind them that food drives the process!

Intense training or heavy training after a layoff, such as when fall athletes return after a sedentary summer, can deplete glycogen stores. That is why training must increase gradually and in conjunction with an individualized eating plan that meets the athlete's needs for his or her sport. (Chapters 5 and 6 provide information for athletes who need to increase muscle mass or decrease body fat.)

Identify which energy systems are most used in your sport and what nutrients fuel them. (Start-Up Activity)

Example

Joe is a speedskater who does short track sprints as well as long events. During short track races he has always felt great, but at longer distances his legs used to ache and he felt more winded. Although he has always tried to eat enough carbohydrate by including cereal, bread, pasta, or rice as part of each meal, he used to keep his fat intake to a minimum. Once he started to add more fat to his diet, by spreading a thin layer of peanut butter on toast or adding a splash of olive oil to his pasta or rice, he had more stamina for his longer races.

TABLE 1.1

Energy Demands by Sport

Sport	Phosphagen system	Anaerobic system	Aerobic system	Primary fuel components
Running				
Sprinting	✘	✘		Creatine, carbohydrate
200-500 m		✘		Carbohydrate
10,000 m elite		✘	✘	Carbohydrate, fat
Jumping	✘	✘		Creatine, carbohydrate
Throwing	✘	✘		Creatine, carbohydrate
Hurdles	✘	✘		Creatine, carbohydrate
Cycling, sprints	✘	✘		Creatine, carbohydrate
Swimming, sprints	✘	✘		Creatine, carbohydrate
Swimming, 200-500 m		✘		Creatine, carbohydrate
Powerlifting	✘	✘		Creatine, carbohydrate
Gymnastics	✘	✘		Creatine, carbohydrate
Sport	Phosphagen system	Anaerobic system	Aerobic system	Primary fuel components
Team sports with sprints				
Football		✘	✘	Carbohydrate, fat
Baseball		✘	✘	Carbohydrate, fat
Basketball		✘	✘	Carbohydrate, fat
Field hockey		✘	✘	Carbohydrate, fat
Ice hockey		✘	✘	Carbohydrate, fat
Lacrosse		✘	✘	Carbohydrate, fat
Rugby		✘	✘	Carbohydrate, fat
Volleyball		✘	✘	Carbohydrate, fat
Tennis		✘	✘	Carbohydrate, fat
Squash		✘	✘	Carbohydrate, fat
Crew*		✘	✘	Carbohydrate, fat*
Speedskating*		✘	✘	Carbohydrate, fat*
Marathon running			✘	Carbohydrate, fat
Triathlon			✘	Carbohydrate, fat
Ultraendurance events			✘	Carbohydrate, fat
Distance cycling events			✘	Carbohydrate, fat

*Crew and speedskating could use both the anaerobic and aerobic systems, depending on the distance rowed or skated.

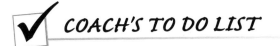

COACH'S TO DO LIST

- Remind your athletes that the only way to provide energy to their bodies is through food.
- Teach your athletes that different activities engage different energy systems, but all sports require that the body be fueled optimally and appropriately.
- Discuss the energy demands of different sports so that your athletes understand what fuels their muscles.
- Tell your athletes that the goal is to be energized and fueled throughout the season. An athlete with sufficient fuel reserves will be more likely to finish strong.
- Make sure your athletes understand that the goal is to create a balance between food consumed to provide energy and to help the body to recover from exercise and calories expended in the process of exercise through the demands for the sport.
- Explain to your athletes that when they train more intensely, or pick up training after a layoff, they need to pay special attention to eating.

SUMMARY

- To be fueled optimally during activity, the body must have adequate stores of the macronutrients used as energy substrates.
- Energy production requires adequate energy substrates, primarily in the form of carbohydrate or fat.
- One or more of three types of energy systems convert the substrate nutrients into energy during exercise: the phosphagen system, the anaerobic system, and the aerobic system.
- The type of system primarily in use at any given time is determined by the intensity and the duration of activity as well as by the athlete's level of training.
- An understanding of the energy systems used during exercise can help you to educate your athletes on which fuel sources will be most beneficial for their sport.

KEY TERMS

adenosine triphosphate (ATP)	catabolism	lactate
aerobic system	creatine phosphate (CP)	lactate threshold
anabolism	glucose	metabolism
anaerobic system	glycogen	phosphagen system
	glycolysis	

GAME PLAN QUESTIONS

1. How can exercise be both catabolic and anabolic?

2. What are the primary fuel substrates for the aerobic energy system?

3. What are the energy systems used in a stop-and-go sport such as football? A sport such as weightlifting?

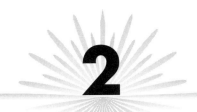

Foods That Fuel

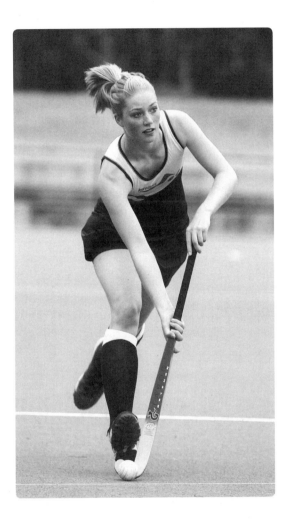

Jill is a high school field hockey player who had great freshman and sophomore seasons. During the first few preseason practices for Jill's junior year, her coach noticed that she tired much more easily and had to sit for the last part of practice. When asked about her summer, Jill said she trained daily, but she also changed her diet in the month before preseason.

One of Jill's friends had told her that carbohydrate-containing foods and high-fat foods would hamper her athletic performance. Jill was worried and decided to change her diet, so she cut out all cereal, bread, pasta, rice, and most fruits and only chose items that were fat free. On a typical day Jill ate fat-free yogurt with unsweetened applesauce for breakfast and a large salad for lunch with beans, chicken, fat-free cheese, and lots of vegetables. Snacks consisted of tuna, vegetables, fat-free bean dip, fat-free cheese or fat-free cottage cheese, or a smoothie made with skim milk, fat-free yogurt, and frozen unsweetened fruit. Dinner would be lots of chicken, ground turkey, or fish; a very large salad; and vegetables. If Jill was hungry at night she ate sugar-free gelatin or sugar-free popsicles. She was surprised that she was so fatigued because she hadn't lost weight. Jill's coach explained that by consuming so little carbohydrate and fat, Jill didn't have enough fuel in her muscles and as a result was slower and weaker and tired more quickly.

At the request of the coach, I talked to Jill's field hockey team. After my talk, Jill told me what had happened with her eating and performance. She said that the coach thought that Jill's diet was too low in fat and carbohydrate, but Jill was afraid to add these foods back to her diet. I stressed that she needed to cut back a little on the protein, add some carbohydrate, and slightly increase fat. Jill tried this for a week; she noticed that she felt better, she had more energy, and her performance improved.

When you finish reading this chapter, you should be able to explain

- what carbohydrate, protein, and fat are and how to determine how much your athletes need;
- which foods are good sources for carbohydrate, protein, and fat;
- what the glycemic index for carbohydrate is;
- which low-carbohydrate foods are healthy;
- which types of fat are "good" or "bad" for your athletes; and
- how your athletes can balance nutrients in their diet.

For athletes to perform their best, their bodies must be fueled optimally. Too often athletes have misconceptions about food choices, sometimes labeling foods as good or bad and eating too much or not enough of the energy substrates for exercise. For many athletes, fueling is low on the priority list, yet a body that does not have enough fuel in the tank will not to be able to maintain high levels of strength, speed, or stamina.

One of your responsibilities is to be the nutrition coach for your athletes. You need to stress nutrition as much as you stress the skills and drills performed in practice. Young athletes need adequate calories for growth in addition to the calories required for sport. The Dietary Guidelines for Americans 2005 (USDHHS & USDA 2005) use the words *balance*, *variety*, and *moderation*, and these terms are important to your athletes as well.

- Athletes should eat balanced amounts of the major nutrients—carbohydrate, protein, and fat—to provide fuel for activity and for muscle growth, development, repair, and recovery from exercise or injury.
- Athletes should consume a variety of foods and fluids to make eating more interesting.
- Athletes should moderate their intake of some high-fat and high-sugar food items that may affect performance and health.

Let's begin by looking at the three major types of macronutrients for the body: carbohydrate, protein, and fat.

Carbohydrate

Carbohydrate is composed of carbon, hydrogen, and oxygen. Carbohydrate can be broken down into glucose, a form of sugar that is the major energy source for the body. Each gram of carbohydrate contains 4 calories.

Carbohydrates are composed of saccharides (sugars) of varying length. Table sugar, or sucrose, is composed of two monosaccharides (glucose and fructose), whereas the sugar found in milk, called lactose, is composed of glucose and galactose (see figure 2.1). Starch is a long chain of glucose molecules. Fiber is another type of carbohydrate, and although fiber is not used as a fuel source, it can help with digestive functioning and regulation of blood cholesterol and blood glucose concentration.

The suffix *ose* in a term indicates that the term describes a saccharide or sugar:

- Glucose: blood sugar
- Fructose: fruit sugar
- Lactose: milk sugar
- Maltose: sugar in starch

Carbohydrates can be classified as simple or complex. Table 2.1 on page 12 lists the classifications of carbohydrates and examples of foods that contain those types of carbohydrates.

People may unnecessarily eliminate foods from their diet assuming that simple carbohydrates are sugar and thus are bad and that complex carbohydrates are healthier and thus good. Some food that contain complex carbohydrates such as sweetened cereals have the fiber, vitamins, and minerals removed, and although some vitamins are added back in, these are referred to as refined carbohydrates and may not be as nutrient dense as unrefined carbohydrates. By comparison, simple carbohydrates can be found in foods such as fruit, which also contains fiber, vitamins, minerals, and phytonutrients (substances in plants that may have health benefits for the body, such as carotenoids, the pigments in fruits and vegetables that may have disease-fighting properties).

The type of carbohydrate eaten is not as important as the total amount of carbohydrate consumed daily. Table 2.2 on page 13 lists the carbohydrate content of some common foods.

Carbohydrate is the preferred fuel source for the brain and nervous system, so for your athletes to learn well, they need to consume adequate amounts of carbohydrate. In addition, carbohydrate, not protein or fat, is stored in the muscles and liver as glycogen, which provides fuel for exercising muscles.

Exercise depletes glycogen stores, which need to be replenished with carbohydrate, not protein or fat! Consuming carbohydrate-containing foods before exercise can help to prevent hunger, delay fatigue, and provide energy during exercise. Carbohydrate consumption after exercise expedites liver and muscle glycogen resynthesis so that the athlete can recover more quickly.

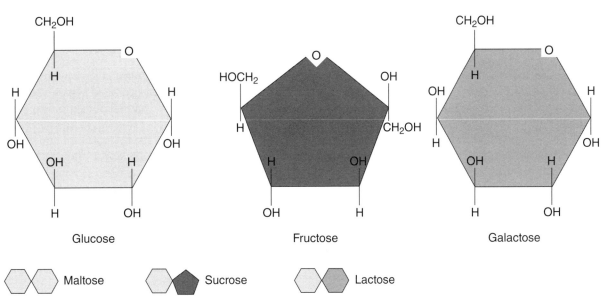

FIGURE 2.1 Molecular composition of three types of carbohydrate.

Adapted, by permission, from A.E. Jeukendrup and M. Gleeson, 2004, *Sport nutrition: An introduction to energy production and performance* (Champaign, IL: Human Kinetics), 3.

TABLE 2.1

Carbohydrate Classifications

SIMPLE CARBOHYDRATES	
Monosaccharides **(glucose, fructose, dextrose, galactose)**	**Disaccharides** **(sucrose, lactose, maltose)**
• Fruit • Honey • Maple syrup	• Table sugar (white, brown, raw) • Dairy foods such as milk and yogurt • Corn syrup and malt
COMPLEX CARBOHYDRATES	
Cellulose (nonstarchy vegetables such as green beans, broccoli, lettuce, tomatoes) • Rice (white and brown) • Root vegetables such as carrots and beets • Tubers (potatoes, yams) • Legumes (dried beans) • Wheat (pasta, bread, crackers, cereals) • Peas • Glycogen (form of carbohydrate stored in the muscles and liver of animals such as poultry and fish)	
HIGH-FIBER FOODS	
• Fruits • Vegetables • Oats • Bran cereal • Bran bread	• Corn • Beans • Peas • Nuts • Potatoes

Isn't it interesting that there are low-carbohydrate sports bars, no-carbohydrate sports drinks, and many so-called energy products with water, caffeine, and artificial sweeteners as the primary ingredients? Although these products may taste sweet, they do not provide the body with adequate fuel for activity.

Each of your athletes will need a specific amount of carbohydrate based on body weight and exercise frequency. In addition, some athletes may ask you about the glycemic index, low-carbohydrate foods, and artificial sweeteners, so read on for more information on these topics.

Carbohydrate Recommendations

The Dietary Guidelines for Americans 2005 (USDHHS & USDA 2005) recommend a diet containing 45 to 65 percent of calories from carbohydrate and not less than 130 grams of carbohydrate per day. By contrast, some of the low-carbohydrate diets recommend an initial carbohydrate intake of 20 grams a day. This would be the equivalent of 6 ounces (180 ml) of orange juice, four gummy-type candies, or two thirds of a cereal bar.

The World Health Organization recommends limiting the intake of free or added sugars and fruit juice concentrate to less than 10 percent of the total daily calories. For a 2,000-calorie diet, this means no more than 200 calories from sugar, the equivalent of a 20-ounce (600 ml) soda. Some athletes may do better with a higher percentage (65 percent) of calories from carbohydrate, whereas others may prefer a more moderate carbohydrate intake, but no athlete will improve performance when the carbohydrate content of the diet is less than 40 percent of the total daily calories.

Your athletes' daily carbohydrate requirements are based on the frequency of exercise:

TABLE 2.2

Carbohydrate Content of Common Foods

Food	Amount	Carbohydrate, g
Bagel	2 oz (60 g)	38
Bagel	4 oz (125 g)	76
Bread	Two slices	32
Cheerios	1 cup (30 g)	23
Pasta	1 cup (140 g)	30
Granola, low-fat	1 cup (110 g)	82
Rice, white or brown	1 cup cooked (200 g)	45
Orange juice	8 oz (240 ml)	27
Coke	12 oz (360 ml)	42
Sports drink	8 oz (240 ml)	14
Sports gel	1 oz (30 ml)	28
Banana	Small	15
Yogurt, fruit	8 oz (230 g)	42
Raisins	1/4 cup (40 g)	31
Pretzels	One handful	22
Baked potato	4 in. (10 cm) long	20
Corn	1/2 cup	15
Corn tortilla	6 in. (15 cm) diameter	20
Green beans	1/2 cup	5

Source: www.calorieking.com and the U.S. Department of Agriculture, Agricultural Research Service. 2007. USDA National Nutrient Database for Standard Reference. Release 20. Nutrient Data Laboratory Home Page, www.ars.usda.gov/ba/bhnrc/ndl

- General training: 5 to 7 grams of carbohydrate per kilogram of body weight (or 2.3-3 g/lb)
- Endurance training: 7 to 10 grams of carbohydrate per kilogram of body weight (or 3-4.5 g/lb)
- Ultraendurance training: 11 grams of carbohydrate per kilogram of body weight (or 5 g/lb)

Glycemic Index

Athletes have recently begun experimenting with manipulating the type of carbohydrate consumed at various points during exercise according to the **glyce-** **mic index** of the food. The glycemic index indicates the effects of carbohydrate-rich foods and fluids on blood glucose and insulin levels. The glycemic index ranks foods by comparing the blood glucose response after ingestion of a test food that provides 50 grams of carbohydrate with the blood glucose response to a reference food such as white bread. The response reflects the rate of digestion and absorption of a carbohydrate-rich food.

Foods with a low glycemic index raise blood glucose slowly, whereas foods with a higher glycemic index raise blood glucose more rapidly. Some scientists believe that the extent to which carbohydrate-containing foods increase blood glucose, the

Example

A 120-pound (54.5 kg) distance runner would require the following amount of carbohydrate daily:

120 pounds × 3 to 4.5 grams = 360 to 540 grams of carbohydrate

(54.5 kg × 6.6 to 9.9 grams = 360 to 540 grams of carbohydrate)

Here's a meal plan that would achieve this carbohydrate intake.

Breakfast
8 ounces (230 g) fruit yogurt
A bagel with 1 tablespoon each peanut butter and jelly
A small banana
Total: 127 grams of carbohydrate

Lunch
Turkey and cheese sandwich on whole-wheat bread
A handful of pretzels
An apple
12 ounces (360 ml) orange juice
Total: 110 grams of carbohydrate

Before Practice
20 ounces (600 ml) sports drink
Total: 37 grams of carbohydrate

After Practice
One cereal bar
Total: 30 grams of carbohydrate

Dinner
2 cups (280 g) pasta
1 cup (240 ml) meat sauce
1 cup of green beans
8 ounces (240 ml) skim milk
Total: 92 grams of carbohydrate

Evening Snack
8 ounces (230 g) low-fat frozen yogurt
Total: 70 grams of carbohydrate

Grand total: 436 grams of carbohydrate

rate of this increase, and the insulin response may increase the risk for obesity, cardiovascular disease, hypertension, and type 2 diabetes. Some of the foods with a high glycemic index are also higher in fat and calories, such as pastries, chips, and sweetened beverages, and are sometimes consumed in larger quantities than foods with a lower glycemic index, such as fruits and vegetables. Overconsumption of foods with a high glycemic index may increase the risk for cardiovascular disease as well as obesity and may be contraindicated in athletes with diabetes or hypoglycemia (see chapter 9 for more on these conditions).

Foods are classified as high, moderate, and low glycemic index. Some examples are shown in table 2.3.

The glycemic index of a food is affected by several factors:

- Large particles take longer to digest than small particles and thus slow the rate of blood glu-

cose increase. For example, regular oatmeal has less of an effect on blood glucose than instant oatmeal, which has smaller-sized oats.

- Soluble fiber (oats, barley, dried beans) takes longer to digest and to leave the stomach than insoluble fiber and thus slows the glycemic response. For instance, fibrous coverings as are found on beans and seeds increase digestion time.

- Acid-containing foods such as fruit, vinegar, or pickled foods take longer to digest than nonacidic foods.

- Fructose takes longer to digest than glucose.

- Fat-containing foods take longer to digest than nonfatty foods.

- Combinations of macronutrients such as protein and carbohydrate or fat and carbohydrate alter the glycemic response.

TABLE 2.3

Sample Foods by Glycemic Index Categories

FOODS WITH A HIGH GLYCEMIC INDEX			
Angel food cake	Sucrose	Pretzels	Sports drinks
Doughnuts and croissants	White bread	Barley bread	Rye bread
Hard candy	Millet	Toaster pastries	Bagels
English muffins	Couscous	Watermelon	Cold cereals
Raisins	Honey and syrup	Ice cream	Pancakes and waffles
Corn chips	Carrots	Molasses	Baked and mashed potatoes
FOODS WITH A MODERATE GLYCEMIC INDEX			
Sponge cake	Mango and kiwi	Banana	Tortillas
Pita	Seven-grain bread	100 percent whole-wheat bread	Oat bran bread
Brown and white rice	Basmati rice	Bran cereal	Pasta
Barley and bulgur	Buckwheat	Citrus juices	Corn
Peas	Sweet potato	Oatmeal and oat bran	Low-fat ice cream
Candy bar	PowerBar	Grapes	Soda crackers
FOODS WITH A LOW GLYCEMIC INDEX			
Milk	Nine-grain bread	Plums	100 percent bran cereal
Yogurt	Citrus fruits	Beans	Nuts
Rice bran	Apples	Apple juice	Raw peaches
Lentils	Tomato soup	Tomato juice	Sports bars such as 　　Zone 　　Balance 　　Power bar, high protein 　　PR bar
Dried apricots	Raw pears	Chickpeas	Hummus

Foods with a high glycemic index produce a greater response from insulin compared with foods that have a moderate or low glycemic index, which enhances glycogen replacement in the muscle. When the goal is rapid repletion, there may be an advantage to consuming foods with a high glycemic index. Moderate and low glycemic index foods take longer to enter the bloodstream and may be preferred for endurance exercise to promote sustained carbohydrate availability.

Manipulating meal choices on the basis of the glycemic index may enhance carbohydrate availability and improve athletic performance. (See chapter 3 for a more in-depth discussion.)

You may have athletes who want to decrease their sugar intake. Although most people can reduce their intake of the "empty" calories of corn syrup and sucrose and still perform well, there is no need to cut out nutritious foods like fruit and yogurt. An athlete might choose to avoid yogurt because it has 40 grams of sugar; however, fructose and lactose compose the sugar content in yogurt. The muscles need carbohydrates to be able to perform well and can break down fructose and lactose to glucose to provide energy for activity. Plus, yogurt provides protein, calcium, and potassium in addition to carbohydrate.

Here are some terms for sugar you might see on a product ingredient list:

Barley malt	Beet juice
Corn syrup	Corn sweeteners
Evaporated cane juice	Fructose
Malt syrup	Maltodextrin
Succanat	Sucrose
Lactose	Maltose
Brown rice syrup	Cane syrup
Crystalline fructose	Dextrose
High-fructose corn syrup	Invert sugar
Maple syrup	Muscavado
Raw sugar	Turbinado sugar

Low-Carbohydrate Foods

Many people mistakenly believe that low-carbohydrate diets or low-carbohydrate foods help with weight loss. The assumption is that carbohydrates make a person fat. The bottom line is that eating any nutrient in excess of need will result in weight gain. Many low-carbohydrate foods are not necessarily low in calories, can be very expensive, and don't always taste great!

Low-carbohydrate foods are everywhere, from health clubs to fast food restaurants. Some of the more popular products include these:

- Beer (calories are from the alcohol, not carbohydrate)
- Pasta
- Candy
- Chips
- Muffins
- Pizza crust
- Bagels
- Cereal
- Milk (the lactose is replaced by artificial sweetener and extra protein)
- Sports drinks

Some of these products are higher in calories and fat than the regular-carbohydrate

versions. Others contain sugar alcohols, such as sorbitol, mannitol, lactitiol, and erythritol, which can have a laxative effect. Some have an unpleasant taste and texture, and most cost significantly more than the regular products. Low-carbohydrate foods such as chips and muffins are not nutritionally equivalent to fruits, dairy foods, and vegetables!

In addition, there is no definition for *low carbohydrate*, and many products may contain the terms *net carbohydrate* or *net effective carbohydrate*. The manufacturers use these terms to make people believe that they are consuming fewer calories. Net carbohydrate content is determined as follows:

Net carbohydrate (g) = total carbohydrate (g) – fiber (g) – sugar alcohols (g) – glycerine (g)

The assumption is that fiber, sugar alcohols, and glycerine do not contribute significant amounts of calories and don't have to be counted. Although the calories derived from carbohydrate-containing foods may be lower, the foods still contain calories, so overall caloric intake may still be appreciable.

There are times when the use of artificial sweeteners may be warranted. Athletes who are trying to lose weight or have diabetes or hypoglycemia may need to curb their sugar intake but still want to enjoy foods with a sweet taste. There is a lot of misinformation surrounding artificial sweeteners. They may help to promote weight loss if the athlete replaces a regular sugar item with an artificially sweetened one, such as choosing diet iced tea instead of sweetened iced tea. But the athlete who chooses a sugar-free cookie may be getting the same number of calories as the regular product, so you should remind athletes that

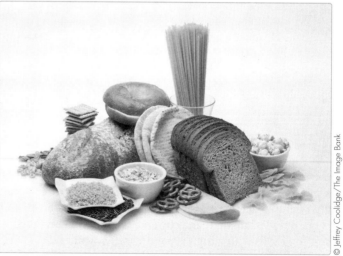

Contrary to what athletes may have heard, foods that contain carbohydrate should be embraced, not avoided. Carbohydrate provides fuel for the brain and the body.

TABLE 2.4

Sweeteners

NONNUTRITIVE SWEETENERS (FEW OR NO CALORIES)		
Sweetener	**What it contains**	**Calories/gram**
Aspartame (Equal, Nutrasweet)	Aspartic acid, phenylalanine	4
Saccharin	Benzoic sulfinate	0
Sucralose (Splenda)	Chlorinated sucrose	0
Acelsulfame potassium (Sweet One)	Potassium salt	0
NATURAL SWEETENERS		
Sweetener	**What it contains**	**Calories/gram**
Sucrose	Glucose and fructose	4.0
Honey and syrup	Glucose and fructose	4.0
Glycerine*	Trihydric ethanol	4.32
Maltitol*	Polyhydric sugar ethanol	2.1
Isomalt*	Polyhydric sugar ethanol	2.0
Erythritol	Polyhydric sugar ethanol	.2
Mannitol**	Polyhydric sugar ethanol	1.6
Sorbitol**	Polyhydric sugar ethanol	2.6
Xylitol**	Polyhydric sugar ethanol	2.4
Lactitol**	Polyhydric sugar ethanol	2.0
Stevia***	South American herb	0

*Mild laxative effect with high use.

** Significant laxative effect with high use.

***Sold as a sweetener and used in ceratin beverages.

sugar-free does not necessarily mean calorie-free. Table 2.4 lists various sweeteners and calories per gram.

Fat (Lipids)

Fat and oils are known as lipids. They are composed of carbon, hydrogen, and oxygen. **Triglyceride,** the main form of fat in the diet as well as for energy storage in the body, consists of a glycerol molecule to which three fatty acids are attached (figure 2.2 on page 18). **Fatty acids** are the building blocks of fat, and there are three types: saturated, monounsaturated, and polyunsaturated. **Fat** is also the most

calorically dense nutrient; each gram of fat supplies 9 calories.

Within every muscle are intramuscular triglycerides, which the body uses as fuel for long-duration exercise. In addition, muscles contain **essential fatty acids,** linolenic acid and linoleic acid, which need to be consumed through food sources.

Dietary fat is an important component for heart health, blood pressure regulation, hair and skin health, and protection of vital organs. Fat is a component of hormones, and it also helps the body absorb fat-soluble vitamins. In addition, fat supplies a concentrated calorie source to provide energy for the athlete.

As shown in figure 2.3 and explained in table 2.5, the structure of saturated and unsaturated fats differs significantly.

Examples of each category of fat are provided in table 2.5. Table 2.6 (on page 20) lists the fat content and type of fat for some common foods.

Inform your athletes about the types of fat and the need for fat in the diet. Otherwise, some athletes may try to minimize fat intake to decrease body fat, not realizing the potentially adverse effect on health and performance.

Fat: Good or Bad?

You may have athletes who say that fat is "bad," specifically saturated fat and trans fat. **Saturated fat** has been linked to increased risk of cardiovascular disease, diabetes, and some cancers. **Trans fat** may lower HDL or good cholesterol and raise LDL or bad cholesterol. **Monounsaturated fat** seems to lower heart disease risk, as do certain types of polyunsaturated fat such those found in as fatty fish, flaxseed, flaxseed oil, and foods fortified with omega-3 fatty acids. The goal is for your athletes to be selective with fat choices rather than to avoid fat in the diet.

Foods with fat provide satiety or a feeling of fullness. How many of your athletes who eat a very low fat diet complain of being hungry? Fat helps us to feel fuller longer, so a slice of toast with peanut butter will stave off hunger longer than toast with jam.

Some of your athletes may believe that eating a diet as low in fat as possible will make them better athletes or help them to lose body fat, but a diet that is too low in fat may limit performance by inhibiting triglyceride storage within muscles, therefore resulting in earlier fatigue during exercise. Inadequate fat intake can also decrease serum testosterone concentration, and lowered testosterone levels may result in decreases in muscle mass and strength. In addition, insufficient fat intake may have a deleterious effect on bone health. So if athletes are trying to eat a diet with no fat, suggest that they add some fat as nuts, nut butter, seeds, or a little oil or dressing. The body doesn't require a lot of fat, but it does require some.

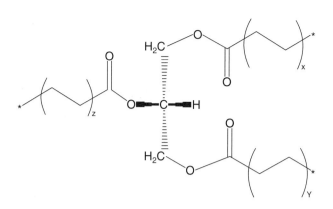

FIGURE 2.2   Molecular composition of triglyceride.

Reprinted from "Triglyceride," Wikipedia, The Free Encyclopedia. [Online]. Available: http://en.wikipedia.org/w/index.php?title=Triglyceride&oldid=255735632 [December 12, 2008].

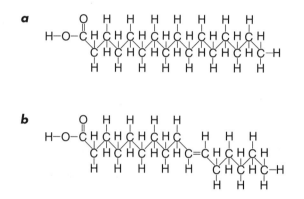

FIGURE 2.3   Molecular structure of (a) saturated and (b) unsaturated fat.

On the other hand, the athlete who eats too much fat from sources like fried foods, fatty meats, or lots of mayonnaise and salad dressing may end with increased fat stores attributable to excess calories. Although eating foods with fat can keep us fuller longer between meals, most athletes will not eat just one chip or one French fry, and because it may require many chips or fries to feel full, the end result could be weight gain. In addition, caution your athletes against eating fatty foods before exercise, especially before competition, because the result can be digestive distress before exercise.

TABLE 2.5

Categories of Fat

SATURATED FAT

In saturated fat, all carbon molecules in the chain are linked by single bonds and attached to hydrogen. This type of fat tends to be more solid (e.g., compared with oils), and excessive intake of this fat has been correlated with increased risk of heart disease.

Sample foods

- Skin on poultry
- Fat on meat or marbled meats (fat within the meat)
- Butter
- Full-fat milk
- Cheese
- Cream
- Ice cream
- Coconut oil
- Palm oil

UNSATURATED FAT

Monounsaturated Fat

The carbon chain in these fats contains one double bond. This fat is derived primarily from plant-based foods such as olive, canola, soybean, sesame, flaxseed, safflower, sunflower, and walnut oils.

* Increased intake of monounsaturated fat has been associated with decreased risk of heart disease.

Sample foods

- Nuts and nut butters
- Olives
- Avocados
- Pesto (olive oil, basil)
- Seeds such as sunflower, pumpkin
- Tahini (sesame seed paste)

* Oils are sources of both monounsaturated and polyunsaturated fat.

Polyunsaturated Fat

The carbon chain in this fat contains two or more double bonds. There are two type of polyunsaturated fat: omega-6, which is correlated with decreased heart disease risk, and omega-3, which may lower heart disease risk and inflammation.

Sample foods (Omega-6 polyunsaturated fat)

Oils or margarines made from these oils:
- Corn
- Safflower
- Sunflower
- Soybean

Sample foods (Omega-3 polyunsaturated fat)

- Fatty fish such as salmon, sardines
- Flaxseed and flaxseed oil
- Walnuts
- Soybean oil
- Purslane
- Borage

TRANS FAT

Trans fat is a polyunsaturated fat where the hydrogen atoms that surround a double bond are on opposite sides of the carbon chain. Trans fatty acids are more similar to saturated fat and may increase the risk for heart disease. Although some trans fat is naturally present in food, the artificial trans fat present in hydrogenated oils is associated with increased risk of heart disease. Hydrogenated oils are polyunsaturated fats which go through an additional step of processing where hydrogen is added; when the hydrogen attaches to the carbon molecules the polyunsaturated fat becomes more similar to a saturated fat.

Sample foods

- Stick margarine
- Baked goods
- Doughnuts
- Some sports bars
- Some ice creams
- Icing
- Frozen confections

TABLE 2.6

Fat Content of Select Foods

Food item	Amount	Fat content, g	Type of fat
Olive oil*	1 tbsp	14	Monounsaturated
Soft margarine*	1 tbsp	11	Polyunsaturated
Mayonnaise	1 tbsp	11	Polyunsaturated
Salad dressings			
Italian*	1 tbsp	7	Polyunsaturated
Ranch	1 tbsp	10	Saturated and polyunsaturated
Blue cheese	1 tbsp	8	Saturated and polyunsaturated
Nuts*	1/4 cup (35 g)	32	Monounsaturated
Peanut butter*	2 tbsp	16	Monounsaturated
Cream cheese	2 tbsp	11	Saturated
Bacon	Two slices	6	Saturated
Chips	1 oz (30 g)	10	Polyunsaturated
French fries	Small serving	12	Polyunsaturated (in the frying oil)
Ice cream	One scoop	20	Saturated
Prime rib	3 oz (90 g)	23	Saturated
Burger	One regular	10	Saturated
Big Mac	One	32	Saturated
Chicken drumstick, fried	One	11	Saturated
Chicken wing, fried	One	15	Saturated

*Healthier choice.

Fat Recommendations

The Dietary Guidelines for Americans 2005 (USDHHS & USDA 2005) recommend a fat intake of 20 to 35 percent of daily calories. If we translate these percentages into numbers, the recommendation for fat intake is weight in pounds × .45 = number of grams of fat per day, or weight in kilograms × 1 (Position of the American Dietetic Association 2000). In addition, the recommended daily intake of each type of fat is as follows:

- Saturated fat: 7 to 10 percent of total daily calories
- Monounsaturated fat: at least 10 percent of total daily calories
- Polyunsaturated fat: 10 percent of total daily calories

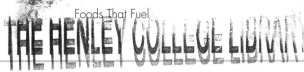

Example

A 140-pound (64 kg) basketball player would require the following amount of fat daily:

140 pounds × .45 = 63 grams of fat

(64 kg × 1 = 64 grams of fat)

Here's a meal plan that would achieve this fat intake.

Breakfast
A bagel with 2 tablespoons of peanut butter
8 ounces (180 mg) skim milk
Fat: 16 grams

Lunch
Baked ham sandwich containing the following:
   Three slices baked ham
   One slice part-skim provolone cheese
   1/2 tablespoon mayonnaise
One apple
Fat: 15 grams

Snack
Pretzels mixed with 1/4 cup (35 g) nuts
Fat: 15 grams

Dinner
4 ounces (125 g) chicken
Broccoli sautéed in a little garlic
   and olive oil
Baked potato with 2 teaspoons of light
   butter
8 ounces (240 ml) skim milk
Fat: 15 grams

Evening Snack
8 ounces (240 ml) low-fat yogurt and
   a banana
Fat: 9 grams

Grand total: 70 grams of fat

Protein

Protein is a macronutrient composed of carbon, oxygen, hydrogen, and nitrogen (and sometimes sulfur). Amino acids are the building blocks of protein, and 10 of them are essential, meaning that we have to consume them in foods because the body cannot manufacture them. The **essential amino acids** are as follows:

- Isoleucine
- Leucine
- Lysine
- Threonine
- Trytophan
- Methinonine
- Histidine
- Valine
- Phenylalanine
- Arginine

When we eat protein-containing foods, we eat a variety of amino acids, not individual amino acids. But your athletes may ask about increasing their intake of individual amino acids to gain mass. For instance, leucine, which is one of the amino acids in whey protein, may help an athlete to maintain or increase muscle mass. Eating foods with whey, such as yogurt, can work equally well. Arginine is an amino acid in many of the nitric oxide stimulator products and is touted to increase muscle mass, although studies have not proven its efficacy.

Protein is necessary for tissue growth and repair, bone health, a healthy immune system, and muscle building and maintenance. Protein also is needed to make hemoglobin, the iron-containing protein in red blood cells that carries oxygen to the cells of the body, and protein is a component of hormones, enzymes, and antibodies. Young athletes who are still growing have higher protein requirements than athletes who have gone through their growth spurt.

Protein can be a source of energy, although it is used by the body for energy much less than is carbohydrate or fat. Each gram of protein supplies 4 calories. Athletes often are confused about how much protein they need and what foods contain protein. Let's look at these areas now.

Sources of Protein

Many athletes think that red meat is the best source of protein and are surprised to find out that ounce for ounce, beef, poultry, and fish have the same amount of protein. In fact, both animal and plant foods contain protein. You may not think of bread or broccoli as foods that contain protein, but they do, although in smaller quantities than meat. Fruits, fat, water, and sugar are the only foods that do not contain protein.

The protein in foods is classified as either complete protein (protein that contains all the essential amino acids) or incomplete protein (protein that does not contain all the essential amino acids).

Foods that contain complete protein include the following:

- Meat (beef, veal, pork, lamb, venison, buffalo)
- Poultry (chicken, turkey, game birds)
- Fish and shellfish
- Eggs
- Dairy foods such as milk, cheese, cottage cheese, and yogurt
- Soy foods (edamame, tofu, soy milk, soy cheese, and meat analogues)

Foods that contain incomplete protein (i.e., that lack one or more essential amino acids) include the following:

- Beans
- Grains such as rice, pasta, bread, and cereals
- Nuts and nut butters
- Seeds
- Vegetables

Commercially available meats such as poultry, beef, pork, veal, and lamb include a Nutrition Facts panel that lists the amount of protein per serving. Packaged foods also list the protein content per serving so that you or your athletes can track protein intake. Protein powders contain a Supplement Facts panel that lists the protein content per serving. Figure 2.4 shows a Nutrition Facts panel.

Athletes have different protein requirements based on age, body weight, training intensity, and body composition goals. They need to know how to meet protein needs daily through food sources that are palatable, affordable, and accessible.

Table 2.7 lists common foods that are sources of protein.

Protein Recommendations

The Dietary Guidelines for Americans 2005 (USDHHS & USDA 2005) recommend a protein range from 10 to 35 percent of the daily caloric requirement. The reason for this range is that some circumstances might warrant consuming a greater percentage of

FIGURE 2.4 Nutrition Facts panel.

calories from protein, such as an athlete trying to increase muscle mass.

During exercise, protein can provide up to 15 percent of the fuel during activity when muscle glycogen stores are low but less than 5 percent when muscle glycogen stores are adequate. (See chapter 1 for a discussion of nutrient use during exercise.)

An athlete who is new to a sport, or who experiences a sudden increase in training frequency, intensity, or duration, can experience muscle breakdown and muscle protein loss. However, as your athletes become better conditioned, the breakdown and loss of muscle protein diminish. This is why protein needs are often higher in the initial phases of training. Be sure to educate athletes about the importance of consuming a diet with adequate amounts of protein.

Athletes who do not meet their protein needs are more likely to have decreased muscle mass, a suppressed immune system (so they get ill more often or take longer to recover from illness), and increased risk of injury. However, excessive amounts of protein can increase the risk for dehydration, increase body fat stores, lead to more fatigue and impaired performance, and result in an unbalanced diet that is often deficient in carbohydrates. Protein requirements are outlined in table 2.8.

TABLE 2.7

Protein Content of Common Foods

Food	Amount	Protein, g
Chicken breast	3 oz (90 g)	21
Chicken thigh	3 oz (90 g)	21
Cod	3 oz (90 g)	21
Hamburger	3 oz (90 g)	21
Steak	3 oz (90 g)	21
Pork chop	3 oz (90 g)	21
Egg	One	7
Soy burger	One	15-18
Nuts	1/4 cup (35 g)	10
Peanut butter	2 tbsp	8
Cheese	One slice	7
Refried beans	1/2 cup	7
Milk	8 oz (240 ml)	8
Yogurt	8 oz (230 g)	9-11
Protein powder	One scoop	32-45
Nonfat dry milk powder	1/4 cup (30 g)	8
Amino acid pills	One serving	10

TABLE 2.8

Protein Requirements for Various Types of Athletes

Type of athlete	Daily protein requirement, g/lb (g/kg) of body weight
Recreational athlete	.5-.75 (1.1-1.6)
Competitive athlete	.6-.9 (1.3-2)
Athlete building mass	.7-.9 (1.5-2)
Teenage athlete	.9-1.0 (2-2.2)
Athlete restricting intake	.7-.9 (1.5-2)
Maximal usable amount by athletes in weight-class sports (e.g., crew, wrestling)	.9 (2.0)

Although most of your athletes know that they need to eat carbohydrate-containing foods as part of a good training diet, their protein intake may range from minimal to excessive. Some athletes believe that they should load up on protein, especially to put on mass, whereas others cut their protein intake because they mistakenly believe that protein can make them fat. Often the athletes who need the most protein consume the least, such as the distance runner, whereas a football player may not always need as much protein as he thinks.

Athletes who strength train regularly and those in power sports sometimes favor protein to excess, resulting in a diet that is deficient in other nutrients. Although muscles need adequate protein to grow, they also need carbohydrate and fat, and eating excess protein will not help athletes get bigger faster. For an athlete who is trying to increase mass, protein intake should not exceed 1 gram per pound or 2 grams per kilogram of body weight.

Endurance athletes often choose carbohydrate over protein, and they may consume too little. Athletes who are increasing their mileage or training intensity, frequency, or duration will need more protein to increase the number of oxygen-carrying enzymes in the blood, to form red blood cells and myoglobin (the protein in muscle cells that carries oxygen), and to replace protein stores that can be depleted during training. These athletes are going to need somewhere between .6 and .7 grams of protein per pound of body weight, or 1.3 to 1.5 grams of protein per kilogram of body weight. For a 130 pound (60 kg) cross country runner, this would be 78 to 91 grams of protein per day.

Getting Your Athletes to Eat Enough Protein

Getting your athletes to consume sufficient amounts of protein can be challenging. Some athletes may say they don't like protein foods or don't know which foods are high in protein. In addition, protein foods are more perishable, so often athletes will consume

---

Example

A 150-pound (68 kg) teenage baseball player who is trying to increase mass would require the following amount of protein daily:

150 pounds (68 kg) × .9-1.0 grams of protein per pound (or 2-2.2 g/kg) = 135 to 150 grams of protein per day

Here's a meal plan that would achieve this protein intake.

Breakfast
Two scrambled eggs
Two slices of toast
12 ounces (360 ml) skim milk
Protein: 30 grams

Lunch
Tuna salad sandwich with 3 ounces (90 g) tuna
Two slices of bread
Pretzels
8 ounces (240 ml) low-fat chocolate milk
Protein: 33 grams

Snack After School
12 crackers with 2 tablespoons peanut butter
Protein: 10 grams

Dinner
6 ounces (175 g) roast chicken
1 cup mashed potatoes
1 cup carrots and peas
12 ounces (360 ml) apple juice
Protein: 50 grams

Evening Snack
2 cups (60 g) cereal
8 ounces (240 ml) low-fat milk
Protein: 12 grams

Grand total: 135 grams of protein

carbohydrate-containing foods as snacks or for a quick breakfast rather than protein foods.

Here are some easy ways for your athletes to add protein to each meal:

Breakfast

Add peanut butter to toast

Add a scoop of nonfat dry milk powder to oatmeal

Have cottage cheese instead of yogurt

Have a hardboiled egg

Lunch

Add two more slices of turkey or ham to the sandwich

Add another slice of cheese

Choose milk instead of juice, water, sports drinks, or carbonated beverages

Snacks

Have a handful of nuts instead of pretzels

Have tortilla chips and bean dip instead of potato chips with sour cream dip

Make a yogurt, milk, and fruit smoothie

Dinner

Have a larger piece of beef, poultry, or fish

Add some cheese to pasta

Choose milk instead of juice, water, sports drinks, or carbonated beverages

Many athletes believe that it's easier to use a protein shake, protein bar, amino acid pills, or protein powder to meet their protein needs rather than eat the right foods. However, shakes can be expensive, they can taste bad, and, unless they are ready to drink, they require mixing in a blender. They need to be refrigerated and may separate when exposed to heat. In addition, protein shakes always have the same sweet taste, whereas a piece of chicken can be sweet, sour, salty, or spicy. And protein shakes won't make athletes feel as full as would a meal with protein.

Protein bars can be too high in protein and too low in carbohydrate, so eating a protein bar before exercise can result in fatigue. In addition, some of these bars are quite high in calories and some have a high fat content. Also, protein bars may be expensive. A peanut butter sandwich is a lot cheaper and tastes better, too.

Although taking amino acid supplements can be appealing because it's easy, no studies have shown that taking amino acid supplements improves sport performance, and these supplements may cause gastrointestinal distress.

Some of your athletes may ask about protein powders. Powders can be fairly costly, they require mixing, and they may not taste good. Of the available protein powders, whey protein isolate is probably the best option. If an athlete wants to use a protein powder, suggest nonfat dry milk powder, which is inexpensive, shelf stable, and tasteless and is an excellent source of calcium.

Now that we've looked at the three main types of nutrients, it's time to consider how to put them together for a balanced diet.

Striking a Nutrient Balance

Most of your athletes are not going to sit down to a meal that is just candy (carbohydrate) or egg whites (protein) or mayonnaise (fat), but many of them may not be eating in a way that optimizes nutrient balance. They need to be reminded that the muscles need enough fuel to perform and that fuel needs to come from various sources. This is why it is a good idea to have your athletes fill out a food frequency form that lists various types of foods and the categories they fall into. Figure 2.5 is an example of a completed food frequency form for Michael, a tennis player. Figure 2.6 is a blank form that you can copy and use.

Have athletes fill out the food frequency form. Also give them the handouts on proper fueling for male and female athletes. Ask the players to compare their food frequency form results to the handouts. (Beginning-of-Season Activity)

Michael's Food Frequency Form

In a week, how often do you eat or drink the following foods and beverages? Place a check in the appropriate column.

Foods and beverages	Daily	Three or four times a week	One or two times a week	Less than weekly
White bread	X			
Whole-wheat bread			X	
Unsweetened cereal	X			
Sweetened cereal				X
Pasta		X		
Rice, white			X	
Rice, brown				X
Baked or mashed potatoes				X
French fries		X		
Fruit		X		
Cooked vegetables			X	
Salad				X
Chips		X		
Cookies				X
Candy	X			
Beef		X		
Pork, ham, or bacon			X	
Sausage, pepperoni, bologna or salami			X	
Poultry	X			
Fish or shellfish				X
Cheese	X			
Cheese, low-fat				X
Yogurt	X			
Eggs			X	
Beans				X
Nut butter	X			
Soy foods				X
Nuts		X		
Butter or margarine		X		
Salad dressing		X		
Juice	X			
Milk	X			
Sports drinks	X			
Carbonated beverages			X	
Coffee or tea			X	
Water	X			

FIGURE 2.5 Sample food frequency form.

Food Frequency Form

In a week, how often do you eat or drink the following foods and beverages? Place a check in the appropriate column.

Foods and beverages	Daily	Three or four times a week	One or two times a week	Less than weekly
White bread				
Whole-wheat bread*				
Unsweetened cereal*				
Sweetened cereal				
Pasta				
Rice, brown*				
Baked or mashed potatoes*				
French fries				
Fruit*				
Cooked vegetables*				
Salad*				
Chips				
Cookies				
Beef, lean*				
Pork, ham, or bacon				
Sausage, pepperoni, bologna or salami				
Poultry*				
Fish or shellfish*				
Cheese, low-fat or light*				
Yogurt*				
Eggs*				
Beans*				
Nut butter*				
Soy foods*				
Nuts*				
Butter or margarine				
Salad dressing				
Juice, 100 percent fruit*				
Milk, low-fat*				
Sports drinks				
Carbonated beverages				
Coffee or tea				
Water*				

* Items are the healthiest carbohydrate, protein, and fat sources.

From L. Bonci, 2009, Sport Nutrition for Coaches (Champaign, IL: Human Kinetics).

FIGURE 2.6 Food frequency form.

Table 2.9 groups some common foods by how well they provide carbohydrate, protein, or fat. The best choices provide the most nutritional value per calorie. As an example, lean and fatty meats both provide protein, but lean meats provide less saturated fat. Oatmeal and cornflakes both provide carbohydrate, but oatmeal is higher in fiber and other health-promoting plant nutrients.

 Post or hand out this table so that your players can make proper food and beverage choices. (Beginning-of-Season Activity)

The goal is for your athletes to choose the best foods 60 percent of the time, the OK foods 30 percent of the time, and the not-so-hot foods 10 percent of the time.

For more guidance, see the handouts for female (pp. 30-31) and male (pp. 32-33) athletes in the next sidebars. Each sidebar includes a food list that is broken down by body weight to make it easy for your athletes to determine whether they are getting the right amount and right distribution of calories throughout the day.

Athletes must fuel their bodies. They should keep charts to get an idea of their current diet so that they can make appropriate performance-boosting changes. Every one of us has particular food likes and dislikes, and although we don't all choose the same foods, we all need to consume enough nutrients every day. This is important for athletes' health, well-being, and sports as well as academic performance. Talk about nutrition requirements so that they understand what their bodies require. Post food lists, encourage athletes to carefully plan what they eat, and make eating a priority for your athletes. The result is that they will do better, feel better, learn better, and be better.

Develop and distribute guidelines for healthful nutrition during the off-season. Remind athletes that by making good choices year-round, they can reduce the amount of work needed to bring their bodies into optimal shape during the pre-season. (Off-Season Activity)

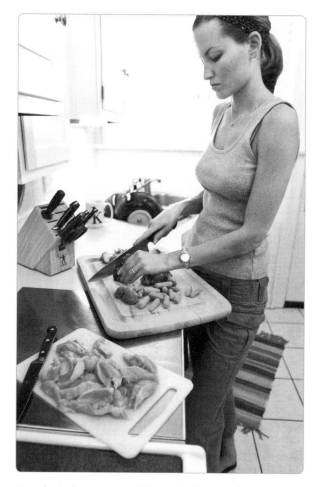

Once they've become aware of their eating habits, athletes can select more healthful foods to meet their nutritional requirements.

TABLE 2.9

Ratings for Food Choices

	Carbohydrate	Protein	Fat
Best	Whole-grain breads	Very lean ground beef	Olive oil
	Brown rice	Pork	Canola oil
	Pasta, white or whole wheat	Veal	Sunflower oil
	Rice	Lamb	Safflower oil
	Barley	Venison	Soybean oil
	Quinoa	Poultry	Corn oil
	Tortillas	Fish	Peanut oil
	Oatmeal	Shellfish	Mayonnaise
	Corn	Soy foods	Nuts
	Whole-grain cereal	Beans	Nut butters
	Whole-grain crackers	Eggs	Seeds
	Fruits	Low-fat milk	Olives
	Vegetables	Low-fat yogurt	
	Baked potatoes	Low-fat cheese	
		Low-fat cottage cheese	
OK	White bread	Low-fat ham	Light salad dressings
	Pretzels	Lean ground meat	Light mayonnaise
	Low-fat crackers	Fish canned in oil	Reduced-fat peanut butter
	Low-fat granola bars	Low-fat hot dogs	Light butter
	Cereal bars	Sliced cheese	
	Low-fat muffins	Light margarine	
	Baked chips		
	Fruit juice		
Not so hot	Pastries	Fried meats	Butter
	Chips (not baked)	Sausage, bacon	Margarine
	Candy	Pepperoni	Cream sauces
	French fries	Burgers	Creamy salad dressing
	Soda	Salami, bologna	Fat-free salad dressings
	Fruit drinks		

A Female Athlete's Guide to Proper Fueling

1. Daily calorie goal

> Weight in pounds × 15-20 or weight in kilograms × 33-44 = number of calories per day for weight maintenance

As a guideline:

15 calories per pound (33 calories/kg) for weight-class or appearance sports such as crew and gymnastics or for athletes who need to lose weight

16 to 17 calories per pound (35-37 calories/kg) for sports such as volleyball, tennis, and throwing sports

18 to 19 calories per pound (39-42 calories/kg) for track and field, basketball, and swimming

20 calories per pound (44 calories/kg) for cross country, soccer, and field hockey

> [Weight (pounds) × 20 or weight (kg) × 44] – 300 = calories for weight loss

> [Weight (pounds) × 20 or weight (kg) × 44] + 500 = calories for weight gain

2. Composition of the diet for optimal performance

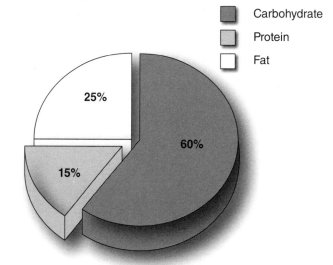

- ▮ Carbohydrate
- ▮ Protein
- ▢ Fat

25%

60%

15%

Carbohydrate: 50 to 60 percent   Protein: 15 to 20 percent   Fat: 20 to 30 percent

Because a gram of carbohydrate or protein has 4 calories and a gram of fat has 9, you can calculate the daily requirements for carbohydrate, protein, or fat like this:

> Carbohydrate requirements in grams = .60 × daily calories divided by 4

> Protein requirements in grams = .15 × daily calories divided by 4

> Fat requirements in grams = .25 × daily calories divided by 9

Example for Female Athletes

A 130-pound (60 kg) athlete would need 1,950 to 2,600 calories per day (weight in pounds × 15-20 or weight in kg × 33-44), which would be made up of the following:

- Carbohydrate needs: .50 to .60 × 1,950 to 2,600 divided by 4 = 243 to 390 grams of carbohydrate
- Protein needs: .15 to .20 × 1,950 to 2,600 divided by 4 = 73 to 130 grams of protein
- Fat needs: .20 to .30 × 1,950 to 2,600 divided by 9 = 43 to 87 grams of fat

 From L. Bonci, 2009, *Sport Nutrition for Coaches* (Champaign, IL: Human Kinetics).

General Recommendations for Females

Weight, lb (kg)	Calories	Carbohydrate selections	Protein selections	Fat selections
100 (45)	1,500-2,000	7.5-12	4-7	3-6
110 (50)	1,650-2,200	8-13	4-7	4-7
120 (55)	1,800-2,400	9-14	4.5-8	4-8
130 (60)	1,950-2,600	9.5-15	5-8.5	4.5-8.5
140 (64)	2,100-2,800	10-15	5-9	5-9
150 (68)	2,250-3,000	11-18	5.5-10	5-9.5
160 (73)	2,400-3,200	12-19	6-10.5	5.5-10
170 (77)	2,550-3,400	13-20	6.5-11	5.5-11
180 (82)	2,700-3,600	13.5-21	7-11.5	6-12
190 (86)	2,850-3,800	14-23	7.5-12	6-12.5
200 (91)	3,000-4,000	15-24	8-12.5	6.5-13

Refer to the lists of carbohydrate, protein, and fat food choices. The selections shown contain the following quantities of nutrients: carbohydrate food choices contain 25 grams of carbohydrate; protein food choices contain 15 grams of protein; fat-containing food choices have 10 grams of fat.

To construct a diet for optimal performance, circle the choices you like from each list and try to include a food from each category every time you eat.

Carbohydrate

1/2 large bagel
1 cup pasta (fist-sized portion)
3/4 rice (fist-sized portion)
1 cup (30 g) plain Cheerios
A low-fat fruit muffin (tennis ball size)
1/2 cup (127 g) applesauce
A 4-inch (10 cm) baked potato
2/3 cup corn
Three fig bars
1 1/2 cups grapes
One English muffin
Two 4-inch (10 cm) diameter pancakes
1/2 cup (110 g) pudding
Two handfuls of pretzels
1 cup (240 ml) juice
3/4 cup (175 g) frozen yogurt
16 ounces (480 ml) sports drink
One packet flavored oatmeal
15 animal crackers
One large banana
One large apple, pear, or orange
One granola bar
10 large marshmallows
1 ounce (30 g) licorice
1/3 cup (41 g) granola
One Nutri-Grain cereal bar
10 jelly beans
16 ounces (480 ml) lemonade or fruit punch
3/4 cup (23 g) sweetened cereal
1/2 bag of microwave low-fat popcorn
Eight vanilla wafers
1/4 cup (40 g) raisins

Protein

Chicken (palm-sized portion)
Beef (palm-sized portion)
Fish (palm-sized portion)
2 ounces (60 g) canned tuna
1/2 cup (112 g) cottage cheese
One soy burger
1 cup pinto beans
Two slices of cheese
Three slices of lunch meat
Two eggs
Hamburger or turkey burger (size of a mayonnaise jar lid)
1/2 cup (180 ml) egg substitute
8 ounces (250 g) tofu

High-Fat and High-Carbohydrate Foods
Try to limit! Not as performance boosting!

Doughnuts
Ice cream
Most cookies
Chocolate chips
French fries

Double-Duty Foods

Carbohydrate + protein
Yogurt 8 ounces (230 g) = 50 grams of carbohydrate + 12 grams of protein
Sports bars: Clif Bar, PowerBar, GatorBar
Certain beverage supplements: Gatorade Nutrition Shake, Boost, Carnation Instant Breakfast
Milk: 16 ounces (480 ml) chocolate milk = 50 grams of carbohydrate, 16 grams of protein
Cheese pizza (two slices = 80 grams of carbohydrate, 16 grams of protein)

Fat

1 tablespoon peanut butter
1/4 cup (35 g) nuts
Two pats butter
2 teaspoons oil
2 teaspoons mayonnaise
Two strips bacon
2 tablespoons cream cheese
4 tablespoons sour cream
1 tablespoon regular salad dressing
2 tablespoons light salad dressing

From L. Bonci, 2009, *Sport Nutrition for Coaches* (Champaign, IL: Human Kinetics).

31

A Male Athlete's Guide to Proper Fueling

1. Daily calorie goal

Weight in pounds × 20-27 or weight in kilograms × 44-59 = number of calories per day for weight maintenance

As a guideline:

20 to 23 calories per pound (44-50 calories/kg) for weight-class or appearance sports such as wrestling and gymnastics, for precision sports such as baseball and golf, or for athletes who need to lose weight

20 to 25 calories per pound (44-55 calories/kg) for football

20 to 27 calories per pound (44-59 calories/kg) for cross country, tennis, swimming, basketball, soccer, lacrosse

[Weight (pounds) × 23 or weight (kg) × 50] − 300 calories for weight loss

[Weight (pounds) × 23 or weight (kg) × 50] + 500 calories for weight gain

2. Composition of the diet for optimal performance

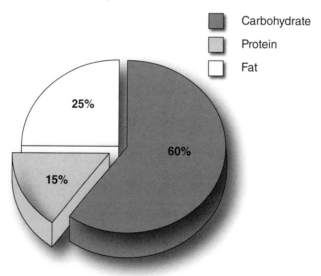

- Carbohydrate
- Protein
- Fat

Carbohydrate: 55 to 60 percent   Protein: 15 to 20 percent   Fat: 20 to 30 percent

Because a gram of carbohydrate or protein has 4 calories and a gram of fat has 9, you can calculate the daily requirements for carbohydrate, protein, or fat like this:

Carbohydrate requirements in grams = .60 × daily calories divided by 4

Protein requirements in grams = .15 × daily calories divided by 4

Fat requirements in grams = .25 × daily calories divided by 9

Example for Male Athletes

A 180-pound (82 kg) athlete would need 4,140 calories per day: weight in pounds × 23 or weight in kilograms × 50, which would be made up of the following:

- Carbohydrate needs: .60 × 4,140 divided by 4 = 620 grams of carbohydrate
- Protein needs: .15 × 4,140 divided by 4 = 155 grams of protein
- Fat needs: .25 × 4,140 divided by 9 = 115 grams of fat

 From L. Bonci, 2009, *Sport Nutrition for Coaches* (Champaign, IL: Human Kinetics).

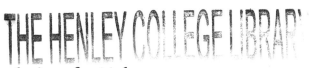

General Recommendations for Males

Weight, lb (kg)	Calories	Carbohydrate selections	Protein selections	Fat selections
130 (60)	2,990	9	5.5	8.5
140 (64)	3,220	9.5	6	9
150 (68)	3,450	10	6	9
170 (77)	3,910	11.5	8	11
180 (82)	4,080	12	8	11
190 (86)	4,270	13	8	11.5
200 (91)	4,600	14	8.5	12

Refer to the lists of carbohydrate, protein, and fat food choices. The selections shown contain the following quantities of nutrients: carbohydrate food choices contain 50 grams of carbohydrate; protein food choices contain 20 grams of protein; fat-containing food choices contain 10 grams of fat.

To construct a diet for optimal performance, circle the choices you like from each list and try to eat a food from each category every time you eat.

Carbohydrate

One large bagel
1 1/3 cups pasta (1 1/2 fist-sized portion)
1 1/2 cups rice
2 cups (60 g) Cheerios
A large low-fat fruit muffin
2 cups (450 g) oatmeal
1 cup (255 g) applesauce
A large baked potato
1 1/3 cups corn
Five fig bars
3 cups of grapes
2 English muffins
Four 4-inch (10 cm) diameter pancakes
1 cup (110 g) pudding
Three handfuls of pretzels
2 cups (480 ml) juice
1 1/2 cups (260 g) frozen yogurt
32 ounces (1 L) sports drink
Two packets of flavored oatmeal
25 animal crackers
Two bananas
Two apples
2 cups of grapes
10 large marshmallows
2 ounces (60 g) licorice
3/4 cup (82 g) granola
Two cereal bars
20 jelly beans
16 ounces (480 ml) lemonade or fruit punch
1 1/2 cups (45 g) sweetened cereal
One bag microwave low-fat popcorn
One Pop-Tart
15 vanilla wafers
1/2 cup (80 g) raisins

Protein

Chicken (computer mouse–sized portion)
Beef (computer mouse–sized portion)
Fish (computer mouse–sized portion)
3 ounces (90 g) canned tuna
3/4 cup (170 g) cottage cheese
One large soy burger
1 1/4 cups pinto beans
Three slices of cheese
Four thin slices of lunch meat
Three eggs
One large hamburger or turkey burger
3/4 cup (180 ml) egg substitute
10 ounces (300 g) tofu

High-Fat and High-Carbohydrate Foods
Try to limit! Not as performance boosting!

Doughnuts
Ice cream
Most cookies
Chocolate
Chips
French fries

Double-Duty Foods

Carbohydrate + protein
Yogurt 8 oz (230 g) container = 50 grams carbohydrate + 12 grams of protein
Sports bars: Clif Bar, PowerBar, GatorBar
Certain beverage supplements: Gatorade Nutrition Shake, Boost, Carnation Instant Breakfast
Milk: 16 ounces (480 ml) chocolate milk = 50 grams carbohydrate, 16 grams protein
Cheese pizza (two slices = 80 grams of carbohydrate, 16 grams of protein)

Fat

1 tablespoon peanut butter
1/4 cup (35 g) nuts
Two pats butter
2 teaspoons mayonnaise
2 teaspoons oil
Two strips bacon
2 tablespoons cream cheese
1 tablespoon regular salad dressing
4 tablespoons sour cream
2 tablespoons light salad dressing

From L. Bonci, 2009, *Sport Nutrition for Coaches* (Champaign, IL: Human Kinetics).

33

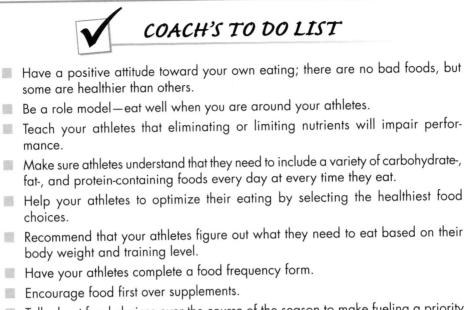

- Have a positive attitude toward your own eating; there are no bad foods, but some are healthier than others.
- Be a role model—eat well when you are around your athletes.
- Teach your athletes that eliminating or limiting nutrients will impair performance.
- Make sure athletes understand that they need to include a variety of carbohydrate-, fat-, and protein-containing foods every day at every time they eat.
- Help your athletes to optimize their eating by selecting the healthiest food choices.
- Recommend that your athletes figure out what they need to eat based on their body weight and training level.
- Have your athletes complete a food frequency form.
- Encourage food first over supplements.
- Talk about food choices over the course of the season to make fueling a priority for your athletes.

SUMMARY

- To perform optimally, one must ingest carbohydrate-, protein-, and fat-containing foods throughout the day.
- Nutrients have specific roles with regard to performance.
- Healthier choices within each macronutrient group can decrease the risk of disease.
- Nutrient requirements will vary depending on body size and level and intensity of training.
- Restricting intake of any nutrient will negatively affect performance.

KEY TERMS

carbohydrate	fatty acids	saturated fat
essential amino acids	glycemic index	trans fat
essential fatty acids	monounsaturated fat	triglyceride
fat (lipids)	protein	

GAME PLAN QUESTIONS

1. Why should athletes eat enough carbohydrate?

2. What are three important functions of protein?

3. What problems can occur when an athlete curtails his or her fat intake?

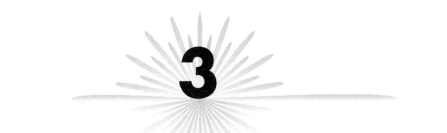

3

Eating Timed for Top Performance

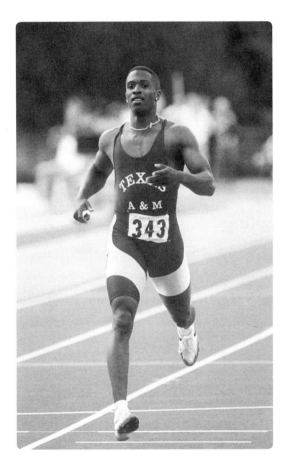

Jordan is a talented collegiate runner who ran well at the beginning of the season but has noticed a significant decrease in his race times and an increase in recovery time as the season goes on. He is very frustrated because he believes he has trained well and can't understand why this is occurring. When we sat down to meet, he told me that he doesn't like the feeling of food in his stomach too close to practice, he is often too tired to eat, and he has no appetite once practice is over. The fact that he is not optimally fueled prior to running and waits too long to eat once he is finished contributes to the fatigue and subpar performance he notices during the season. The good news is that with a little bit of tweaking and consistency with timing of meals and snacks, he should be able to finish strong.

When you finish reading this chapter, you should be able to explain

- what and when your athletes should eat before exercise,
- what and when your athletes should eat before and during an athletic event, and
- what and when your athletes should eat after exercise.

Too often, eating is an afterthought for many athletes. The reality is that when one eats is as important as what is consumed, and the proper timing meals can go a long way toward optimizing performance. This chapter focuses on strategies to help your athletes develop a fueling plan for before, during, and after workouts and competition.

Pre-Exercise Eating

Regular pre-exercise eating and hydration (see chapter 4) are recommended so athletes take in what they need daily to keep muscles fueled and hydrated, optimize performance, and ensure adequate recovery. During exercise, athletes rely mostly on the glycogen stored in the muscles and liver and on fat stores. Although a pre-exercise meal is not immediately available for energy, it can contribute when exercise or athletic events go on continuously for more than an hour.

The other goal of the pre-exercise meal is to lessen the feeling of hunger, which can distract an athlete.

Send out a letter to all athletes one week before the start of preseason reminding them to eat and drink before practice and to bring snacks and fluids to practice. (Off-Season Activities)

A hungry athlete cannot focus fully on the task at hand. A pre-exercise meal containing carbohydrate will elevate blood glucose and serve as an additional fuel substrate during exercise for the muscles.

Athletes in sports such as soccer, hockey, track and field, and short-distance swimming must consume enough carbohydrate to fill muscle and liver glycogen stores. Because these sports involve high-intensity bursts of activity that require carbohydrate as the primary fuel, carbohydrate needs are higher. A pre-exercise meal that contains a significant amount of carbohydrate (200 grams) improves endurance but may also be beneficial for athletes who are exercising after an extended period of time without food, such as athletes who have early-morning practice or competition. A carbohydrate-dense morning meal will restore liver glycogen stores that are low after an overnight fast and can increase suboptimal muscle glycogen stores to improve performance. There is never a reason for athletes to stop consuming carbohydrate, because they will never be able to perform at their best without it.

Another issue in planning the pre-exercise meal is preventing gastrointestinal distress. Low-fiber foods that empty more rapidly and cause less bloating than high-fiber foods are recommended. Consuming a high-fiber food such as a large bowl of raisin bran is probably not a great idea before exercising. If athletes are concerned that they will experience gastrointestinal upset by competing after a pre-event meal, they can try liquid meals. Carnation Instant

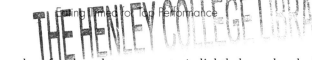

Breakfast, Boost, a smoothie, or low-fat chocolate milk can provide necessary nutrients that leave the stomach more quickly. For lactose-intolerant athletes or those with milk allergies, a soy-based smoothie, soy milk, or shakes such as Amazishake can be used.

The closer the meal is consumed prior to the practice or competition, the smaller the meal should be. More food in the stomach means more blood being diverted to the gut, which can be uncomfortable. Athletes who compete in morning events, such as track athletes in all-day meets or swimmers or rowers who have to be in or on the water at 6 a.m., are probably not going to wake up several hours ahead of time to eat, so liquid meals present a viable alternative. Gelatin, yogurt, and puddings can be used by athletes who complain of being too tired to chew!

Two concepts that often come up when discussing pre-exercise nutrition are carbohydrate loading and the glycemic index of foods. Let's examine those briefly now.

 Arrange for students to eat in the period before practice during the school year. (Preseason Activities)

Carbohydrate Loading

You may be familiar with the concept of **carbohydrate loading,** where over a seven-day period leading up to competition the athlete depletes muscle glycogen stores through exhaustive exercise and simultaneously decreases carbohydrate intake, so that when a large amount of carbohydrate is consumed the muscles can supersaturate with glycogen. The rationale for this type of nutrient manipulation is to prevent fatigue associated with glycogen depletion. The downside of this method is a feeling of stiffness and heaviness in the muscles, which is very uncomfortable for the athlete and potentially impairs performance in short-term events.

A better way of achieving these results is to have athletes eat a little more carbohydrate as part of every meal in the three days leading up to competition. In addition, they should decrease exercise during the taper period because the rest will encourage glycogen resynthesis. Carbohydrate loading does not have to be accomplished by wolfing down a pound of jelly beans. It can be done by eating or drinking the following:

- A slightly larger bowl of cereal at breakfast
- A bagel instead of bread at lunch
- A larger serving of rice, pasta, or potato at dinner
- Carbohydrate-containing juice, lemonade, and sports drinks
- Carbohydrate supplements such as gels

If your athletes choose to consume carbohydrate supplements, make sure these athletes consume water simultaneously to prevent any digestive issues.

Glycemic Index of Foods

Athletes might ask you whether there are some carbohydrate-containing foods that should be preferentially consumed prior to exercise. This is based in part on the glycemic index of foods, or the ability of a food to affect blood glucose (as discussed in chapter 2). There are three categories: high glycemic index, moderate glycemic index, and low glycemic index carbohydrate-rich foods. Examples of foods in each category appear in table 3.1.

Ingesting low glycemic index foods before competition may result in sustained availability of carbohydrates during exercise and prevent an insulin surge and subsequent decrease in blood glucose. This may be most useful for the athlete who experiences hypoglycemia during competition or fatigues early. However, some athletes may find these foods to be unappealing or too heavy prior to exercise.

Another option is to have the athlete wait to consume carbohydrates a few minutes before exercise and preferably to consume a liquid form, such as sports gels, sports drinks, or gelatin. The reason is that once exercise begins, there is an increase in the hormones epinephrine, norepinephrine, and growth hormone, which inhibit insulin's release and the blood glucose–lowering effect of insulin. This way the athlete will not have the surge and drop in blood glucose.

For your athletes who are not sensitive to changes in blood glucose, consuming foods from the high glycemic index list one hour before exercise may be advantageous. This is probably best for the athlete who has a morning practice or event after an overnight fast. Starting the day with a corn-, wheat-, or rice-based cereal, a bagel or toast with jam, or a sports drink will fuel the athlete who has a one- to two-hour practice or endurance event early in the day.

TABLE 3.1

Common Foods Grouped by Glycemic Index Rating

Low glycemic index	Moderate glycemic index	High glycemic index
Beans	Rice	Glucose
Plums	Vanilla wafers	Carrots
Dairy foods	Bagels	White potatoes
Apples	Crackers	Honey
Dried beans	Soda	Corn flakes
Pastas	Cakes and cookies	White bread
Peaches	Wheat bread	Corn chips
Fructose	Sugar	Sports drinks
Nuts	Low-fat ice cream	Ice cream
	Sweet potatoes	Rice cakes
	High-fiber cereal	
	Potato chips	

Example

Joan is a cross country athlete who is gearing up for the end-of-season meets. In the past she has felt more depleted than she wanted even though she does a good job with fueling during the season. She decided to make the following changes to her eating and exercise one week before a meet.

Three days prior to the meet Joan cut her mileage significantly. She also adjusted her diet as follows:

Typical Day	**Additions three days before her meet**
Breakfast	
1 cup (30 g) cereal	Increase to 1 1/2 cups (45 g) cereal
A banana	Add 6 ounces (180 ml) juice
6 ounces (180 ml) skim milk	
Lunch	
Sandwich on two slices of whole wheat bread	Change to a whole-wheat bagel
A piece of fruit	Two handfuls of pretzels
A small handful of pretzels	
Water	
Snack	
Granola bar	Two granola bars
Water	Sports drink
Dinner	
2 cups of pasta with meat sauce	3 cups of pasta
Salad	
A slice of bread	
Glass of milk	

Pre-Event Eating

It would be great if athletes had three to five days to rest and fuel optimally prior to competition. Reality dictates that for many sports, tournaments or invitationals consist of all-day activity or back-to-back days, and practices are two per day. If the body is given 24 to 36 hours to fuel before events, performance can be maintained at a high level.

When it comes to pre-event eating, tell your athletes to stick with familiar foods. If they have never eaten a food before, they don't know how their body is going to react. Nothing puts a damper on sport performance like a digestive issue. Caution your athletes to steer clear of the following foods if they have never used them before:

- Caffeine in large doses: Energy drinks can be loaded with caffeine.
- Carbonated beverages: They can cause bloating.
- High-fiber cereals (e.g., bran): These cereals take too long to empty from the digestive tract.
- Dried beans: Beans may cause bloating, gas, and a feeling of heaviness, so your athletes will need to experiment with the amount consumed to determine tolerance levels.
- Cabbage family vegetables, such as broccoli, cabbage, and coleslaw: These can cause gas and bloating and do not provide enough calories for activity.
- Fatty foods, such as pepperoni, salami, hot dogs, sausage, and bacon: These foods can take too long to empty from the stomach.
- Fried foods, such as fried chicken and French fries: These can take too long to empty from the stomach.
- Dried fruit, such as raisins, apricots, and dried plums: In large quantities, they can have a laxative effect (but a small amount may work well).
- Juices: They are high in fructose, which is used by the liver as a fuel source and takes too long to convert into available muscle fuel.

Eating the right foods and staying properly hydrated before an event can make the difference between winning and losing. The timing of meals is also important. Here are some recommendations for pre-event eating, on the night before and the day of the event, including the time of day the event is held.

Night Before an Event

The night before an event, have your athletes consume the following:

- An additional two glasses of fluid or a bowl of soup in the early evening.
- An evening meal that's about two thirds carbohydrate. Here are some examples:
  - Pasta with marinara sauce (if tolerated), olive oil and garlic, or a small amount of margarine and Parmesan cheese and a slice or two of bread
  - A turkey or ham hoagie
  - Stir-fry with chicken or beef and vegetables over a lot of rice
  - Fajitas with chicken or beef, lettuce, and salsa, and rice on the side
  - Thick-crust plain or vegetable pizza

If the team is traveling and eating out, pick a restaurant with a varied enough menu to satisfy the majority of the team's food preferences. A buffet is always a good bet to satisfy the vegetarians as well as the meat eaters on your team.

If fast food is the option, suggest to the athletes that they choose from the following items:

- Grilled chicken sandwich and a baked potato
- Fajitas or soft tacos and rice
- Turkey, chicken, or ham and cheese hoagie with baked chips

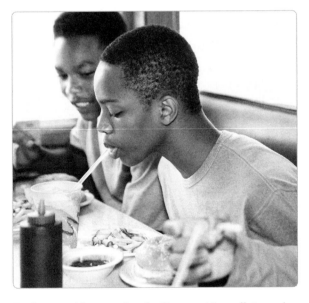

Teach your athletes to select familiar, nutritious offerings when eating out before an event.

- A burger or grilled chicken sandwich and a shake
- Bagel sandwiches and juice
- Wrap sandwiches and lemonade
- Low-fat shakes and smoothies

Athletes should eat something about one hour before bed and drink about 16 to 20 ounces (480-600 ml) of liquid to top off fluid requirements. When you travel, either provide snacks for the team or suggest that each athlete pack snacks. Better yet, arrange an evening meeting solely for the purpose of making sure that everyone on your team eats something before going to bed. Appoint a snack coach to make sure that every athlete brings her fluid bottle and snacks on the trip.

If your athletes are at home or go out for an evening snack, they can choose perishable items such as these:

- Low-fat shake
- Soft-serve ice cream, sorbet, sherbet, or fruit ice
- A smoothie
- Chocolate milk
- Yogurt
- Pudding

Here are some items that travel well and can be packed in athletes' bags:

- Cereal bars
- Popcorn
- Cereal
- Bagel with peanut butter
- Crackers
- Pretzels
- Dried soup packets

Day of the Event

On the day of the event, ask your athletes to drink these amounts:

- 16 to 20 ounces (480-600 ml) of water two hours before the event
- Another 16 ounces (480 ml) of water or a sports drink 30 minutes before the event

Serve meals or ask athletes to eat meals such as the following, depending on how close the meal is to the event:

Four hours before an event

- Turkey, ham, tuna, or roast beef sandwich and soup
- An omelet
- Scrambled eggs and toast
- A grilled chicken sandwich or a turkey burger
- Yogurt and a bagel
- Spaghetti with sauce, olive oil and garlic, or a small amount of margarine

Two to three hours before an event

- Cereal and milk
- Bagel with a small amount of peanut butter or a slice of cheese
- English muffin with jelly and a small amount of margarine
- Waffles or pancakes with syrup
- High-carbohydrate sports bar such as Clif Bar, LaraBar, Odwalla Bar, or PowerBar

One hour before an event

- 8 ounces (230 g) yogurt
- 10 ounces (300 ml) fruit smoothie
- Handful of crackers
- Cereal bar or granola bar

Smoothie Recipe

It is easy to make a smoothie rather than buy one ready to drink, but this requires a blender.

Smoothie recipe
4 ounces (115 g) yogurt
4 ounces (120 ml) skim milk
1/2 cup fruit (fresh or frozen) or a small banana

Or
A packet of instant breakfast
8 ounces (240 ml) low-fat milk
1/2 cup frozen fruit or a small banana

Athletes who are traveling and have early-morning events should pack some snacks to eat when they wake up, to get some fuel into the body. Consider doing a bag check to see if your athletes have come prepared! If you can, work with your high school or college food service department to put together a list of portable snacks, such as these:

- Dry cereal
- Cereal bars
- Trail mix
- Granola bars
- Bagels
- Crackers
- Pretzels
- Sports bars

Time of Day of the Event

The optimal meal for a given event may depend on the time it is held. Here are suggestions for various times of the day.

For morning competitions The athlete should be up two to three hours before the competition. He should eat and drink something with calories 60 to 90 minutes before the event, such as the following:

- A small muffin with a glass of milk
- A smoothie or breakfast shake and a slice of toast with jelly
- Cereal and milk
- One or two waffles with syrup

The athlete should also consume 16 ounces (480 ml) of fluid at this meal.

For midday events (1-2 p.m.) Athletes have the opportunity to eat twice prior to competition, so encourage them to eat breakfast.

Meal at 8 a.m.
- Cereal
- Cereal bar and yogurt
- Smoothie and toast with jelly
- Waffles, French toast, or pancakes with syrup
- 16 ounces (480 ml) fluid

Meal at 10:30 to 11:00 a.m.
- A 6-inch (15 cm) hoagie with turkey, ham, cheese, roast beef, or light tuna or chicken salad
- An omelet with a bagel or a low-fat muffin

- A bowl of oatmeal with fruit
- 16 to 20 ounces (480-600 ml) fluid

Athletes who have nervous stomachs before events can choose a liquid meal as their second meal of the day, such as the following:

- A smoothie
- Yogurt
- High-carbohydrate sports drink
- Sports bar and 16 ounces (480 ml) fluid
- Soup with noodles and meat or poultry

For evening events (7 p.m. or later) on a weekday Athletes can eat breakfast, have lunch between noon and 1 p.m. (this should be the largest meal), and take a mid-afternoon snack around 3 to 4 p.m.

Lunch
- Pasta with marinara sauce and bread
- Baked chicken with rice, rolls, and vegetables
- Stir-fry with lots of rice
- A hoagie with pretzels or baked chips and fruit
- 16 to 20 ounces (480-600 ml) fluid

Midafternoon snack
- A peanut butter and jelly sandwich and milk
- Cereal and milk
- Sports bars
- Peanut butter crackers and milk
- 16 to 20 ounces (480-600 ml) fluid

For evening events (7 p.m. or later) on a weekend Athletes can eat brunch around 11 a.m. or noon, have a major meal around 4 p.m., and then have a snack around 6 p.m.

Major meal
- Pasta
- Chicken, potatoes, vegetables, rolls
- Stir-fry
- Fajitas
- 16 to 20 ounces (480-600 ml) fluid

Snack
- A few crackers
- A cereal bar
- A granola bar
- A handful of cereal
- 16 ounces (480 ml) fluid

For all-day events Because turnaround time is minimal between events, the goal is to have athletes eat small amounts of easily digestible foods that are available all day, such as these:

- Dry cereal
- Cereal bars
- Pretzels
- Cut up fruit
- Yogurt
- Cheese sticks
- Trail mix, Chex mix, or mix of cereal, pretzels, and chocolate chips

You can also have the following foods available:

- Honey wands or sticks—These are made of crystallized honey and are sold at places like Sam's Club, Costco, and Trader Joe's. They are not messy or sticky and not overly sweet, so they are palatable.
- Gels (such as Gu or Clif Shot)—Gels come in foil packages and are single-serving portions of carbohydrate. They are available at sporting goods stores, supermarkets, and on-line but are fairly pricey.
- Gelatin—Use 4-ounce (112 g) containers of Jell-O, or find a parent who is willing to make gelatin cubes, which can be a refreshing source of carbohydrate on a hot day.
- Sugar cubes—Five or six cubes constitute a serving. They are available at grocery stores and are not overly sweet.

Offer liquids at every opportunity.

Although athletes may think about the need to eat during all-day events, what about sports with breaks, such as soccer, basketball, hockey, and football? Most athletes do not eat a lot before they play, and meals are usually four to five hours before competition, so the athlete may feel strong at the beginning of competition but may tire quickly. Athletes need to consume 30 to 60 grams of carbohydrate per hour of exercise. This can be accomplished by consuming more than just water at breaks. A better choice is a sports drink or sports gels with water. As a longtime soccer mom, I have cut up my share of oranges for halftime, but most soccer players won't eat enough orange wedges to get adequate fuel or fluid. You can offer orange wedges with a sports drink, but because time is limited, I suggest gels, honey sticks, sugar cubes, or sports drinks instead.

Postexercise Eating

Your athletes will always have more training sessions in a week than competitions, so postexercise eating plays an essential role in helping the athlete recover quickly so that she can get out there and do it again the next day. Timing is the key factor in expediting recovery and assisting in muscle tissue repair. Athletes need to be reminded about the importance of fueling after exercise and making this a priority. Make sure that before they shower, text message, put on the i-Pod, or drive home from practice, they eat to replete! Cool-down is a perfect time to have your athletes stretch and eat something. This way, you know they've refueled!

Tell your athletes "within 15." You want them to eat or drink something containing calories within 15 minutes of completing exercise to optimally **replete** muscle and liver glycogen stores. If they don't, they will need up to 24 additional hours to recover, and they do not have that kind of time!

Some athletes will tell you they are too tired to eat during this period of time and are not hungry anyway; they may tell you that they will eat when they are hungry, but that is too late. Your athletes need fuel the most when they want it the least! Figure 3.1 illustrates the need to bracket athletic activity with food and fluid.

Make food and beverages readily available to athletes so that refueling is not an afterthought. Your athletes need to bring a bottle of sports drink or a water bottle containing a powdered sports beverage to practice. They should also have nonperishable food in their bag such as granola or cereal bars, a small bag of cereal, some pretzels, trail mix, or a package of peanut butter crackers. At the high school level, parents and booster clubs can supply the postgame snacks. At the university level, handing a bottle of water or sports drink and a sports bar to athletes after

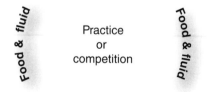

FIGURE 3.1 Emphasize the importance of eating and drinking before and after every practice and every competitive event.

workouts, or having food available and visible, can be a great reminder to refuel.

There has been some recent research on the benefit of chocolate milk as a recovery beverage (Karp et al. 2006). However, milk must be stored at a temperature of 40 degrees F or colder to prevent harmful bacteria from growing in the milk. If coolers are available, consider a sports shake, chocolate milk, smoothies, or yogurt for postexercise repletion.

When your athletes exercise in cold weather, consuming warm foods after exercise can expedite blood flow to the extremities. Hot cocoa, instant soup, or instant oatmeal can provide a warming, nourishing postexercise fuel. This can be helpful for skaters and ice hockey players or during cold-weather football and soccer practice. Consider getting the high school booster clubs involved; at the collegiate level, consider working with your food service department.

As a sports dietitian, I often am asked why athletes can't just have fruit or drink fruit juice after exercise. The carbohydrate in fruit is fructose, which takes longer to resynthesize muscle and liver glycogen than does glucose or sucrose. Your athletes can have fruit as long as they also consume another carbohydrate source to expedite muscle glycogen recovery. Orange juice and pretzels, or a banana with a granola bar, would be fine. The goal is to drink or eat at least 50 grams of carbohydrate as soon as possible after exercise. Listed in table 3.2 are 50-gram carbohydrate equivalent food choices.

For athletes who don't want something sweet, suggest Chex mix, Goldfish crackers, or pretzels—about a cup and a half of any of these.

Should athletes consume protein with carbohydrate after exercise? Specific amino acids such as glutamine and arginine may hasten the body's ability to resynthesize glycogen after exercise (Ivy et al. 2002; Varnier et al. 1995; Yaspelkis and Ivy 1999). In addition, protein plus carbohydrate may assist in the repair and synthesis of muscle proteins after endurance exercise (Levenhagen et al. 2002). These studies suggest a more rapid recovery from exercise with some protein, but the amount required is small, about 15 grams, and the body still needs more carbohydrate than protein. Chocolate milk, trail mix, a peanut butter sandwich, or a high-carbohydrate sports bar would all work well.

Remind your athletes that they do not have to consume a full meal in the 15 minutes after exercise. They can wait until they are hungry to eat, but the meal should still have a significant amount of carbohydrate, so a steak, salad, or chicken wings alone is not going to cut it. Breads, pasta, or rice should be part of this meal to help the athlete to recover fully. It is not necessary for the athlete to consume huge quantities, because that may lead to unwanted weight gain. The most important consideration is for your athletes to eat a little something right after each bout of exercise.

TABLE 3.2

Foods That Contain 50 Grams or More of Carbohydrate

Food	Amount	Carbohydrate, g
Sweetened cereal	2 cups (60 g)	54
Pretzels	Two handfuls	60
Gatorade energy drink	8 oz (240 ml)	78
Bagel with jelly	4-oz (112 g) bagel, 1 tbsp jelly	52
Clif Bar	One	52
Gatorade Bar	One	49
Nutri-Grain Bar	Two	52

Getting Athletes to Eat

The hardest thing about the timing of meals and snacks is getting athletes to buy into the concept that correct timing will benefit them. They need to be proactive, because they can't fuel for an event or practice if it has already occurred. As the coach, you must be proactive as well; make a rule that the athlete who is not fueled can't practice or compete.

If you have students who help with the teams, designate one or more of these helpers as snack coaches to make sure all of your athletes have access to food and fluid during and after practice and competition. Make it a team effort, rewarding those who come to practice and competition fueled and hydrated. In the college setting, work with the athletic director to set up a snack budget, or work with the food service to provide some portable items for the athletes, especially for travel.

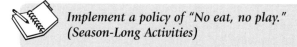 *Implement a policy of "No eat, no play." (Season-Long Activities)*

A season is not one event, and competition gets tougher as the season goes on. What your athletes eat throughout the season can make the difference between ending your season early and advancing to postseason play. Timing can be the deal-maker or -breaker, so remind athletes, make them accountable, and see that they eat and replete. You will get more out of your athletes if they do this consistently.

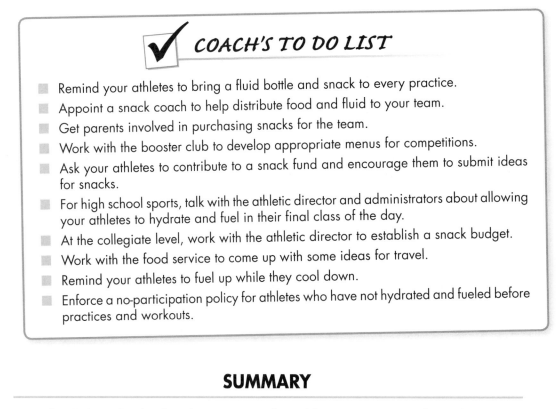

✔ COACH'S TO DO LIST

- Remind your athletes to bring a fluid bottle and snack to every practice.
- Appoint a snack coach to help distribute food and fluid to your team.
- Get parents involved in purchasing snacks for the team.
- Work with the booster club to develop appropriate menus for competitions.
- Ask your athletes to contribute to a snack fund and encourage them to submit ideas for snacks.
- For high school sports, talk with the athletic director and administrators about allowing your athletes to hydrate and fuel in their final class of the day.
- At the collegiate level, work with the athletic director to establish a snack budget.
- Work with the food service to come up with some ideas for travel.
- Remind your athletes to fuel up while they cool down.
- Enforce a no-participation policy for athletes who have not hydrated and fueled before practices and workouts.

SUMMARY

- The timing of eating is as important as what athletes eat in terms of providing energy for practice, competition, and recovery.
- Fueling for sport must occur before, during, and after practices, not just for competition.
- Each of these fueling times is equally important.
- Athletes must be educated on proper timing and food choices for events.
- Athletes need to come prepared for practices and competition by bringing foods and fluids to fuel their body for sport.

KEY TERMS

carbohydrate loading   replete

GAME PLAN QUESTIONS

1. What can you do to make sure your athletes come to practices and workouts hydrated and fueled?

2. What should your athletes do right after practices and workouts?

3. What recommendations will you give your athletes regarding pre-event fueling?

4

Hydrating for Top Performance

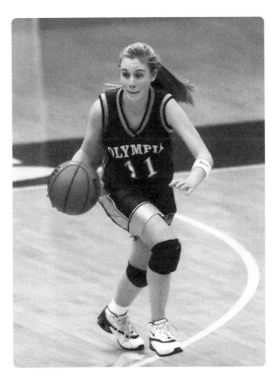

Jessica is a high school basketball star who plays for a school team, plays for an AAU team, and attends summer camps. This past summer at camp she was winning all the medals, outscoring everyone, and in line to win the "hustle" award, when she started to feel lightheaded, got very dizzy, felt faint, and passed out. The athletic trainer determined that she was dehydrated. When she was feeling a little better, I asked her what she had had to drink that day during camp. Her answer: "8 ounces (240 ml) of water in the morning and a few sips from the water fountain during warm-ups." When I asked her why she didn't drink more, she said she didn't want to take time away from the court. Jessica missed a few days of practice because she needed to rest and replete, but now she always has her bottle at practice and drinks on a regular basis.

When you finish reading this chapter, you should be able to explain

- how athletes become dehydrated or overhydrated;
- the effects of dehydration or overhydration on your athletes' health and performance;
- what, when, and how much your athletes should drink;
- what "salty sweaters" are and how they need to monitor their salt balance; and
- how caffeine and alcohol fit into a hydration plan.

Fluid balance is essential for cardiovascular function, body temperature regulation (thermoregulation), injury prevention, and recovery from activity. A body that is not optimally hydrated cannot perform to the maximum. In addition, most athletes sweat when they exercise. Fluid needs are always going to be higher in a physically active person than in someone who is sedentary. And most athletes are going to do some, if not all, of their training in warm or hot weather or a warm room, such as basketball court or wrestling gym.

An athlete who loses 2 percent of his weight attributable to water loss will see a decrease in performance. As an example, a 185-pound (82 kg) cornerback who loses 3.7 pounds (1.7 kg) during practice or competition could see as much as an 8 percent decrease in strength, speed, and stamina. The 2007 ACSM Position Stand on Exercise and Fluid Replacement discusses the performance and health issues associated with **dehydration,** including these:

- Increased heart rate
- Impaired ability to appropriately regulate body temperature
- Early-onset fatigue
- Increased perceived effort of exertion
- Decrease in sustained attention

Every liter of sweat loss results in an eight beat per minute increase in heart rate, so the athlete who does not replace the fluid she loses is forcing her heart to work harder earlier in the exercise bout, increasing the likelihood of early-onset fatigue. In addition to having physiological effects, dehydration can affect mental functioning. Athletes who are dehydrated will be less likely to pay attention, which can affect learning in the classroom as well as on the playing field. Their error rate increases, their response time and task accuracy decrease, and they're more likely to be injured. These effects do not contribute to optimal performance!

Every summer we hear and read about cases of heat illness. Heat-related injury is associated with body water loss, so it is imperative that athletes consider their size, sweat rate, pace, and environmental conditions when deciding how much to drink. An athlete becomes acclimatized by exercising in the heat and hydrating correctly, with a plan in place.

Why Do Athletes Become Dehydrated?

Although we tell our athletes all the time about the importance of being hydrated, most of them are not. A study of recreational exercisers (Stover, Petrie et al. 2006) and a study of high school athletes (Stover, Zachwieja et al. 2006) showed that in both cases, more than 50 percent of the subjects arrived at the gym or field dehydrated. It can only go downhill from there because dehydrated athletes cannot drink enough to rehydrate during exercise. In addition, athletes can become dehydrated because of changes in altitude, increases in training intensity and frequency, sudden climate changes, and long plane flights.

So why don't athletes drink enough? Many factors affect fluid consumption:

- Beverages that are too concentrated in sugars, such as carbonated beverages, fruit juice, fruit punch, and energy drinks, take too long to empty from the gut and make their way into the muscles.
- Some athletes are superstitious and stick with the product that they believe improved their performance in the past; others might have tried a new beverage, ended up with an upset stomach, and blamed the beverage.
- Athletes are influenced by beverage advertising and packaging, but that doesn't mean what they drink will be the appropriate product for them.

- Athletes who eat only once a day are probably going to be somewhat dehydrated because food is a way to help meet fluid needs, and most people drink something when they eat.

- The more dehydrated people are, the less they may want to drink, and when they do drink, they may feel too full and uncomfortable.

- Most of us drink when our mouth is dry, but some beverages may taste better than others. A study has shown that taste preferences may change during activity, and therefore the beverage choices or flavors may need to change as well (Passe et al. 2000).

- Athletes may experience stomach fullness or distention when they are dehydrated, because it takes longer for the fluid to leave the stomach, and if they sip fluid instead of gulping, this also delays the gastric emptying time. Carbonated beverages take longer to empty from the stomach because of the carbonation.

- Accessibility is the most important reason and the reason most often cited for why athletes don't drink enough. If fluid isn't around, they don't think about it and consequently don't hydrate well.

Many athletes have been told to drink when they are thirsty, just as we all know we are supposed to eat when we are hungry. However, thirst isn't an adequate indicator, especially during exercise. Exercise can blunt the thirst mechanism, so voluntary fluid consumption may be insufficient to meet fluid needs. Behavior and habits, rather than thirst, are primarily responsible for determining fluid intake. So as a coach, you need to make fluid intake a practiced and learned behavior that occurs on a schedule. If you stress the importance and allow for fluid breaks, your athletes will be more likely to buy in.

What Should Athletes Drink?

A lot of misinformation is out there concerning fluid choices and what actually constitutes a fluid. All liquids except alcohol count toward the daily fluid requirement. Water, juice, sports drinks, milk, coffee, and tea count fully as fluids. Caffeine is not a **diuretic** (a substance that causes increased urine output); therefore, drinks with caffeine can be part of the fluid allotment for the day. Alcohol is a diuretic and is not considered to be part of the daily fluid intake. Liquid foods such as soup, gelatin, sorbet, sherbet, and popsicles, and foods that have a high water content, such as fruits and vegetables, can

count as part of the daily fluid intake. Too often athletes say that they are not getting enough fluid because they drink very little water, so they need to be reminded of the other choices. However, for the athlete who is trying to lose weight, calories should come from foods, not beverages. Beverages do not make athletes feel full, because beverages leave the gut fairly quickly. Food requires chewing, takes longer to digest, and does a much better job of suppressing hunger. Conversely, those who are trying to gain weight should drink something other than water to provide extra calories.

Some beverage choices are better than others, especially around the time of exercise. Carbonated beverages are not a good choice because they take too long to leave the stomach. This is also true of energy drinks and highly sugared fruit drinks, as well as fruit juice. The goal of drinking fluid before and during exercise is to move the fluid out of the gut fast so it can get to the muscles. That is why water and sports drinks are the top two choices.

Sports drinks are appropriate during exercise, perhaps even more so than water. Why? Many athletes arrive at practice without having eaten anything. How long does practice last—a few hours? If they haven't eaten anything prior to practice, they are going to get hungrier and more fatigued as practice goes on. A sports drink supplies not only liquid but also fuel and electrolytes, especially sodium. **Electrolytes,** which include sodium, potassium, and chloride, dissolve into charged particles or ions that are used by the cells to regulate the electric charge and flow of water molecules across cell membranes. Electrolytes also help to maintain fluid balance so that an athlete will not dehydrate or overhydrate during exercise. More fluid

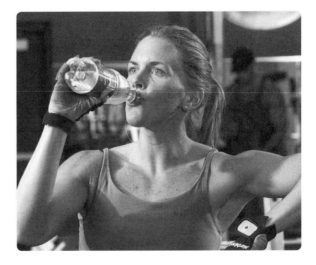

Although there are many ways athletes can increase their overall fluid intake, water and sports drinks are the best options for hydrating before, during, and after exercise.

is absorbed into the muscles from a carbohydrate–electrolyte-containing beverage than from plain water alone, and again, this provides some fuel to the active muscles as well as to the brain. If your athletes use sports drinks, discourage the athletes from diluting these beverages. They already are dilute and are not as effective if they are watered down.

You may wonder why sodium is added to these products. Sodium is in sports drinks primarily to make athletes thirstier, so they'll drink more. However, sodium in a sports drink also helps to reduce urine production and speeds rehydration because the water and glucose in these beverages can be delivered to the muscles faster than plain water. Some of you will have salty sweaters or salt losers on your team, and these athletes need to be vigilant about drinking something other than water (see the section on salty sweaters later in this chapter).

How Much Should Athletes Drink?

When you talk with your athletes about hydrating, you want them to think about what they need during the day and what they might need for exercise.

Daily Maintenance

In 2004, the Institute of Medicine released updated fluid guidelines. Gone are the recommendations for

Explain the importance of hydration to your athletes. Educate them on appropriate fluid choices. (Beginning-of-Season Activities)

eight glasses of water day; instead, there are specific guidelines based on age and gender (see table 4.1).

Keep in mind that these are baseline requirements and do not include the additional fluid needed for exercise.

Exercise Guidelines

Follow four rules to get your athletes to hydrate properly before, during, and after exercise. Have your athletes arrive at practice, conditioning, and competition well hydrated. When the body is sufficiently hydrated, urine will flow in large quantities and look light yellow rather than dark. Tell your athletes to look for this! The National Athletic Trainers' Association (NATA) 2000 position paper on hydration contains a urine color chart that you may want to post in the bathroom.

To ensure that your athletes are hydrated, have them focus on drinking liquids the hour before practice. It takes 60 minutes for 20 ounces (0.6 liters) of fluid to empty from the stomach and be absorbed by the intestine, so drinking ahead of practice makes sense. For example, if your practice is at 3 p.m., have your athletes drink 20 ounces of fluid starting around 2 p.m. so that they don't feel bloated once practice

TABLE 4.1

Fluid Guidelines (Institute of Medicine 2004)

Population		Fluid requirement
Children ages 4-8		5 cups (1.2 L) per day
Children ages 9-13		
	Male	8 cups (1.8 L) per day
	Female	7 cups (1.6 L) per day
Adolescents ages 14-18		
	Male	11 cups (2.6 L) per day
	Female	8 cups (1.8 L) per day
Adults		
	Male	13 cups (3 L) per day
	Female	9 cups (2.2 L) per day

Adapted from National Academy of Sciences, 2004, *Dietary reference intakes for water, potassium, sodium, chloride, and sulfate* (Washington, DC: Author), 143-146.

begins. You may have to talk with not just the athletes but also their teachers to make sure the athletes are allowed to drink during class. This leads to Rule 1:

Rule 1 Players must drink 20 ounces (about 0.6 liters) of fluid one hour before practice or competition.

 Give players multiple fluid breaks during practice. (Season-Long Activities)s)

What about fluid intake during practice or competition? A larger fluid intake during exercise leads to greater cardiac output, greater skin blood flow, lower core temperature, and reduced perceived effort of exertion. Fluid requirements can range from 14 to 40 ounces (420 ml to 1.2 L) per hour depending on sweat rate, although most athletes consume less than 8 ounces (240 ml) of fluid per hour of activity. Why is that? They don't have access to fluid, or they don't get fluid breaks. I hope that after reading this you put breaks into your practices! Other reasons may be that athletes put water in their mouths, swish it around, and spit it out. On a hot day, see what your athletes are doing. Pouring water on their heads? Not a route of entry into the body. Remind them that the slogan for Gatorade is "Is it in you?" not "on you"!

Another issue concerns how athletes drink fluid. If they bring a water bottle or sports bottle with a pop top, they are more likely to sip fluids rather than gulp. Sipped fluids take longer to empty from the stomach, so the result is inadequate fluid being consumed. Gulps are preferred over sips, so athletes should use a cup or unscrew the sports bottle and chug. Cool fluids may be preferred over ice-cold or room-temperature fluids, and your athletes may drink more. Thus, Rule 2 is as follows:

Rule 2 Players must drink 14 to 40 ounces (420 ml to 1.2 L) of fluid, depending on their sweat rate, per hour of exercise.

What about after exercise? Because everyone sweats and most don't drink enough fluid to replace all the losses that occur while they are active, they are going to need to drink enough after exercise to replete. None of us can tell by looking at ourselves how much fluid we lose when we sweat. The only way to know is to weigh before and after exercise. This is done routinely in certain sports, such as football, but not as much in tennis, soccer, cross country, or hockey. In addition, some people are really uncomfortable having to weigh. Try to obtain a few scales for your athletes, at least one for the males and one for the females if you coach both (perhaps parents may be willing to donate or purchase scales). Have athletes weigh before and after exercise (ideally nude or with little clothing on, because sweat-soaked clothes weigh more) three to four days in a row so they can see what their fluid losses are. If athletes are not comfortable weighing in public, put the scales in a private place. Remind them that the most important number is the difference, not the actual number. In other words, an athlete who begins practice at 150 pounds (68 kg) and weighs 147 pounds (67 kg) at the end has lost 3 pounds (almost 1.4 kg), all of it water, which he is going to need to replace. How much fluid is needed to replace this? The goal is 24 ounces (720 ml) of fluid for every pound lost or 52.8 ounces for every kilogram lost. So this particular athlete is going to need to drink 72 ounces (about 2.25 L) of fluid—3 times 24 ounces or 1.4 times 52.8—to replace the fluid lost during sport. This gives us Rule 3:

Rule 3 After exercise, players must drink 24 ounces (480 ml) of fluid for every pound (.45 kg) lost during exercise.

 Make sure that players rehydrate after exercise. (Season-Long Activities)

To curb excess drinking after exercise, have your athletes figure out their sweat rate and drink accordingly during exercise so they have less to replace afterward. This will also help to prevent overdrinking. Taking in too much fluid is just as dangerous as not consuming enough, because it usually results in water overload and potential sodium loss. **Hyponatremia,** or low blood sodium, is becoming more common. It is caused by a combination of excess fluid intake, inadequate sodium intake, and excess sweat sodium losses. A hyponatremic athlete can suffer from headaches, nausea, vomiting, swelling in the extremities, and fatigue. If severely hyponatremic, an athlete can become comatose, have seizures, or develop pulmonary edema, and any of these events can be fatal.

To determine how much fluid they need to drink to replace what was lost during exercise, athletes should use this equation:

$$\frac{\text{Pre-exercise weight} - \text{postexercise weight} + \text{fluid consumed during exercise}}{\text{Hours spent exercising}}$$

= Hourly sweat rate and number of ounces (or ml) to consume per hour

Let's look at an example.

Example

A 125-pound [58 kg] runner practices for two hours and drinks a total of 20 ounces [60 ml] of fluid during practice. After practice, he weighs 123 pounds [57 kg].

125 pounds (preweight) – 123 pounds (postweight) = 2 pounds [1 kg] or 32 ounces [960 ml]

32 ounces [960 ml] + 20 ounces [60 ml] (fluid consumed during practice) = 52 ounces [1020 ml]

52/2 [1020/2] (hours spent exercising) = 26 ounces [510 ml] per hour

Thus, 26 ounces is the runner's hourly sweat rate.

This leads us to Rule 4.

Rule 4 Have athletes figure out their sweat rate so they know how much to drink per hour and have them bring a water or sports bottle!

Sources are available that provide additional hydration guidelines for athletes. The American College of Sports Medicine published a position stand on fluid replacement in 2007 providing the rationale and the guidelines for hydration (ACSM 2007). The National Athletic Trainers Association position stand on fluid was released in 2000 (NATA 2000), and USA Track and Field has released fluid guidelines for competition (Casa 2003).

What Are Salty Sweaters?

In addition to losing fluid, some athletes, called salty sweaters or salt losers, will lose significant amounts of sodium during exercise. These athletes are more likely to experience muscle cramps, their sweat stings their eyes, and they may notice salt on their skin or clothes after exercise. These athletes must consume enough salt throughout the day to replace sodium losses. Many athletes and coaches mistakenly believe that eating bananas or drinking orange juice will alleviate or prevent cramps, but these foods are high in potassium, which is lost in small amounts during exercise compared with sodium losses, which can exceed 8 grams in a two-hour practice. This is true for many sports, not just football; sodium losses can be huge in tennis, running, and basketball.

Some athletes may voluntarily restrict sodium intake to lower their risk for hypertension, but most athletes require a liberal salt intake to maintain blood volume. An athlete will most likely require more than the 2.3 grams of sodium per day recommended

Have athletes weigh themselves before and after exercise to determine their sweat rate. (Beginning-of-Season Activities)

Have returning athletes check their sweat rate a few days before the start of pre-season. (Off-Season Activities)

in the 2005 Dietary Guidelines for Americans (U.S. Department of Health and Human Services and U.S. Department of Agriculture 2005). The athlete who unnecessarily restricts sodium may impair her performance. Tell your athletes that sodium added to a beverage such as a sports drink helps with fluid retention and prevents sodium loss but will not have an adverse effect on blood pressure. Remind your athlete of the acronym SALT—Sodium Advances the Level of Training.

The athlete who drinks only water loses significant amounts of sodium in sweat, and if she does not consume adequate sodium, she may be at risk for hyponatremia. Although this is more likely to occur during endurance events, athletes who participate in other sports have suffered from inadequate sodium intake. Sodium consumption during and following dehydrating exercise will maintain or restore blood volume more completely than plain water. Suggest that salty sweaters do the following:

- Consume sports drinks rather than water during more exercise.
- Add 1/4 teaspoon of salt to 20 ounces of sports drink.
- Add extra salt to food.
- Consume salty condiments such as Worcestershire sauce and soy sauce.
- Eat salty foods like pickles, crackers, pretzels, soup, and broth.
- Drink salty beverages like V8 or tomato juice.

If you have meetings after practice, consider having a big tub of pretzels or Chex mix (provide a cup or scoop for hygiene purposes) so your salty sweaters can start to replace their sodium losses.

Encourage salty sweaters to consume salty foods or drinks following exercise. (Season-Long Activities)

What About Caffeine and Alcohol?

Although caffeine is not a diuretic, it is not an energy source either; it is a stimulant. And some caffeine-containing beverages are too concentrated in carbohydrate. In addition to the carbonation and caffeine in a cola beverage, excess sugar makes cola an inappropriate fluid choice before, during, or after activity. An energy drink can contain more than 300 milligrams of caffeine, can contain too much sugar, or might have no calories whatsoever so that it is not a source of energy at all.

The main issues with alcohol are that it is a diuretic, delays muscle glycogen resynthesis, is a major source of calories, and can be an appetite stimulant. It is imperative that you talk with your athletes about the effects of alcohol and stress the performance effects:

- Delayed rehydration
- Delayed muscle recovery from exercise
- Potential delay in healing from soft tissue injury
- Restless sleep patterns
- Excess calories
- Overly active appetite

How Can You Get Athletes to Hydrate?

Athletes must follow fluid strategies before, during, and after exercise. Being the hydration enforcer will help you get the most out of your athletes. The time you allot for fluid breaks will come back to you in a big way, with athletes who are healthier, happier, and better able to perform. So encourage them to drink early, often, and enough. They will have fewer injuries, less fatigue, and better concentration, and they will be able to give you more effort.

✓ COACH'S TO DO LIST

- Remind your athletes to drink when they wake up in the morning.
- Encourage them to consume 20 ounces (600 ml) of fluid with every meal.
- Make sure athletes calculate sweat and fluid losses so they can determine their individual sweat rate.
- Remind them to hydrate one hour before practice.
- Enforce a no-participation policy for athletes who are dehydrated when they come to practice or don't bring fluid bottles.
- Remind athletes to carry fluid or mixes to add to water such as lemonade, powdered Propel, or sports drink powder.
- Provide cups at practice.
- Schedule fluid breaks during every practice.
- Remind your athletes to swallow rather than spit fluids.
- Make sure they rehydrate before leaving practice or workouts.
- Encourage them to drink even if they are not thirsty.
- Tell athletes to drink enough before exercise to have a full stomach. Gastric emptying is more rapid and efficient when the stomach is somewhat full rather than empty.
- Discourage the use of energy drinks around the time of exercise.
- Talk with your team about the performance-detracting effects of alcohol.

SUMMARY

- Athletes who are not well hydrated are a liability to themselves, the team, and the coach.
- Dehydration impairs performance and jeopardizes health.
- Athletes need to understand how important it is to have a positive fluid balance so they are neither dehydrated nor overly hydrated.
- Athletes must be educated about appropriate fluid choices and should know that some fluids are better during exercise than others.
- Athletes should limit use of caffeine during exercise and should know that alcohol can impair performance.
- Athletes need to pay attention to fluid timing and to the quantity of fluid they need to consume.
- Athletes need to know how to calculate sweat rates.
- Salty sweaters must make sure that they meet their sodium needs to prevent hyponatremia.

KEY TERMS

dehydration	electrolytes	hyponatremia
diuretic		

GAME PLAN QUESTIONS

1. When is it important for athletes to consume fluids?
2. What are some of the effects of dehydration?
3. How can athletes learn to drink the right amount of fluid for activity?
4. What are the best ways to prevent excessive sodium losses during exercise?

5

Reducing Body Fat

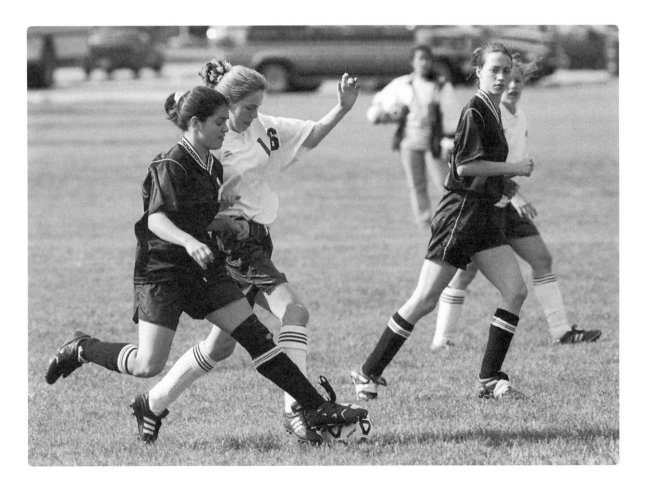

Laura, a high school soccer and basketball player, had always been praised for her agility and speed. Between her junior and senior year she grew three inches (7.6 cm) but also gained weight. Although the weight gain did not happen overnight, she added 15 pounds (5.6 kg) from the end of basketball season to summer training camp for soccer. She noticed that her clothes were tighter, and her coach remarked that she was not as quick to the ball. She also felt a little more winded during practices and sluggish, a feeling she had never experienced before.

With fall season three weeks away, Laura felt a little panicky. Her aunt, trying to help, gave her a high-protein diet book. Laura decided to cut out all fruits, bread, rice, pasta, and cereal from her diet and just have chicken, tuna, low-fat cheese, and salad.

The first few days she was tired but thrilled by the number on the scale. However, her coach and other teammates remarked that she was not giving 100 percent in practice, saying, "Where is the old Laura?" Laura thought that the excess weight was still the problem, so she continued with the high-protein diet but added a fat-burning supplement to give her energy and speed up the weight loss.

Laura took a synephrine-based product, and although her fatigue went away, her rapid heart rate before and during practice left her feeling winded. She also found it hard to fall asleep and hard to concentrate fully in class, but she saw a drop on the scale so kept taking the supplement. Three weeks into the high-protein diet and fat burner supplement she had lost 12 pounds (4.5 kg), but to her dismay her performance had worsened. She wasn't sleeping, she was tired, she watched longingly as teammates ate the foods that she didn't allow herself to have, and, worst of all, she couldn't perform to her potential on the soccer field.

Her friends encouraged her to eat more carbohydrates to help with her performance and recovery. Laura was too afraid to do this for fear of gaining the weight back. Tearfully, she approached her parents for help. They set up an appointment with a sports dietitian, who gave Laura the appropriate advice for an athlete desiring weight loss. Laura changed her diet, finished her soccer season strong, and was excited, well fueled, and ready for her basketball season.

When you finish reading this chapter, you should be able to explain

- the different body composition techniques used to assess the overly fat athlete's body;
- how to assess what and how the athlete eats;
- what foods, diets, and pills really help athletes lose weight;
- how to create an action plan for weight management; and
- how to make referrals to weight management professionals.

We and our athletes are bombarded with information about weight loss from magazine articles, Web sites, and television commercials that guarantee fast and easy weight loss. These are words that make the books, products, and diets too good to resist. Too bad they're not true! It's not easy to understand how to help your athletes realize their weight-loss goals while maintaining their competitive edge.

One of the main reasons that athletes come to dietitians for help is to lose weight. For some, it may be a matter of dropping a few unwanted pounds, whereas others may have much more to lose. No matter what the starting point, some ways to lose weight just don't work. Your athletes probably have, in an attempt to lose weight,

- not eaten all day;
- eliminated all the foods they like;
- eaten on the run, without sitting down;
- eliminated an entire group of foods;
- consumed only liquids instead of food;
- eaten a lot less and exercised a lot more; or

- relied on fat-burning or weight reduction supplements.

With so much advice about weight loss out there, it is easy to get caught up in the hype, and quite honestly some of these wild claims do seem to make sense. Following are some of the weight-loss myths that athletes have heard and sometimes believe. What about you?

- It's all mind over matter. Diets fail because someone doesn't have willpower.
- Eating after 6 p.m. will make you gain weight.
- Eating carbohydrate-containing foods will increase body fat.
- You should cut your fat intake to a minimum to burn fat.
- You can change fat into muscle, and if you don't exercise, muscle turns into fat.
- There are "bad" foods.
- If you eat sweets, you will get fat.
- Some foods burn fat.
- Alcohol is not a major calorie source.
- Only food affects your weight, not beverages.

Your athletes probably want to lose weight to enhance their sport performance. To use a race car as an analogy to the body, drag translates to a decrease in speed. If the goal is weight loss to get rid of some of the drag, your athletes need to get rid of some of the excess baggage, or body fat, but not the entire engine. So they need to have a plan to maximize loss of body fat while minimizing decreases in lean muscle mass.

You may assume that losing body fat is just a matter of eating less or exercising more. In a sense, that is true; however, to be successful athletes must determine how much fat must be lost and find the appropriate calorie level. After considering ways to cut calories, you and your athletes must develop an action plan.

Assess Where the Athlete Is

If an athlete is interested in losing body fat, she needs to know her starting weight, starting percentage of body fat, and estimated caloric expenditure. Having this information will help your athlete develop a realistic weight-loss plan.

Your role in this process is twofold. First, you must choose someone to weigh your athletes and assess their body composition and second, you need to be part of your athlete's support system. If you are a high school coach, get the school nurse or the athlete's physician to weigh the athlete. If you have an athletic trainer who works with your team, that person can do the weigh-ins. If you are a collegiate coach, your athletic trainer, consulting sports dietitian, or student health service personnel should monitor the athletes' weight and help them to set appropriate body weight goals.

Your main role is to provide education and support to help your athletes reach their goals. If your athletes have decided they are ready to lose weight, they are 90 percent there, because they will make the effort. If they think it can be done, it will be done. Your job is to remind your athletes that weight loss is going to take a lot of time and effort on their part. You can't eat or work out for your athletes.

Your athletes need to know what they can and cannot change about their bodies, accept these limitations, and focus positively on the areas where they can make a difference. Talking to your athletes about these facts can help them as they work on their weight goals.

Athletes can change the following:

- Fluid balance (They should approach this with caution because rapid fluid loss can lead to dehydration and impaired performance. For a more in-depth discussion of hydration, see chapter 4.)
- Fat content
- Muscle mass

Athletes cannot change these things:

- Height
- Frame size

If you don't have access to a sports dietitian, you will need to assess what and how the athlete eats, which includes

- estimated daily caloric intake,
- patterns of types of foods eaten, and
- eating habits.

Assessing the Athlete's Body

Start by having someone measure the athlete's weight and body composition.

Weight

A health professional will weigh the athlete on a scale, in the morning after the athlete has voided; the athlete should wear minimal clothing, preferably only underwear. Most scales have a maximum of 350 pounds (159 kg). Athletes who weigh more than this may need to go to a local hospital, which usually has scales to measure larger individuals.

Body Composition

As a starting point, the person assessing the **body composition** of younger athletes can use the Centers for Disease Control and Prevention growth charts (2002), found at www.cdc.gov/growthcharts. The body mass index (BMI) charts can also be a starting point in determining athletes' appropriate weight. The BMI is a measure of body weight in kilograms divided by height in meters squared (kg/m^2). The BMI takes body fat into account. A BMI of less than 18.5 kilograms per square meter is considered too thin and greater than 25 kilograms per square meter is considered overweight.

You can find a BMI calculator for children and adolescents on the Centers for Disease Control and Prevention Web site: http://apps.nccd.cdc.gov/dnpabmi/Calculator.aspx. Measuring BMI can help to determine if someone is overfat or underweight, and it is helpful for the general population as a screening tool to assess who may be at risk for certain diseases. However, the BMI is of limited usefulness for most athletes, because this tool is not applicable for the athlete with a high muscle mass.

When an athlete needs to decrease body fat, the health professional will need to know the athlete's initial body fat percentage and lean muscle mass before making recommendations. This will prevent loss of fat-free mass in athletes who already are within an acceptable body fat range.

> *Have a health professional assess the athletes' weight and body composition. (Activities for Athletes Who Want to Lose Fat)*

Various methods are used to assess body composition. Even though you will not conduct the assessment yourself, you should understand the various techniques.

Two methods commonly used to assess body fat are measurement of skinfold thickness and bioelectrical impedance (BIA) testing. Skinfold thickness is used to assess body composition by measuring subcutaneous fat at various sites on the body. Although skinfold calipers are not as exact as other methods to measure body fat, they are inexpensive, they provide a baseline, and they can be used periodically to assess progress. If you work with an athletic trainer, ask her to take these measurements on your athletes. If not, perhaps the school nurse or the athlete's physician or

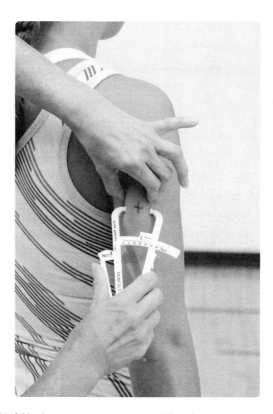

Skinfold caliper measurements are a quick and easy way to measure an athlete's progress in losing body fat.

nurse practitioner can do this assessment. You should not be the one to assess your athletes.

Bioelectrical impedance measures the conductivity of different body tissues. Blood has high conductivity, whereas fat and bone have low conductivity, so BIA measures the resistance or impedance of the current flow as it passes through the body. The Tanita body scale uses a similar technique. However, the accuracy of body fat assessment using either BIA or the Tanita scale is questionable in very muscular athletes, who may have more fluid in their fat-free mass, or in athletes who are dehydrated.

More sophisticated body composition measuring methods include dual-energy X-ray absorptiometry (DEXA). This provides estimates of bone mineral, fat-free soft tissue, and fat mass through the attenuation (loss) of X-ray energy on different body components. DEXA also provides information on body composition by quadrants—arms, legs, and trunk—as well as a total estimate. However, this method is very costly and is typically not covered by insurance. For college coaches, your university may have access to DEXA. If you are a high school coach, see whether a nearby medical facility or a local university has DEXA available and would be willing to test your athletes.

Hydrodensitometry, or underwater weighing, is another high-tech method used to calculate fat-free and fat mass. Body density is determined by dividing body weight measured on a scale by body volume, assessed with underwater weighing. Body fat percentage is then calculated using equations. People with more body fat are more buoyant in the water and weigh less. People who are leaner will sink in the water and weigh more. This is a very accurate technique for assessing body fat in young white males but is not as accurate for women and other races. Plus, many athletes find it difficult to be submerged under water!

Air-displacement plethysmography also assesses body composition by body density. The BOD POD is the equipment most often used. Body volume is determined by how much air the athlete displaces when seated in the BOD POD, and then body fat percentage is calculated using the same equations as those used for underwater weighing. Many athletes prefer this technique, because they do not have to be submerged under water. The equipment is expensive, however, so find out whether a local facility or health club has a BOD POD and would be willing to test your athletes.

Not all of your athletes will have access to a DEXA machine, an underwater weighing tank, or a BOD POD, but they will all require some method of body composition estimation. It is impossible for you to estimate body fat or lean muscle mass by eyeballing your athletes. If you're near a university with an exercise science department or a medical center that does obesity or osteoporosis research, find out what body composition assessment tools are available. Often graduate students or researchers are looking for research subjects and will be willing to assess your athletes.

Assessing Calories Spent Daily

An assessment of **metabolic rate** (often referred to as resting metabolic rate, or RMR) can tell you how many calories an athlete expends at rest. If you and your athletes know how many calories are being burned at rest, appropriate calorie recommendations can be made to help your athlete lose body fat without impairing performance.

Although devices such as the MedGem and metabolic carts assess metabolic rate by measuring the rate of oxygen consumption and carbon dioxide gas production, they may not be readily available to you or your athletes. Use table 5.1 to estimate your athletes' RMR.

To get a more precise idea of an athlete's energy expenditures, ask her to keep an activity log so you can determine the number of calories she uses throughout the day. By knowing both of these numbers, you will be able to help your athlete determine

TABLE 5.1

Estimating RMR

Body weight (lb) × 10 or weight (kg) × 22 = number of calories the body requires at rest
If your athletes are injured or cannot exercise: Body weight (lb) × 13-15* or weight (kg) × 29-33*
If your athletes exercise three or four days per week: Body weight (lb) × 14-17* or weight (kg) × 30.8-37.4
If your athletes exercise five or six days per week: Body weight (lb) × 17-27* or weight (kg) × 37.4-59.4*

*Lower numbers are for females, higher numbers for males.

a daily calorie level to promote body fat loss without sacrificing muscle mass.

Your athletes need to determine their energy expenditure for the entire day, not just for the time they spend exercising. The body burns calories 24 hours a day, so when the goal is weight loss, athletes need to find ways to burn more calories over the course of the day beyond what they expend in practice. For instance, an athlete who spends two hours a day in front of the computer may be able to reduce the sitting time to one hour by substituting another activity such as taking the dog for a walk or going for a bike ride. At the end of the day, he will have expended more calories.

Encourage your athletes to track their energy expenditure over one day. They need to keep track of everything they do, and the number of minutes they spend doing it, from the time they wake up until they go to bed. Figure 5.1 shows a sample activity log for Kristin, a 150-pound (56 kg) softball player. Figure 5.2 is a blank form you can copy for your athletes to use.

As you can see by this example, our 150-pound athlete expended 2,415 calories a day, a total of calories for light activities (eating, sitting, walking to school) and calories expended for sport.

If your athlete records this by hand, you'll need to supply him with a source for determining the number of calories used such as one of the resources shown on page 60.

Assess your athletes' calorie expenditure by having them keep an activity log. (Activities for Athletes Who Want to Lose Fat)

Book

McArdle W (ed). *Exercise Physiology: Energy, Nutrition, and Human Performance.* 5th ed. Malvern, PA: Lea & Febiger; 2006.

Web site

www.aolhealth.com/tools/calories-burned?s em=1&ncid=AOLHTH00170000000022& s_kwcid=calories%20burned|1939849520

Example

A 150-pound athlete exercises five days per week.

$$150 \times 17 = 2{,}550 \text{ calories per day or } 68 \text{ kg} \times 37.4 = 2{,}550 \text{ kcal/day}$$

To lose weight by decreasing body fat, the athlete should subtract 300 calories from her estimated daily needs.

$$2{,}550 - 300 = 2{,}250 \text{ calories per day to achieve weight loss without fluid loss or muscle or bone loss.}$$

Kristin's Activity Log

Activity	Time spent	Calories expended
Brush teeth, wash face, shower, get dressed	10 min	27
Eat breakfast	5 min	10
Walk to school	5 min	20
Sit in classes	180 min	368
Eat lunch	25 min	51
Sit in classes	90 min	184
Sit in study hall	25 min	51
Get ready for softball practice	5 min	13
Run 1 mile (1.6 km; 8 min mile)	8 min	120
Participate in softball practice	2 hr	565
Walk home	5 min	20
Eat dinner	10 min	20
Do homework, sitting, online	3 hr	367
Brush teeth, wash face, get ready for bed	5 min	27
Sleep	7 hr	572
		Total: 2,415

FIGURE 5.1 Sample activity log.

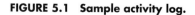

Activity Log

List all your activities and the amount of time you spend doing them over the course of the day. Use a resource such as those listed on page 60 to calculate the calories expended for each activity.

Activity	Time spent	Calories expended
		Total:

From L. Bonci, 2009, *Sport Nutrition for Coaches* (Champaign, IL: Human Kinetics).

FIGURE 5.2 Activity log.

An easier way to do this recording is to use MyPyramid Tracker, an online tool developed by the United States Department of Agriculture and the Center for Nutrition Policy and Promotion, found at www.mypyramidtracker.gov. When the user enters the activities into the application, it calculates the number of calories automatically. Figure 5.3 shows an example.

Although recording this information takes time, it is the only way to figure out how many calories are

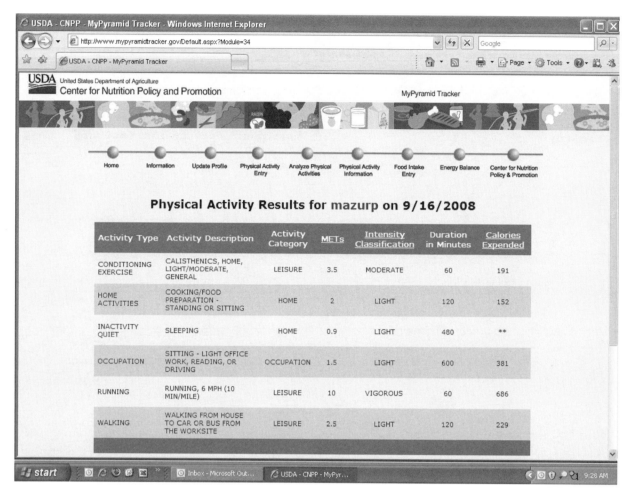

FIGURE 5.3 Sample MyPyramid report.

expended every day so that you can help your athlete accurately determine how much he or she should eat to lose body fat.

Assessing What and How the Athlete Eats

To reduce weight, athletes must focus more on diet, rather than exercise, because it will be extremely difficult for them to lose weight by simply adding more activity to their day. Although successful body fat loss requires expending both more energy and calories, your athletes need to also change the amount of food they eat to decrease overall caloric intake. Many athletes believe that exercise burns huge amounts of calories, but consider how long (in minutes) someone must work out to burn the calories from these foods:

- A pastry = 30 minutes on the treadmill
- Four chicken wings = 20 minutes on the elliptical
- A cheeseburger = one hour of soccer practice

- A 20-ounce (600 ml) soda = 30 minutes of basketball
- A small bag of M&Ms = a three-mile (4.8 km) run

In some cases, it may be warranted to recommend an additional cardiovascular workout for the overweight athlete to expedite weight loss, but you should specify the frequency and duration of the additional activities so that the athlete does not end up with an overuse injury or show up for practice too tired to perform.

What should your athletes do to lose weight? They need to get a very good idea of how they are eating now. Then they need to examine the types of foods they normally eat, and finally they should think about how they usually go about eating.

Food Diary

Athletes who keep a food diary record what they eat, how much, the time of day they eat, how fast they eat, any activity they do while eating, and the number of calories consumed. Your athletes will probably

Example

Toby, a pole vaulter I worked with, gained 20 pounds (7.5 kg) in his first two months as a college freshman. I asked him to keep a food diary for a week, and then we met to review it. The food diary showed that he ate 50 chicken wings and a 2-liter bottle of soda two nights per week. This added up to about 16,000 extra calories a week, or the equivalent of about three to four pounds (1-1.5 kg) per week. Writing down his intake made him aware of what he was doing, so that we could come up with some goals to reduce intake and decrease weight.

complain that this takes too much time. However, think about it: If I asked you what you ate yesterday, unless you had written it down, you wouldn't be able to tell me everything you had.

When we have to monitor our eating, we think about it more and are more accountable to ourselves. If your athletes balk at this suggestion, they are probably not going to be successful with long-term weight loss.

To get an accurate idea of what your athletes eat, ask them to keep a food diary for a week. Tell them to eat the way they normally do because the goal of this exercise is to figure out what they are doing now in order to decide what to change. They may eat differently during the week than on the weekend or differently on a practice day than a game day. Remind them to write down everything, from a sip of soda to a meal. Figure 5.4 shows a sample food diary. Your athletes should write down not only what they eat but how much. A glass of milk can range from 6 to 16 ounces (180-480 ml), and obviously there will be a big difference in calories. This figure shows a diary of a typical day's intake for Anthony, a high school basketball player. Copy figure 5.5 to use with your own athletes.

Once the athletes have written down the foods they have eaten, should they worry about the fat content, sugar, calories, or all of these? The most important consideration is the number of calories consumed; the athletes must eat fewer calories to lose weight. If your athlete decreases only her fat intake, she may not decrease caloric intake and will not lose weight. The same thing may happen if the only focus is to decrease sugar. Many low-fat, non-fat, reduced-sugar, and sugar-free products are not lower in calories than the full-fat or full-sugar versions.

You and your athletes can determine the number of calories they have eaten in several ways. First, you can use the Nutrition Facts panel from the food label. This is based on the serving size, so your athlete must measure what she eats, compare the amount consumed to the serving size on the label, and multiply or divide accordingly. If foods don't have the Nutrition Facts panel, check your school or local library for the books listed next or any computerized nutrition programs. You also can access the listed Web sites, which list nutritional information.

Books

Pennington JAT, Douglass JS, Bowes AP, Church HN. *Food Values of Portions Commonly Used.* 18th ed. Baltimore: Lippincott Williams & Wilkins; 2004.

Netzer, C. *Complete Book of Food Counts.* 5th ed. New York: Dell; 2000.

Web sites

www.calorieking.com

www.nutrax.com

www.ediets.com

www.usda.gov/cnpp (Healthy Eating Index)

www.nutritionassistant.com

Example

One of my professional football players came to my office because he wanted to lose a few pounds. He ate very well, but I found out that he was drinking roughly 3,000 calories of fruit punch daily. We came up with some ideas for lower-calorie but flavorful beverage options including flavored waters, diluted juice, and iced tea sweetened with a little fruit juice. He was able to drop the weight in about 6 weeks and didn't have to give up flavor.

Anthony's Food Diary for Losing Weight

Time	Food and beverages consumed	Amount consumed	Time spent eating or drinking	Activities while eating or drinking	Calories consumed
7 a.m.	Pop-Tart	One package	5 min	Getting ready for school	400
	Orange juice	8 oz (240 ml)	1 min	Rushing out the door	120
12 noon	Ham sandwich with cheese and mayonnaise	Two	15 min	Sitting with friends	600
	Apple	One half			40
	Chips	Two small bags			200
	Orange drink	20 oz (600 ml)			240
	Chocolate chip cookie	Large			400
3 p.m.	Granola bars	Two	5 min	Getting ready for practice	240
	Gatorade	20 oz (600 ml)			125
6 p.m.	Fried chicken thighs	Three	15 min	Having dinner with family	600
	Fried potatoes	Two large handfuls			400
	Applesauce, sweetened	1/2 cup (128 g)			100
	Corn	1 cup			140
	Soda	24 oz (720 ml)			300
9 p.m.	Chips	One half of a large bag	20 min	Doing homework on the computer	500
	Fruit punch	12 oz (360 ml)			200
					Total: 4,605

FIGURE 5.4 Sample food diary for losing weight.

The food diary provides valuable information not only about what your athletes eat and drink but also about their eating patterns. They may discover that they always eat a chocolate bar at 4 p.m. or skip lunch five days a week. Many athletes are surprised to find out that they eat a lot more food on Saturday and Sunday than Monday through Friday.

Lead by example: If you keep a food diary, your athletes will be more likely to do it too. Make this a team effort, so that those who are trying to lose weight are not singled out; plus, there are probably several athletes on your team who could use a dietary tune-up even if their weight is fine.

Food Diary for Losing Weight

Time	Food and beverages consumed	Amount consumed	Time spent eating or drinking	Activities while eating or drinking	Calories consumed
					Total:

From L. Bonci, 2009, *Sport Nutrition for Coaches* (Champaign, IL: Human Kinetics).

FIGURE 5.5 Food diary for losing weight.

Food Patterns

Another essential step is to get your athletes to focus on what they are eating so that they can identify food patterns, that is, foods that they eat frequently or not at all, and foods they find hard to stop eating.

Instruct your athletes to use figure 5.6 on pages 66-67 to identify the foods they eat frequently, foods they find too tempting or eat too much of, and foods they never consume. They should place an X in the appropriate columns.

After your athletes complete this chart they will have a good idea of the items they consume most regularly as well as those that they rarely eat. If an athlete notices that he is only picking high-calorie

Food Pattern Form

CARBOHYDRATE-CONTAINING FOODS			
Food item	**Frequency eaten (times per week)**	**Trigger foods (hard to control)**	**Foods never eaten**
Bread			
Bagels			
Cereal			
Pasta			
Rice			
Fruit			
Vegetables			
Juice			
Sports drinks			
Soda			
Candy			
Cookies			
Cake and pies			
Pastries			
Crackers			
Pretzels			
Chips			
Potatoes			
Yogurt			
Ice cream and frozen desserts			
PROTEIN-CONTAINING FOODS			
Food item	**Frequency eaten (times per week)**	**Trigger foods (hard to control)**	**Foods never eaten**
Beef			
Veal			
Lamb			
Pork			
Fish			
Shellfish			
Chicken			
Turkey			
Eggs			
Cheese			
Nuts			

From L. Bonci, 2009, *Sport Nutrition for Coaches* (Champaign, IL: Human Kinetics).

FIGURE 5.6   Food pattern form.

PROTEIN-CONTAINING FOODS, *continued*			
Food item	**Frequency eaten (times per week)**	**Trigger foods (hard to control)**	**Foods never eaten**
Nut butter			
Dried beans (kidney beans, lentils)			
Soy products (tofu, soy milk, veggie burgers)			
Milk			
Yogurt			
FAT-CONTAINING FOODS			
Food item	**Frequency eaten (times per week)**	**Trigger foods (hard to control)**	**Foods never eaten**
Margarine			
Butter			
Salad dressing			
Mayonnaise			
Oil			
Bacon			
Cream cheese			
ALCOHOLIC BEVERAGES			
Food item	**Frequency eaten (times per week)**	**Trigger foods (hard to control)**	**Foods never eaten**
Beer			
Wine			
Mixed drinks			

From L. Bonci, 2009, *Sport Nutrition for Coaches* (Champaign, IL: Human Kinetics).

FIGURE 5.6 *(continued)*

foods, suggest that he add some lower-calorie items and decrease the frequency of some of the high-calorie foods. Trigger foods are items that people have trouble limiting, so identifying these foods can help athletes determine which items they should remove from the house, desk, locker, or dorm room to make it easier to achieve weight goals.

The list of foods never eaten is also important. For example, one recommendation for those who are trying to lose weight is to eat a lot of fruits and vegetables. If an athlete has identified several fruits and vegetables on the list of foods never eaten, suggest other low-calorie foods that she would be willing to eat.

For many athletes, snacks are the problem. Meal-time may be somewhat controlled by the size of the plate, but who eats just one chip or cookie? When trying to lose weight, people tend to eliminate all favorite foods, and this can be a recipe for disaster. Ask athletes to identify the foods they like to snack

on and figure out a way to fit them in. If they like pizza, how about half of the pie instead of the whole thing? (Pizzas do come in sizes other than large.) And athletes can order pizza without extra cheese or with half the pepperoni. Athletes who love fries can choose the regular size instead of super or split a large order with a friend or family member. At the movies, athletes can order a small popcorn and a regular-sized soda instead of the super-sized versions. Because the candy boxes sold in movie theaters are large, athletes can save calories and money by bringing a snack-sized plastic bag filled with their favorite treats.

Eating Habits

The other component of successful weight loss is identifying eating habits. It is not just about the food. How do your athletes eat? Do they sit down to meals or eat on the run? Do they eat quickly or slowly? Have your athletes complete the questionnaire shown in figure 5.7. If athletes are to be successful in the long

Check yes or no to the statements listed below

I prefer to stand to eat.	Yes ☐	No ☐
I eat on the run.	Yes ☐	No ☐
I eat at fast food restaurants often.	Yes ☐	No ☐
A meal is not complete without meat.	Yes ☐	No ☐
A meal is not complete without pasta, potatoes, rice, or bread.	Yes ☐	No ☐
I am not satisfied unless I have a lot to eat.	Yes ☐	No ☐
I have better control of eating when I eat out.	Yes ☐	No ☐
I don't eat a lot around other people, but when I am alone I tend to overeat.	Yes ☐	No ☐

From L. Bonci, 2009, *Sport Nutrition for Coaches* (Champaign, IL: Human Kinetics).

FIGURE 5.7 Eating style questionnaire.

run, their individual eating styles must be taken into account.

If your athletes answer yes to any of the questions in figure 5.7, here is some useful advice:

I prefer to stand to eat.

Suggest to your athletes that they sit down, preferably at a table, so they can focus on what they are eating; they will probably eat less.

I eat on the run.

Recommend to your athlete or the athlete's family that the meal be split, so that half is eaten before practice, school, or a music lesson, and the rest is eaten later, so that the athlete is not gulping food and then running out the door.

I eat at fast food restaurants often.

Advise your athletes to reduce the frequency of fast food dining by 50 percent or choose healthier items if fast food is the only option available.

A meal is not complete without meat.

Athletes don't have to quit eating meat, but they should have other items on their plate; perhaps the amount of meat can be decreased to one third of the plate to leave room for grains and vegetables.

A meal is not complete without pasta, potatoes, rice, or bread.

Remind your athletes that carbohydrate-containing foods are important fuel sources for exercise, but the athlete who is trying to lose weight should eat one of these foods at a meal instead of several.

I am not satisfied unless I have a lot to eat.

Some of your athletes are volume eaters. Decreasing the amount of food that they eat at each meal by half is going to leave them feeling unsatisfied and more likely to overeat at the next meal or snack. Recommend that they add high-volume, low-calorie items to meals to help them feel fuller. Salads, fruit, broth, tomato-based soups, and chili can be filling.

I have better control of eating when I eat out.

Some of your athletes may find it too hard to practice portion control at home if they have access to unlimited amounts of foods. Suggest that they purchase measuring cups and spoons or consider buying food in single-serving packages to make it easier to control the amount consumed.

I don't eat a lot around other people, but when I am alone I tend to overeat.

Suggest that this athlete eat as much as possible with friends, roommates, or family members or that she identify an eating buddy who can eat with her and help her to be mindful of the amount of food she consumes.

The purpose of this analysis is to help the athlete identify her eating patterns and trouble areas so that she can improve them. For instance, the athlete who wants to try a carbohydrate-restricted diet but feels that a meal is not complete without pasta, potatoes, rice, or bread is probably not going to be able to stay on the diet for long. Perhaps this athlete can reduce the amount of carbohydrate-containing foods rather than eliminate them.

> *Have the athletes keep a food diary for one week. Also, ask them to fill out a food pattern form and the eating style questionnaire. Review the results with the athletes. (Activities for Athletes Who Want to Lose Fat)*

Getting Lean and Ripped at the Same Time

You may have athletes who want to both increase muscle mass and decrease body fat; do they need to eat differently than those who are trying only to increase muscle mass or only to lose body fat? First they need to prioritize their goals. If they have a little extra around the middle or on the hips, it is probably more important to work on decreasing body fat than adding size to the biceps. Remind your athletes that muscle doesn't turn to fat or fat to muscle, but they will still look and probably feel better no matter whether they focus on the muscle mass increase or the body fat decrease. We can't just look at a number on a chart or the scale to determine which to focus on.

If your athlete increases the amount of time spent lifting, there is a chance that his weight may not change at all, even though he may look more "cut" or toned. The reason is that muscle is more dense and weighs more than fat. So your athletes need to assess progress by noticing how their bodies are changing and how clothes are fitting, not just by the number on the scale.

If an athlete tries to decrease body fat by cutting large number of calories and exercising excessively, she may end up not only burning fat but also losing muscle mass. Remember, exercise is catabolic, requiring fuel for the muscles. If an athlete has a higher energy output (through excess exercise) compared with energy intake (food consumed), the body may have to use its own muscle as a fuel source during exercise.

No matter what the focus is, it is important to have a plan.

Tell your athletes to do the following to increase muscle mass and decrease body fat:

To increase muscle mass

Eat enough to stimulate muscle growth.

Eat before and after lifting.

Eat enough protein.

To decrease body fat

Limit serving sizes.

Eat enough to fuel your workouts.

Don't skip meals.

Eat enough protein.

Finally, if your athletes want to lose weight, they must be consistent with the number of meals eaten every day. Many of them will say, "If I skip meals, I'll eat less and lose weight faster." This approach usually backfires because when they do eat, they will be hungrier and more likely to overeat. To keep your athletes on track, suggest that they try the following tips:

- Establish an eating schedule. Think about your classes, work, practices, lessons, and all the things you do, and plan your eating around your activities.

- Eat breakfast every day.

- Eat lunch. If you don't like what is offered at school or at work, bring something with you.

- If late afternoon is your hungry time, plan to eat more at breakfast and lunch; also plan a snack to have at this time of day.

- Sit down to eat, even if you get fast food. And no eating in the car! Either eat at the restaurant or take the food home, unwrap it, put it on a plate, and take the time to eat. You'll feel much more satisfied!

There are times in your athlete's lives when they are more likely to experience weight changes. Prepuberty is a time of increased fat and muscle mass, so the previously rail-thin athlete may now notice curves in areas that were previously flat. Injured athletes may gain weight because their appetite does not always decrease even though their exercise is curtailed, so it is extremely important to work with these athletes to prevent excessive weight gain or caloric restriction, which may delay healing. Athletes entering college may notice that they gain weight during their first semester. If you are a college coach, have a sports dietitian talk to your team about healthy eating, late-night eating, snacks, and alcohol use, because all of these can affect your athletes' weight.

Consider Diet Options

A lot of myths are floating around about food and weight gain, so let's review some common questions coaches have, then examine whether fad diets are worthwhile, and finally, consider whether weight-loss pills are worth what they cost.

Common Questions About Food

Let's look at some common questions that coaches have about food and weight loss.

Common Questions About Food and Weight Loss

What about fat-burning foods?

Sorry, but there are no fat-burning foods. Athletes need to eat a variety of foods to optimize performance. Even with weight loss as a goal, athletes still have to eat enough to fuel their participation in their sports. But they may need to change some of their food choices and quantities.

Some foods help you to feel more full for a longer time. Part of this is the way the food tastes and the "mouth feel" as well as the comfortable feeling you get after eating a meal. It is also the "chew" factor. No one feels full after a beverage, at least not for an extended period of time, but when you eat a small steak, or a small plate of pasta, or soup and a sandwich, you need to chew, which is part of the fill factor.

Shouldn't carbohydrate intake be restricted?

Carbohydrate-containing foods such as fruits, vegetables, bread, rice, cereal, pasta, and sweets are fuels for exercise. Eliminating these foods will not make one a better athlete and may lead to cravings that will sabotage weight-loss efforts. However, some carbohydrate-containing foods are more satisfying than others. It takes time to eat a salad if one doesn't want to choke on the lettuce! A piece of fruit requires chewing, whereas juice doesn't take any work at all. A bowl of a high-fiber cereal such as Kashi or Raisin Bran will keep one feeling full for longer than corn flakes.

The bonus of high-fiber carbohydrate is threefold:

* Some high-fiber foods take longer to eat.
* The feeling of fullness lasts longer.
* The body has to expend a few more calories to digest high-fiber foods.

Shouldn't protein be the focus?

Many athletes believe that it is necessary to eat a lot of protein if the goal is to increase muscle mass and decrease body fat. That isn't always true, and if one eats a lot of protein but doesn't cut back on other foods, he will gain weight, and not just muscle weight.

With all of the high-protein diets and products on the market, some athletes think that a high-protein diet is the best approach to weight loss. Unfortunately, these diets and foods are all too low in carbohydrate, so they may impair performance and they are incredibly monotonous as well!

Foods that contain high-quality protein are an essential part of a good body-fat reduction plan. Meat, poultry, fish, eggs, cheese, soy products, and beans such as kidney beans, navy beans, and chickpeas are all examples of protein foods that require chewing. Some require cooking, which delays the hand to mouth action, and some require the use of a knife and fork, so they take longer to eat. Beans, soy foods such as veggie burgers and soy nuts, and nuts and seeds also contain fiber in addition to protein, which makes one feel more full for a longer time.

It takes about three to four hours for protein-containing foods to leave the gut, compared with one to two hours for carbohydrate-containing foods and six hours for fat-containing foods. The longer the food takes to empty, the longer one feels satisfied and less likely to eat. This is really important when the goal is weight loss. In addition, the body uses slightly more calories to digest protein than other types of nutrients, so athletes should include some protein as part of every meal and snack.

To lose weight, low to no fat intake is best, right?

Many athletes believe that to lose body fat, it is necessary to cut out all dietary fat. This belief is wrong. Fat-containing foods such as butter, margarine, mayonnaise, salad dressing, oil, and peanut butter not only make foods taste good but make one feel fuller longer. Fat-free does not equal calorie-free, so if your athletes polish off a bag of fat-free pretzels, they are still consuming a lot of calories and are not going to lose weight. Reduced-fat peanut butter has the same number of calories per serving as regular peanut butter and doesn't taste as good. Some fat-free foods actually have more calories than the regular item. In addition, fat-free foods aren't as satisfying, so one will be more likely to eat more. Fat is a fuel source for endurance exercise, and if an athlete's fat intake is too low, he will experience increased fatigue earlier on in exercise.

To drink or not to drink: Is this a question?

Water is essential for active people, but it does not flush fat or curb appetite. If an athlete doesn't drink enough fluid, her body will not burn fat as effectively, but drinking gallons of water won't make her any thinner.

Athletes seem to forget that liquids can pack a powerful caloric punch. With beverages from Starbucks to energy drinks, carbonated beverages, and fruit juice or fruit drinks, buyer beware. It is very easy to tack on an additional 1,000 calories in beverages every day without feeling full.

Help your athletes cut calories by suggesting they limit intake of the following beverages:

- Sweetened iced tea
- Fruit juice (even though it is natural, it is still high in calories)
- Fruit drinks
- Two percent or whole milk
- Sweetened seltzer waters, unless calorie-free
- Flavored waters, unless calorie-free
- Energy drinks
- Coffee beverages such as cappuccino and lattes
- Alcohol (low-carbohydrate beer still has calories!)
    - Beer, 12 ounces (360 ml): 90-150 calories
    - Glass of wine, 4 to 5 ounces (120-150 ml): 100 calories
- Mixed drinks
    - Gin and tonic: 200 calories
    - Hurricane: 400 calories
    - Martini: 300 calories
    - Margarita: 330 calories
    - Pina colada: 300 calories
    - Rum and Coke: 360 calories

It is a much better idea to get calories from food than from fluids, because one will feel more full for a longer period of time. However, there are some low-calorie liquid choices:

- Sports drink (but only during exercise)
- Fitness waters that average 10 calories per serving
- Water
- Flavored low-calorie or calorie-free water
- Sugar-free fruit drink mix
- Sugar-free iced tea
- Herbal tea
- Tomato juice or vegetable juice
- Skim milk
- Soups like tomato soup and vegetable soup
- Sugar-free carbonated beverages
- "Light" juice or regular juice that is diluted to one part juice and three parts water

 Encourage athletes who want to lose body fat to work on their goals in the off-season under the supervision of a health professional. (Off-Season Activities)

Foods on the Road

Athletes often have to travel to competitions and end up eating at restaurant chains that may offer tempting, calorie-laden foods. Appendix A provides recommendations for eating healthy food at restaurants.

Don't Use Body Weight Charts!

Do not set weight goals for your athlete, especially goals based on body weight charts. Body weight is a combination of frame size, body shape, muscle mass, and fat content, and weight charts are not necessarily applicable to athletic bodies. It is possible for five individuals of the same height to have different, healthy body weights based on frame size and body composition.

Fad Diets: Yes, No, Maybe?

The Zone, South Beach, Atkins, high fiber, no sugar—the list of diets is endless. There are as many different diets as there are types of sports, and it seems that every day a new diet plan appears on the Internet, in newspapers or magazines, or on television. Not one of these diets is designed for athletes; the calories are just too low, which means performance will suffer!

Just as there are clothing fads, there are diet fads. Right now, the most popular diets recommend that we eat a lot of protein and fat but cut back on bread, cereal, rice, pasta, fruits, sweets, and some vegetables. But active bodies require carbohydrate to fuel the muscles, so if your goal is to keep your athletes in the game, they should stay away from these diets. Table 5.2 lists the different categories of diets and some of the issues that affect athletes.

Fad diets result in a drop on the scale that is usually caused by water loss because of a restriction in calories or carbohydrate intake. Most of these plans are very boring and are hard to follow when the athlete is out with friends, is traveling, or is at all-day sports events. Just eating two subs a day or drinking Slim Fast gets old fast, and if your athlete follows a beverage-only diet, she won't get the chew factor and thus won't feel satisfied for long. When athletes are tempted by any of these plans, just ask whether they could see themselves eating this way for more than a week. If the answer is no, the program isn't the right one!

Preparing for Weigh-Ins

For athletes who are in weight-class sports such as wrestling, crew, and boxing, weigh-ins can be a time fraught with worry and performance-detracting diet behaviors such as dehydration and fasting. The goal is to get these athletes to within one to two pounds (.38-.75 kg) of their competition weight a week before the start of season. Three to four days before a match, the following strategies can be used:

* Decrease sodium in the diet to help decrease fluid retention.
* Focus on low-fiber foods a couple days before weigh-ins; examples include low-fat yogurt, sugar-free Jell-O, unsweetened applesauce, and low-calorie shakes.
* Educate athletes about proper hydration strategies (see chapter 4). If they take in more fluid than they need in an attempt to lessen hunger, they may end up with more water weight, which will increase the number on the scale.

As you have probably guessed by now, for athletes there are no effective shortcuts to losing weight. You want your athletes to lose weight safely and to stay on the field.

TABLE 5.2

Fad Diets

GENERAL PLANS		
Diet	**Facts**	**Issues for athletes**
High protein, high fat, low carbohydrate	These diets promote weight loss.	These diets don't provide enough calories to meet the energy demands of exercise.
	They may dehydrate the body.	Such a diet doesn't provide enough carbohydrate to meet the energy demands of exercise.
	These diets may lead to a greater feeling of fullness than do lower-fat, lower-protein diets.	Foods with protein are not always portable.
	Such a diet is very monotonous.	
	These diets may cause constipation.	
High carbohydrate, low fat	These diets may lead to weight gain.	They are not as satisfying as higher-protein diets.
	These diets may not contain enough protein or fat for growing athletes.	These diets may not supply enough fat as an energy source for exercise.
	They may cause digestive distress.	A low protein intake may have a negative effect on the immune system.
	These dietary plans don't guarantee that one will pick healthier food items.	
	Fat-free does not mean calorie-free.	
SPECIAL COMBINATIONS		
Zone diet	Weight loss occurs because of a low calorie level.	This diet may be too high in protein and too low in carbohydrate for athletes.
	There is nothing magical about this combination.	The calorie level is too low for athletes.
	The Zone does promote a mix of nutrients at every meal and snack.	
BALANCED EATING PLANS		
Weight Watchers	This plan does promote weight loss.	This plan is too low in calories for athletes.
	It is not a restrictive plan.	By adding calories for exercise, the athlete could find this plan effective.
	Athletes can choose the foods they like.	
BIZARRE AND UNTRUE		
Food combination diets: Eat Right 4 Your Type Subway diet	Weight loss occurs because of restricted calories.	Such a diet gets really boring after awhile.
	These diets are too low in calories for athletes.	
Liquid diets: Slim Fast LA Weight Loss	Weight loss occurs because of lower calories.	These diets get boring quickly.
		These plans are too low in calories for athletes.

What About Pills?

A number of products on the marketplace claim to burn fat or result in weight loss. These products do one or more of the following:

1. They act as a stimulant so the consumer feels more energized. Your athletes may notice that their heart is racing, they feel more awake, and they are breathing more rapidly. If they think that this results in weight loss, they are wrong. Avoid Ephedra, ma huang, synephrine, zhi shi, citrus aurantium, and products such as Xenadrene and Thermadrene that may contain these ingredients.

2. They act as a laxative or diuretic. The lower number on the scale reflects loss of water weight, not body fat. Avoid products with cascara, senna, and herbal diuretics.

3. They are absolutely useless. Products in this category include cayenne pepper, which claims to boost fat burning; starch blockers, which claim to reduce weight by preventing carbohydrate calorie absorption; quercetin, which is an antioxidant that may help to lower heart disease risk but has no effect on weight; or chitin, which is claimed to block fat absorption.

None of these products has been tested in young athletes, and some of them may impair performance. For instance, dieter's tea contains some pretty powerful laxatives. You wouldn't be too happy if one of your athletes drank it just before a basketball game and ended up in the restroom rather than on the court when the starting whistle blew!

Now that you understand more about how athletes can reduce calories and follow good eating habits, we can turn to developing an action plan.

Create an Action Plan

When an athlete expresses interest in losing weight, sit down with him and gather some information prior to goal setting. A few key questions can help you determine the athlete's level of commitment and whether his desired results are realistic. This line of questioning also helps you identify some red flags that the athlete may be facing body image issues or pressure to lose weight. Questions to ask might include these:

- Why are you interested in losing weight?
- Has anyone told you that you have to lose weight?

- Do you have particular health concerns?
- Have you lost weight in the past? If so, how?
- What performance effects do you expect to notice as a result of weight loss?
- How much time do you have to commit to working on weight goals?
- What are obstacles that may hinder your efforts to lose weight?
- Do you have a support system in place?
- Do you have a time frame for weight loss?

You must address the athlete's concerns as well as temper any unrealistic expectations. The athlete needs to understand the realities of weight loss:

- Weight loss is more like gradual steps than a slide.
- Body fat loss does not happen quickly.
- Once an athlete loses weight, to maintain the new lower weight, she has to eat less than she did at the higher weight; otherwise the weight returns.

A qualified health professional should set the weight range goal for your athlete. A reasonable short-term weight loss goal is one to two pounds (.38-.75 kg) per week, but for your athletes who are hard losers, even one-half pound per week is a realistic and achievable goal for weight loss. There is not a specific weight that is best for an athlete but more a weight range. Your objective observations of strength, speed, stamina, and recovery are the tools you should use to assess your athletes' progress.

You may also want to have your athletes sign a student-athlete weight contract. In this contract they acknowledge that it is their responsibility as a team member to maintain a healthy weight and that they agree to seek treatment if they need help in doing this. Figure 5.8 is an example of such a contract.

Tell the athlete that you will not be the one doing the initial physical assessment or ongoing monitoring, but encourage her to let you know how she is progressing. Praise the athlete for positive changes in sport performance attributable to weight loss.

Once your athletes have weight goals, assemble a weight-loss team to help them achieve their goals and take steps to create an individualized action plan for each of them.

Set up individual meetings with athletes to discuss their reasons for wanting to lose weight. (Activities for Athletes Who Want to Lose Fat)

Player Name _____

(print)

Student-Athlete Weight Contract

I realize that as a student athlete, I have a responsibility to my team, my school, and my coach to make sure that I am healthy and able to perform. If I experience problems attributable to being overweight, being underweight, or having eating or body image issues, I am willing to seek treatment.

   I understand that treatment may involve the following:

   Meeting with a physician and school nurse to evaluate medical status

   Meeting with a sports dietitian for nutritional counseling

   Meeting with a sport psychologist or therapist for psychotherapy if indicated

   Meeting weekly with one of my coaches or the athletic trainer

   I understand that if I do not comply with this contract, I may not be able to participate in practices and competition.

_____   _____

Athlete's signature   Date

From L. Bonci, 2009, *Sport Nutrition for Coaches* (Champaign, IL: Human Kinetics).

FIGURE 5.8   Sample weight contract.

Choose the Weight-Loss Team

To increase the likelihood that your athletes will lose the desired amount of weight, they need to be accountable. You should know how your athlete is progressing, but the day-to day issues surrounding weight goals should be someone else's responsibility.

   You do not want to be the diet enforcer. This will take time away from your coaching responsibilities, resulting in animosity toward the athlete and disrupting the team dynamics. So you should create a weight-loss team, including the following people:

- The point person to whom the athlete will report weekly. The athletic trainer is ideal because she often has the most frequent contact with the athlete. If the athlete is seen by a registered dietitian, nurse, physician, or therapist, the athletic trainer can reinforce what the health professional has recommended and also report back to the health professional on how the athlete is progressing.

- The athlete's support system (teammates, roommates, friends, parents). If a parent is responsible for buying and preparing the athlete's food, she definitely should be part of the action plan, so that the athlete will have a greater chance for success.

- Others who need to be kept in the loop (you, the team physician). The point person should report to you at least monthly.

The weight-loss team members should remember that although they may have found the meal plan and lifestyle pattern that works for them, the athlete trying to lose weight must find her own individualized plan to meet her needs. Team members should provide support and guidance and help the athlete to modify her eating plan to achieve weight-loss goals.

   If you have several athletes who are trying to lose weight, it may be advantageous for them to meet as a group. This uses time more effectively and allows them to support each other.

Example

Steve, a goalkeeper for his high school soccer team, believed that he was carrying too much weight and complained of feeling sluggish during practices. He had missed the prior season because of shoulder surgery, and the inactivity coupled with overeating resulted in a 20-pound (7.5 kg) weight gain over a year. When I saw him, he weighed 180 pounds (67 kg) and believed that he would be more comfortable at 160 pounds (60 kg), his usual playing weight. Successful body fat loss is considered to be 10 percent of starting weight over six months, or for Steve about one-half to one pound (.22-.45 kg) per week.

I told Steve that to lose one-half to one pound of fat per week, he would need to cut about 375 calories from his daily intake. When we looked at his food diary, he said he could change his beverages and decrease the size of his snack choices. His action plan was to cut 375 calories from his daily intake by choosing lower-calorie beverages and decreasing the size of snack items.

In the first month, Steve lost eight pounds (3 kg). I told him that often weight loss is faster earlier on and then it starts to slow, so to keep the momentum going, I had him continue to keep food records, and he added an extra conditioning session, such as 30 minutes on the treadmill, elliptical trainer, or stationary bike after practice, to burn additional calories. In the second month, Steve lost four more pounds (1.5 kg).

Over the remaining four months, Steve continued to watch his portions, but he did allow himself some treat items, just not as frequently as he used to. And because he was exercising more, he was burning more calories every day than when he was injured. He reached his goal of 160 pounds at the end of five months and was able to maintain the weight loss and play well.

Select and form a weight-loss team to monitor and support your athletes. (Activities for Athletes Who Want to Lose Fat)

Because the focus for sport performance is body fat loss, not just weight loss, the athlete will have to consume enough calories to meet the body's basic requirements. Too few calories consumed will translate to more lean muscle mass lost. The amount of body fat an athlete should lose is around one-half to one pound (.19-.38 kg) per week. Remember, fat is what should be lost, not water or muscle. An athlete who skips breakfast to save calories and has early morning practice is going to end up losing muscle, not fat, and although weight may be down, this type of weight loss impairs performance and is unacceptable.

Take Steps to Create a Plan

To help your athletes achieve their weight-loss goals, follow these steps to create an action plan for each athlete:

1. Have a health professional do the baseline measurements of weight and body composition and set a weight-loss goal.

2. Assess RMR and determine baseline caloric requirements.

3. Determine the amount of calories that the athlete consumes daily (Activity Log) and then reduce that amount by around 300 calories a day.

4. Track daily activity to identify ways the athlete can burn more calories.

5. Have the athlete fill out the Food Diary, Food Pattern Form, and Eating Style Questionnaire.

6. Help the athlete find ways to eat fewer calories daily by looking at his completed forms and making suggestions.

Having your athletes fill out the Activity Log and other forms engages them in the process, heightens their awareness of their activity levels and eating habits, and helps them find ways to change those patterns in order to lose weight.

Here are some things your athletes can do to reduce their calorie intake:

1. Limit or get rid of foods and beverages they can do without:

   - High-calorie beverages
   - Large portion sizes of anything
   - Condiments such as mayonnaise, salad dressing, butter, and margarine

2. Right-size plates, mugs, and glasses, and consider using small spoons or salad forks instead of soup spoons and larger forks.

3. Add foods that require more work:

   - Food that has to be chewed
   - Food that has to be cut
   - Hot foods that take more time such as soup and oatmeal

4. Add liquid-based foods and foods with a high moisture content to meals, because they increase satiety:

   - Stew
   - Chili
   - Soup
   - Unsweetened applesauce
   - Salads

5. Space meals out:

   - Have the salad or soup and then the sandwich instead of both together.
   - Have the salad first and then the meal.

6. Create an eating environment that is conducive to success:

   - Include foods that make one feel more full for a longer period and are nutrient rich:
     Fruits
     Vegetables
     Beans
     High-fiber cereals
   - Have fewer tempting foods around.
   - Include foods that are easily portioned:
     One half of a chicken breast
     A piece of string cheese
     A container of yogurt
     A piece of fruit
     A 100-calorie snack pack
     A snack-size bag of microwave popcorn

7. Replace easy-to-eat large-volume foods with finite portions:

Instead of	*Choose*
crackers out of the box	a package of peanut butter crackers
several scoops of ice cream	an ice cream sandwich
cookies	a cereal-sized bowl of sweetened cereal with milk

8. Focus on times of the day when it's difficult to control eating instead of the whole day.

9. Eat breakfast. Studies show that breakfast eaters are lighter and burn calories more efficiently!

Because high school athletes are in a time of rapid growth, they must not cut calories too much. Athletes need to eat enough for activity, basic body needs, and growth. Consuming too few calories will not help your athletes to reach their goals.

Talk with athletes about how to decrease their number of calories eaten daily. (Activities for Athletes Who Want to Lose Fat)

Seek Referrals

Helping athletes reach their weight goals requires a lot of time and effort on your part as well as the athletes'. It is hard to be the team coach and the nutrition coach. Seek out dietitians in your area, and consider having one talk to your team about healthy eating and achieving weight goals. You can find registered dietitians through your local hospitals. Dietitians in private practice are listed in the phone book or online, or go to the American Dietetic Association Web site, www.eatright.org, and follow the Find a Dietitian link. Dietitians charge a fee for this kind of service; perhaps the school's booster club would underwrite the cost. In some cases, health care insurance will cover the costs of nutrition counseling. This might include athletes who have not only weight issues but also health issues such as diabetes and hypertension (see more on these issues in chapter 9).

Develop a list of dietitians and other health professionals in your area to whom you could refer your athletes. (Activities for Athletes Who Want to Lose Fat)

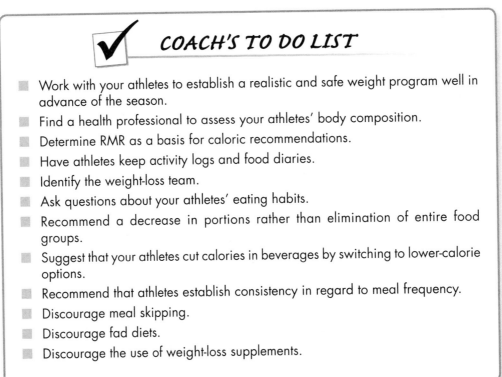

SUMMARY

- Inappropriate weight-loss strategies are not successful in the long run and may compromise performance in the short term.
- Athletes need to understand what they can and cannot change about their bodies.
- Body composition assessment is important to prevent muscle mass loss and to set appropriate weight goals.
- Someone other than the coach should perform body composition measurements.
- Assessing resting metabolic rate will provide a better way of estimating caloric requirements.
- Athletes need to monitor food intake and amounts as well as activity levels to get a baseline estimate of calories consumed and expended.
- Identifying food patterns can help athletes to discover which foods may be problematic.
- Understanding eating habits and working to change them can contribute to the success of a weight management program.
- A good weight-loss program incorporates carbohydrate-, fat-, and protein-containing foods.
- Limiting calories from fluids can help with body fat loss.
- To decrease body fat and increase muscle mass, athletes must have a plan of action.
- Fad diets result in temporary weight loss, and their low calorie level may adversely affect athletic performance.
- Weight-loss supplements are not effective and may be harmful.

- Athletes need to be educated on how to prepare for weigh-ins for sports in which they have to make weight.
- Creating a weight-loss action plan with athletes increases the likelihood that they will be successful.
- A weight-loss team and referrals to weight-loss experts can help the athlete achieve his body composition goals.

KEY TERMS

body composition   metabolic rate

GAME PLAN QUESTIONS

1. What are four important factors to consider in helping an athlete to lose weight?
2. Why do athletes need to assess their activity levels?
3. Why is it important for an athlete to keep a food diary?
4. Why do eating habits make a difference?
5. Why are fad diets not recommended for athletes?

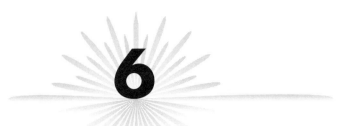

Increasing Muscle Mass

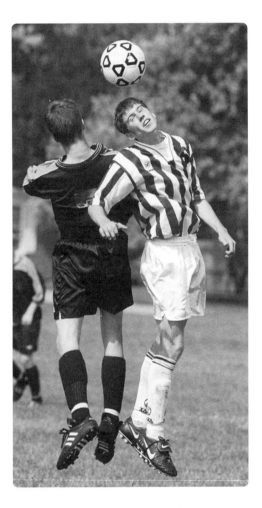

Gregory, a soccer player, is a freshman in high school. He was thrilled when he found out he had made the varsity squad. However, many of his teammates and opponents were a lot bigger and stronger, so that despite his speed and agility, he often found himself being outmuscled and pushed off the ball. This did not escape the coach's watchful gaze. Gregory spent the rest of the season on junior varsity with the coach's words echoing in his ears: "Gain 20 and you'll be back."

Greg decided he needed a plan. The day after the season ended, he decided to spend three or four days per week in the weight room, still continuing to run but swapping soccer practice times for lifting. He also knew he needed to eat more. He enjoyed food but was never overly hungry and was often teased by his friends who were incredulous that he could exercise so much and be satisfied with so little. Some of the older kids and adults in the weight room talked a lot about protein powders and weight-gain supplements. Greg was curious, but because he didn't have a lot of money to spare and his parents weren't keen on these products, he decided to increase his food intake by eating more frequently and eating a larger amount at each meal.

Although his weight didn't increase quickly and several weeks went by where he stayed the same weight despite lifting and eating, he was able to achieve his goals. At the end of his freshman year soccer season, he weighed 120 pounds (54 kg) and was five feet, five inches (1.65 m). By August of the following year, he had grown two inches (5 cm) and had put on 20 pounds (9 kg), to 140 (63 kg). The growth spurt, increased eating, and weight training paid off. He felt great on the field, the coach was delighted, and his performance didn't suffer at all!

When you finish reading this chapter, you should be able to explain

- what an athlete needs to have or do to increase muscle mass,
- how to determine the athlete's current weight and body composition and the number of calories needed to gain mass,
- where to get help in developing an exercise regimen,
- how to create an action plan to increase muscle mass,
- how to determine what and when your athlete should eat, and
- when supplements can help increase muscle mass.

If your goal is to increase athletes' weight, the more specific goal is to have them increase lean muscle mass. The last thing you want is for athletes to pack on body fat. If the increase is done right, when an athlete gains weight, he or she may gain a little bit of body fat in the process but the weight increases primarily because of an increase in muscle. It's going to take much more than Cheetos, Krispy Kremes, and milkshakes for your athletes to get the body they want.

How Can Athletes Add Muscle Mass?

An increase in muscle mass will only occur if

1. enough testosterone is available,
2. the muscles work maximally, and
3. the athlete consumes enough fuel through food and beverage to support everyday activities plus extra calories for weight gain.

First, athletes who have not yet attained puberty are not going to see significant muscle gain until testosterone levels are optimal. The team physician or the athlete's pediatrician can help you determine each athlete's stage of growth and developmental progress.

Second, your goal is for the athletes to work on getting stronger as well as bigger. To accomplish this, they need to lift weights. Athletes who cannot devote a lot of time to lifting weights during the season will need to put in some quality time in the weight room after the season is over.

Third, you need to measure the athlete's daily caloric intake and energy expenditure to determine how many calories he or she will have to consume in order to gain weight. To use these calculations to formulate a goal that is appropriate for your athlete and to get a baseline of the athlete's current weight and body composition in order to measure progress toward that goal, you and a qualified health professional need to do some assessments.

Determine a Starting Point

When an athlete is interested in adding mass, he needs to begin with baseline measurements. Measurement of weight and body fat and the determination of metabolic rate and daily energy expenditure give the athlete a clear picture of his own body composition and caloric expenditure so that a plan can be customized to reflect his specific needs.

What Is the Athlete's Weight and Body Composition?

Appoint a health professional to weigh the athlete and assess her body composition. Body composition yields valuable information on the percent body fat and fat-free mass. As mentioned in chapter 5, many methods are used to assess body composition, from relatively inexpensive skinfold calipers, handheld scales that assess body fat (such as Tanita), and bioelectrical impedance analysis (BIA) to the state-of-the-art methods such as air displacement (e.g., the BOD POD), hydrostatic or underwater weighing, and dual energy X-ray absorptiometry (DEXA). Table 6.1

Have a health professional assess the athletes' weight and body composition. (Activities for Athletes Who Want to Gain Mass)

lists the most common and least expensive methods used to assess body composition.

Although skinfold calipers, body fat scales, and BIA machines are not exact, they are inexpensive methods that are generally available. They provide a baseline and can be used periodically to assess progress.

As mentioned in chapter 5, another way to assess athletes is to have an athletic trainer or other health professional measure body mass index (BMI). The BMI charts can help to determine whether your athletes are underweight. For most people, a BMI less than 18.5 is considered to be underweight.

When an athlete expresses interest in increasing mass, he needs to realize that if he has a small frame, he may not be able to put on a lot of mass. An athlete with a small frame is probably not going to become a hulking lineman no matter how much time he spends in the weight room. Your athletes need to accept what they cannot change about their bodies and instead focus on the areas they can change.

The good news is that athletes can increase muscle mass through a combination of strength training and increased caloric intake. An athlete who is trying to gain weight may also experience a slight increase in body fat as a consequence of a greater caloric intake. However, gains in body fat can be kept to a minimum by being selective about foods consumed and incorporating strength training into a weight-gain program.

TABLE 6.1

Methods to Assess Body Composition

Method	What is measured	Advantages	Disadvantages
Bioelectrical impedance analysis (BIA) or Tanita scales	Conductivity of body tissues	Easy, convenient, inexpensive	Hydration status affects accuracy
Skinfold calipers	Subcutaneous fat as a predictor of total fat	Easy, convenient, inexpensive	Must use correct equations and proper technique
BOD POD	Air displacement	More accurate than calipers, BIA, or body fat scales	Expensive and not readily available
Hydrostatic weighing	Body fat and lean mass	More accurate than skinfold calipers, BIA, or body fat scales	Expensive and not readily available
Dual-energy X-ray absorptiometry (DEXA)	Body fat, lean mass, and bone density	More accurate than BODPOD, BIA, body fat scales, and skinfold calipers	Expensive and not readily available

How Many Calories Does the Athlete Need?

One of the themes of this book is that there is no one meal plan, weight, or calorie level that is appropriate for every athlete. You must determine an individual calorie level that will result in the desired changes in the body while providing enough energy for the demands of exercise. Athletes who are trying to increase mass need to know their baseline caloric requirements so that they can add enough calories to gain weight. They must know not only what they take in but what they burn. If an athlete expends the same number of calories per day as he consumes, his weight will stay the same. The goal is to eat more than what is expended, and athletes who need to gain weight usually burn as many calories as they take in.

You or a dietitian needs to help your athletes determine their baseline caloric requirements so that they can add the appropriate number of calories to promote weight gain. To get a better idea of your athletes' caloric requirements, you can approximate your athletes' resting metabolic rate (RMR) from the equations in table 6.2.

TABLE 6.2

Estimating RMR

Body weight (lb) × 10 or weight (kg) × 22= number of calories the body requires at rest
If your athletes are injured or cannot exercise: Body weight (lb) × 13-15* or weight (kg) × 28.6-33*
If your athletes exercise three or four days per week: Body weight (lb) × 14-17* or weight (kg) × 30.8-37.4*
If your athletes exercise five or six days per week: Body weight (lb) × 17-27* or weight (kg) × 37.4-59.4*

*Use lower numbers for females and higher numbers for males. Sports such as soccer or hockey may have higher calorie expenditures.

Example

In sports such as hockey, soccer, and lacrosse, caloric requirements can be up to 27 calories per pound (59.4 kg) of body weight.

A 150-pound (68 kg) soccer athlete exercises five days per week.

150 × 27 (68 x 59.4) = 4,050 calories per day

For weight gain, the athlete should add 1,000 calories to his estimated daily requirement to result in a weight increase of 1 pound.

4,050 + 1,000 = 5,050 calories per day to achieve weight gain

---

This is a rough estimate of basic needs. For a better estimate, have your athletes keep an activity log so that they can better estimate how many calories they need to consume daily. Encourage your athletes to keep a paper log, or use the computer, to track their energy expenditure over the day. They need to record everything they do and the number of minutes spent

 Assess the athletes' caloric expenditure by having them keep an Activity Log. (Activities for Athletes Who Want to Gain Mass)

doing it from the time they wake up until they go to bed. Figure 6.1 shows a sample activity log for Brian, a soccer player. Figure 6.2 is a blank form you can copy for your own athletes to use.

As you can see by this example, our 150-pound athlete expended 3,690 calories a day, a total of calories for light activities (eating, sitting, walking to school) as well as those calories expended for sport.

If your athlete records this by hand, you'll need to supply him with a source for determining the number of calories used. Here are a few:

Brian's Activity Log

Activity	Time spent	Calories expended
Wake up; get out of bed; do crunches, pull-ups, and push-ups	10 min	54
Brush teeth, wash face, shower, get dressed	10 min	27
Eat breakfast	5 min	10
Walk to school	15 min	61
Sit in classes	90 min	184
Play basketball and shoot hoops in gym class	45 min	343
Sit in classes	90 min	184
Eat lunch	25 min	51
Sit in classes	90 min	184
Sit in study hall	25 min	51
Sit in band practice	45 min	91
Get ready for soccer practice	5 min	13
Run 3 miles (4.8 km) (8 min mile)	8 min	360
Go to soccer practice	2 hr	986
Walk home	15 min	61
Eat dinner	30 min	61
Do homework, sitting	2 hr	245
Sit at the computer, watch TV, snack	2 hr	245
Brush teeth, wash face, get ready for bed	5 min	27
Sleep	7 hr	572
		Total: 3,690

FIGURE 6.1   Sample activity log.

Book

McArdle W (ed). *Exercise Physiology: Energy, Nutrition, and Human Performance.* 5th ed. Malvern, PA: Lea & Febiger. 2006.

Web site

www.aolhealth.com/tools/calories-burned?s
  em=1&ncid=AOLHTH00170000000022&
  s_kwcid=calories%20burned|1939849520

An easier way to keep a log of physical activity is to use MyPyramid Tracker, an online tool developed by the U.S. Department of Agriculture and the Center for Nutrition Policy and Promotion. The Web site is www.mypyramidtracker.gov. When the user enters data into the application, it calculates the number of calories automatically. Figure 5.3 on page 62 shows an example.

Although recording this information takes time, it is the only way to figure out how many calories are expended every day, so that you can help your athlete more accurately determine how much more she needs to eat to gain muscle mass.

Activity Log

List all your activities and the amount of time you spend doing them over the course of the day. Use a resource such as those listed on page 85 to calculate the calories expended for each activity.

Activity	Time spent	Calories expended
		Total:

From L. Bonci, 2009, *Sport Nutrition for Coaches* (Champaign, IL: Human Kinetics).

FIGURE 6.2   Activity log.

Set Up an Exercise Regimen

To build muscle, athletes will need to devote some quality time to lifting. The number of hours they spend in the weight room is not as important as the efficiency of the workout. Several excellent resources provide guidelines for setting up a program:

National Strength and Conditioning Association, Brown LE (ed). *Strength Training*. Champaign, IL: Human Kinetics; 2007.

Kraemer WJ, Fleck SJ. *Optimizing Strength Training*. Champaign, IL: Human Kinetics; 2007.

Gambetta V. *Athletic Development*. Champaign, IL: Human Kinetics; 2007.

Kraemer WJ, Fleck SJ. *Strength Training for Young Athletes.* 2nd ed. Champaign, IL: Human Kinetics; 2005.

Enlist the help of a strength coach if possible; this individual is a valuable resource for you and for your athletes.

You might have athletes who are already lifting weights several times a week, but their bodies aren't changing. How can that be?

They may be

- lifting weights that are too light;
- doing the same exercises and not working all muscles;
- eating insufficient protein to support muscle growth;
- eating insufficient overall calories; or
- still going through puberty, so that their testosterone production is not sufficient to result in an increase in muscle mass.

Develop a strength training plan for athletes who want to increase muscle mass. (Activities for Athletes Who Want to Gain Mass)

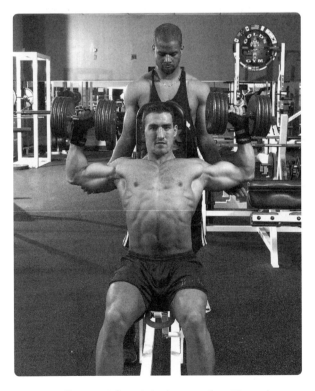

Frequent, efficient weight training is a must for athletes who want to gain muscle.

Implement an Action Plan

Once you have gathered baseline weight and body composition information and have an activity log and a food diary from your athlete, you can determine the number of extra calories she probably needs to eat and consider what type of weightlifting exercises she needs to do. Here is an action plan:

1. Have a health professional conduct the baseline measurements of weight and body composition and set a weight-gain goal.
2. Assess RMR and determine baseline caloric requirements.
3. Assess daily energy expenditure (Activity Log).
4. Develop a strength training plan.
5. Assess daily energy intake (see Food Diary in next section).
6. Work with your athlete to find a way to add at least 500 extra calories per day, up to 1,000 calories per day if she can.

Before you work out a plan with the athlete, you must decide who will monitor her. If you have to be the diet enforcer, you won't be able to focus fully on the other players, which can result in animosity toward the affected athlete and disrupt the team dynamics. Yet accountability is a huge part of goal setting. All people work harder and better when they know they have to answer to someone other than themselves. Your athlete needs to have a point person to report to, rather than rely on himself for support and encouragement. Set up a point person and a weight-gain team as described in chapter 5. The point person should report to you on the athlete's progress at least once a month.

Weight-gain team members should remember that the athlete trying to make weight must find his own individualized plan to meet his needs. They should provide support and guidance but not expect that the athlete should do exactly what they do.

During practices or conditioning time, do not single out the athlete who is trying to make weight. If you belittle or criticize him, even though you are trying to help, your efforts may backfire. Making weight is hard to do no matter what end of the scale someone is on. Both the athletic environment and the support system need to be conducive to success, and positive approaches always work best.

Your athletes need to be willing to devote the time to getting bigger. Just as they have homework assignments for school or designated practice times, they need to make this effort a priority and work on it every day. You may want to have your athletes sign a student-athlete weight contract. In this contract they acknowledge that it is their responsibility as a team member to maintain a healthy weight and that they agree to seek treatment if they need help in doing this. (Figure 5.8 on page 75 is an example of such a contract.

> *Select and form a weight-gain team to monitor and support your athletes. (Activities for Athletes Who Want to Gain Mass)*

Praise your athletes and acknowledge their efforts at modifying their diet and lifestyle to alter their body composition. Remind them to focus on their short-term weight goals, which are much easier to achieve and provide more immediate feedback than long-term goals. For example, a goal of gaining three to five pounds (1.4-2.3 kg) in a month is more realistic than focusing on the 30 pounds (14 kg) that the athlete is trying to gain. An athlete who gains even a little weight might notice that she feels stronger and less fatigued during practice and is able to recover more quickly. Some athletes may report that their clothes don't hang off their bodies once they've put some weight on. Gaining weight is not going to happen overnight, and the recommendations that you make at the outset may need to be modified over time.

Have your athletes take some baseline measurements and track their progress. Some athletes experience an increase in the size of the chest, biceps, or thighs without a change in weight, and they become discouraged, assuming they have done something wrong. This is precisely why it is so important to have many different outcome measures rather than just the number on the scale.

A reasonable expectation for weight gain is one-half pound (.23 kg) per week. Your athletes also need to understand that everybody responds differently to resistance training. This is in part attributable to sexual maturation and the presence of hormones that help an athlete to increase mass. The athlete may see very little change in body size in a month's time, but after three months it would be reasonable to expect an increase of up to one-half inch (1.3 cm). To keep your athletes motivated and engaged in gaining mass, suggest that they keep a chart as shown in figure 6.3.

Chest and arm circumference will not change overnight, but your athletes may be surprised at how well they are doing when they start to monitor the changes. For instance, you may have an athlete who adds one-half inch (1.3 cm) to the size of his upper arm over a three- to four-month period, yet his weight may not change much.

Weight gain is best accomplished in the off-season, when the athlete has time to devote to eating and lifting more. Make sure that you or whomever you designate as the point person has regular meetings with the athlete to make sure he is making forward progress. Even athletes who don't put on a lot of weight will still improve their fueling and hydration

Monitoring Body Changes Chart

Measure	Oct	Nov	Dec	Jan	Feb	Mar	Apr	May	Jun	Jul	Aug	Sep
Weight												
Chest												
Waist												
Hips												
Thigh												
Calves												
Upper arms												

From L. Bonci, 2009, *Sport Nutrition for Coaches* (Champaign, IL: Human Kinetics).

FIGURE 6.3 Monitoring body changes chart.

habits, which ultimately will help them to optimize their performance, which in turn will make you and your athletes feel great!

Once you and your athlete have set your calorie and strength training goals, you'll need to discuss what foods to eat and how to alter eating habits to increase caloric intake.

Decide What and When Your Athlete Should Eat

Athletes need to realize that eating to gain weight involves not just putting food into their mouths but also deciding when to eat and how much. It's the combination of food choices and eating habits that will bring about weight gain and improve their mental and physical well-being and sport performance.

No matter what your athletes' body goals are, eating is supposed to be a pleasurable, not punitive experience. Work with them to find foods and times to eat that are reasonable and take their likes and dislikes into account.

What Should Athletes Eat to Build Muscle Mass?

Is there one sports diet for all? The answer is no. First of all, everyone has particular food preferences and certain times of the day that they are most or least hungry; second, your athletes may need to alter their diets for their sport.

People eat food, not just nutrients, and most foods that people eat are a mix of one or more nutrients. For instance, milk is composed of carbohydrate, protein, and, in some cases, butterfat. Unless people eat table sugar (all carbohydrate) or cooked egg whites (all protein) or drink vegetable oil (all fat), they're going to get a mix of nutrients from the foods they consume. This is why it is very important to emphasize food more than the nutrients that compose foods.

Do certain foods help an athlete to gain muscle? Yes, but more important than eating specific foods is eating a larger volume of food. Remember that only one of these three eating and exercise patterns will result in weight gain:

Energy intake = Energy output → Weight stays the same

Energy intake < Energy output → Weight decreases

Energy intake > Energy output → Weight increases

The goal here is not just to increase weight but to increase muscle mass as well. With that in mind, what and how much does your athlete need to eat?

Adding Calories

If the goal is to increase muscle and weight, your athlete needs to eat more to take in more calories. A useful rule is to add 500 to 1,000 calories per day. Athletes sometimes say that they can't understand why they aren't gaining weight because they eat all day, but when you ask them what they eat, they say chips and soda, not a lot of nutrient-rich food. It is OK to include some low-nutrient snacks as part of an eating plan, but muscle needs more than those types of food to grow. A 500 to 1,000 calorie increase is doable, and it will not make your athletes feel so stuffed that they are ready to burst! If they eat too much, your athletes are more likely to want to take a nap than go to lift or practice. Athletes should increase calories strategically and comfortably so that they can sustain this way of eating as long as is necessary to get to the desired outcome.

 Have the athletes keep a food diary for one week. (Activities for Athletes Who Want to Gain Mass)

Your athletes must be willing to thoroughly and truthfully record everything they eat and drink so that they can determine current intake and see what times of the day they could add food and where calories are coming from. Strongly suggest that your athletes keep a food diary for a week. Figure 6.4 shows a typical day's intake for Veronica, a volleyball player who wants to gain mass. Copy figure 6.5 and give it to your athletes to track their daily food consumption.

You and your athletes can determine the number of calories in a given food in several ways:

- Use the Nutrition Facts panel from the food label. The calorie counts given in this panel are based on the serving size, so your athlete will need to measure what she eats, compare the amount consumed to the serving size on the label, and multiply or divide accordingly.

- Consult books or Web sites that list the calories in foods, such as those listed on page 85.

Once the athlete has recorded the information, sit down with her to review the food diary and make suggestions. For instance, you may notice that the athlete eats very little during the day or nothing before or after practice. Using the information you see in the food diary, you may be able to give her recommendations on how to increase protein intake in meals, add calories in beverages, or add an extra snack. In the sample food diary in figure 6.4, this athlete could change to a beverage with more calories and add more turkey and cheese to the sandwich to

Veronica's Food Diary for Gaining Mass

Time	Food or beverage consumed	Amount	Calories
7 a.m.	Orange juice	6 oz (180 ml)	90
	White toast	Two slices	160
	Peanut butter	2 tbsp	190
9 a.m.	Cereal bar	One	140
12 noon	Turkey sandwich	One sandwich with three slices of turkey and one slice of cheese	560
	Chips	Small bag of chips	160
	Apple	Small apple	80
	Chocolate chip cookie	Large cookie	210
	Water	20 oz (600 ml) water	0
3 p.m.	Sports drink	20 oz (600 ml)	120
6 p.m.	Spaghetti with marinara sauce	3 cups (710 ml)	550
	Bread, Italian with butter	Two slices of bread 2 tsp of butter	160 90
	Salad with ranch dressing	1 cup of salad 2 tbsp of dressing	25 90
	Water	12 oz (360 ml)	0
9 p.m.	Chocolate ice cream	1 cup (130 g)	240
			Total: 2,865

FIGURE 6.4 Sample food diary for gaining mass.

add calories and protein. Reviewing the food diary is much more effective than just asking the athlete what she eats during the day. When the athlete takes the time to record food and beverage intake and calculate the calories consumed, she will be better able to identify areas where she can change her diet.

Choosing Foods

People should eat foods that they like. If food doesn't taste good, it's going to be hard to get it down and hard to stay with the food plan over time. Your athletes need to build their plans around foods that they like, but they will need to eat more of those foods to get the best results. Remind them to eat some protein-, carbohydrate-, and fat-containing foods at every meal and snack.

Table 6.3 on page 92 is a chart of common foods that contain carbohydrate, protein, and fat. Make sure that your athletes have at least one serving of an item from each category every time they eat. Some foods are a source of more than one nutrient, such as nuts, which are a source of protein and fat, and beans, which are a source of carbohydrate and protein.

Food Diary for Gaining Mass

Time	Food or beverage consumed	Amount	Calories
			Total:

FIGURE 6.5   Food diary for gaining mass.

TABLE 6.3

Common Food Sources for Carbohydrate, Protein, and Fat

FOODS THAT CONTAIN ONE MAIN NUTRIENT		
Carbohydrate	**Protein**	**Fat**
Bagel	Beef	Bacon
Bread	Cheese	Butter
Cake	Chicken	Cream
Cereal	Egg	Cream cheese
Crackers	Lamb	Margarine
Fruit	Milk	Mayonnaise
Milk	Pork	Oil
Pasta	Shellfish	Salad dressings
Rice	Soy foods	Nuts
Sweets	Nuts	Nut butters
Ice cream	Nut butters	
Vegetables	Dried beans	
Dried beans		

FOODS THAT CONTAIN MORE THAN ONE MAIN NUTRIENT	
Protein + carbohydrate	**Protein + fat**
Milk	Nuts
Yogurt	Seeds
Beans	Nut butters

When Should the Athlete Eat?

The main reason athletes do not always successfully gain weight is because their eating is too erratic. One day they may eat all day long, another day, only once. The number on the scale won't rise unless they are consistent with their eating, so they need to find a number of meals and snacks that they can reasonably eat on a daily basis and stick to their plan. Athletes need to be reminded to train with eating just as they train with practice. Encourage your athletes to think of increasing their weight as a homework assignment; gaining weight means they aced the final!

If athletes currently eat twice a day, it is unrealistic to expect that five meals a day will be comfortable at first, so for the first week, they may want to start with three meals a day, the next week increase to four, and

the third week increase to five. If they can do more after three weeks, great.

 Encourage athletes to gradually increase the number of times a day they eat. (Activities for Athletes Who Want to Gain Mass)

Athletes who don't allow enough time to eat in the morning often find themselves dashing for the bus or car without putting anything in their stomach. They need to make an adjustment. If they can't get up earlier, they should keep a few granola bars, cereal bars, or packages of peanut butter crackers by the bed so they can eat as soon as they wake up.

It takes all of five minutes to eat a bowl of cereal, a yogurt, or a peanut butter sandwich. There are

Increasing an Athlete's Calories by Meal

Here is an example of how to increase calories meal by meal.

Regular meal	Enhanced meal
Breakfast	
Two eggs	Three eggs
Two slices of toast with butter and jelly	Bagel with melted cheese and two slices of ham
Two sausage patties	Large glass of juice
Orange juice	12 ounces (360 ml) low-fat chocolate milk
Lunch	
Two bologna sandwiches	Two roast beef sandwiches with four slices of roast beef and one slice of cheese on each Kaiser roll
Chips	One large blueberry muffin
Two cupcakes	12 ounces (360 ml) grape juice
One can of soda	12 ounces (360 ml) low-fat milk
Snack before practice	
Nothing	20-ounce (600 ml) sports drink
	One package of peanut butter crackers
Dinner	
Two Big Macs	One milkshake
Large fries	One quarter pounder with cheese
Large soda	One grilled chicken sandwich
	Regular fries
Evening snack	
Chips	Bowl of cereal, a mix of flake type and granola with milk, fruit, and nuts
Cookies	

Here are some ideas for food substitutions to add more calories.

Instead of	Try
Corn flakes	Granola
Cheerios	Frosted Mini-Wheats
Toast	Bagel
6 ounces (180 ml) juice	12 ounces (360 ml) juice
Butter and jelly on toast	Peanut butter and jelly on toast
Pretzels	Nuts
Cookies	Muffin
Water at practice	Sports drink

Besides changing the item eaten, the athlete can add something to the food, such as nuts, mayonnaise, butter and jelly, or cheese, or he can put the food or drink in or on a larger glass, plate, or bowl and increase the amount.

premixed fruit yogurt smoothies that go well with cereal or granola bars and take minimal time to eat. If athletes don't eat something in the morning, they have missed an opportunity for food, and they'll be playing catch-up the rest of the day.

For weight training, have the athlete consume protein before lifting to maximize the anabolic effect of protein. It may be that 12 to 15 grams of protein are enough. That would be a 12-ounce (360 ml) glass of chocolate milk, or a container of yogurt with some nuts, or a turkey sandwich. Notice that carbohydrate as well as protein is important. Muscle growth also occurs after lifting, but rather than rushing for just the protein, athletes should include some carbohydrate, as in these foods:

- 32 ounces (~1 L) Gatorade and a handful of nuts
- A PowerBar, Zone Bar, Clif Bar, Odwalla Bar, or Gatorade Nutrition Bar
- Yogurt with granola added
- Two handfuls of trail mix with cereal, dried fruit, and nuts

Eating a carbohydrate-containing food after lifting can help stimulate growth hormone release. Remind your athletes to bring a carbohydrate-containing food to practice.

The high school athlete who has an early lunch period with practice right after school from 3 to 5 p.m. must have a snack before practice. It is hard to keep a sandwich in a knapsack or locker all day, but it is possible to have a package of peanut butter crackers, trail mix with some nuts added, or a sports bar that contains protein, carbohydrate, and fat.

Set up individual meetings with athletes to discuss how to increase the number of calories eaten daily. (Activities for Athletes Who Want to Gain Mass)

Eating a lot more food may seem overwhelming to your athletes at first. They need to understand that sometimes they will need to force themselves to eat even when they are not hungry.

You may also want to recommend that your athletes implement the following strategies:

- Plan on eating something every three to four hours. This means no skipping breakfast or lunch, and it means including midmorning and midafternoon snacks and something at night after dinner.
- Aim to eat one fourth more food at every meal and snack, such as an extra slice or two of meat on a sandwich or an additional scoop of rice, pasta, or potato.
- During nontraining times (such as meals and snacks), make sure that what you eat or drink has calories. But during workouts, be careful to not consume too much sugar, because it can cause cramps and bloating. A sports drink is the best choice during workouts, because it provides some calories but not too much sugar.
- Aim for a gradual weight gain, because this is much more comfortable for your body than a rapid gain.

What About Supplements?

It would be great if all your athletes had to do to increase muscle was to take a pill, drink some water, go to sleep, and wake up ripped. Nice theory, but I don't think so! There are several **supplements** on the market that claim to build muscle, and some have pretty creative and hard-to-resist ads. For the most part, their claims are too good to be true.

Although some athletes benefit from a protein powder or creatine, I always tell my athletes that supplements are the dessert, whereas the food and strength training are the meal. The dessert is sweet

Example

I had the opportunity to work with a former Heisman trophy winner who decided that after his senior year, he needed to add some weight to be a more attractive candidate for the NFL draft. He told me that he had to triple his food intake and often felt like food was going to shoot out of his nostrils! He made it a point to add calories at every opportunity, both in food and beverages, and never took one supplement. He also increased the time and effort he put into strength training. He was able to add 10 pounds (4.5 g) in about three months, he felt strong, and the added weight didn't slow him down. Best of all, he was drafted in the first round!

and tastes great going down, but ultimately you'll get much more out of the whole meal!

Table 6.4 lists various types of muscle-building products, the claims, and the facts and suggests some food alternatives. See chapter 7 for more on supplements.

Your athletes must be not only responsible but also committed. If they really want to see an increase in muscle mass, they need to spend more time eating and lifting than they are right now. In addition, they are ultimately responsible for what they put into their bodies and must avoid taking a **banned substance**, any product that is illegal in the governing bodies that oversee collegiate, Olympic, and professional sports. Many collegiate and professional athletes have paid the price for taking a banned substance and have been suspended from competition, or in some cases barred from sport. These athletes sometimes state that they didn't know what was in their supplements. That is never a problem with food. What you see is what you get.

Your high school athletes may think that substance bans don't apply to them. However, some schools are starting to do drug testing. And the National Colle-giate Athletic Association (NCAA), which historically has only tested football and track-and-field athletes, is contemplating expanding drug testing to more sports, for both men and women. So why not stop the use of those products in high school and encourage athletes to really make an effort with food instead?

The two other big issues with supplements are the taste and the cost. Some of the products taste nasty, and by the time your athletes mix up the powder in a large glass of water and force it down, they may be nauseated or too full to eat a meal. Either way, they are not going to consume enough calories. A far tastier and cheaper alternative would be to mix two packets of Carnation Instant Breakfast in a large glass of milk, or make a shake with milk, yogurt, and fruit and add a small packet of instant pudding powder to add more calories.

Encourage athletes who want to gain muscle mass to work on their goals in the off-season under the supervision of a health professional.

TABLE 6.4

Supplements and Food Alternatives

Supplement	Claims	Facts	Food alternatives
Protein powders	Increase mass and strength	They may achieve claims but are very pricey.	Milk, cheese, eggs, nuts, poultry, meat, fish, beans, soy foods
Weight gainers	Increase mass and strength	They are high calorie, and some are very high in fat.	Carnation Instant Breakfast, peanut butter, any calorie-containing food
Creatine	Aids with recovery, increases fat-free mass	It doesn't work for everyone and is very costly. Protein can work as well.	Meat, chicken, fish
Steroid prohormones	Increase muscle mass, decrease body fat	They do not increase muscle size or strength in the amounts sold over the counter.	Nutritious food
Plant sitosterols	Increase mass	They don't achieve their claims.	Dietary fat, such as margarine, mayonnaise, oil, nuts, and seeds
Myostatin blockers	Increase mass	They don't achieve their claims in humans.	More calories

Don't Try These!

Here are some of the ineffective things that many high school, collegiate, and professional athletes do when trying to get bigger:

- Eat infrequently
- Lift more but don't eat more
- Just try to eat more protein
- Eat more only a few days a week
- Eat and lift normally but add a weight-gaining supplement

High school athletes, coaches, and parents of athletes need to be aware of the following:

- Most high schools do not test for supplement use; however, some schools randomly test for steroids. Some over-the-counter anabolic products can contaminate steroid testing results. Products that contain nandrolone, which is an anabolic steroid, may result in a failed drug test.
- No studies have examined the effectiveness of supplements in high school athletes.
- The dose given on the product label is an adult dose.
- High school athletes often are inconsistent with supplement use.
- Some athletes may be inclined to use supplements in place of food.
- Too much protein results in too little carbohydrate.
- A muscle-building supplement does not replace time spent in the gym.

But what about vitamins and minerals? Although these can help the body to optimally digest and absorb the calories from the foods we eat, athletes do not gain muscle by taking a chewable vitamin! To get vitamins, an athlete can take a multivitamin–mineral supplement, which has no calories, or eat a bowl of Total cereal, which is fortified with 100% of the daily requirements for vitamins and minerals, with milk and fruit for 300 calories—more if the athlete uses a large bowl!

It is as hard for some athletes to gain weight as it is for others to lose weight; for some it is harder. Weight gain requires effort on the athlete's part and a lot of encouragement from you and the athlete's support system (friends, family, teammates). There are only two tried and true methods for increasing weight, especially when the goal is to increase lean mass. One is to eat more, and the other is to lift weights. Remind your athletes that there are no quick fixes when it comes to weight gain, and always emphasize food over supplements.

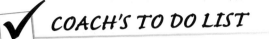

COACH'S TO DO LIST

- Well in advance of the season, sit down with your athletes who need to gain weight and help them determine realistic goals and a timetable.
- Remind your athletes that someone else will monitor their weight progress.
- Assign someone to assess the athletes' weight and body composition.
- Have athletes complete food diaries and activity logs to get a baseline estimate of caloric intake and energy output.
- Have athletes meet with the strength coach to develop a goal-focused weight-training plan.
- Make sure athletes track weight and body changes.
- Have them report to someone on the weight management team at regular intervals.
- Encourage them to eat more food more often.
- Recommend that they replace low-calorie foods with higher-calorie items.
- Emphasize food over supplements.
- Encourage adding calories through beverages as well as through food.
- Monitor, assess, and tweak the weight-gain program as needed.

SUMMARY

- The primary objective is to help the athlete increase muscle mass, not body fat.
- An increase in muscle mass requires adequate testosterone, strength training, and sufficient calories.
- Body composition assessment is necessary to help the athlete set appropriate goals.
- Keeping an activity log and food diary will help you and the athlete determine the calories required to increase muscle mass.
- You should help the athlete in setting up an effective strength training program.
- The weight-gain team will work with athletes to help them increase muscle mass.
- Athletes must understand the importance of monitoring changes in the body in addition to numbers on the scale.
- Athletes need to increase the caloric density of food as well as the quantity consumed and the number of meals consumed daily to achieve an increase in muscle mass.
- Weight-gain supplements may contain banned substances, are quite costly, and are not always effective.

KEY TERMS

banned substance   supplements

GAME PLAN QUESTIONS

1. What baseline measurements should you take before helping an athlete develop a weight gain plan?

2. What are some of the mistakes athletes make with eating when they are trying to gain weight?

3. Why should athletes keep track of body changes?

4. Why is it important for your athletes to keep food and exercise diaries?

5. Why should athletes shy away from weight-gain supplements?

Sizing Up Supplements

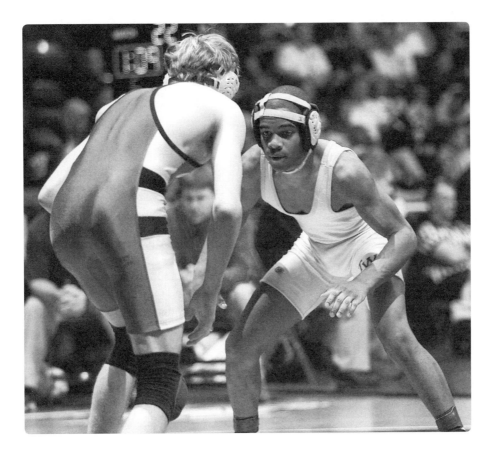

Mickey, a high school wrestler, wanted to compete at a lower weight class. He began to cut weight by decreasing his caloric intake and adding some extra cardiovascular workouts. Although his weight was dropping, he wanted to see more rapid loss with the season approaching. He ordered a "fat burner" supplement online using his parents' credit card.

A few days after he started taking the supplement, he noticed he was not as hungry, but he also noticed that his heart was beating faster and he was having trouble falling asleep. However, he was losing weight, so he was pleased. Some of his teammates became concerned because Mickey, always the team clown, had become very moody and would lash out instead of joking with his teammates. The coach also noticed this change in behavior and sat down with Mickey.

After much reluctance, Mickey admitted to taking a fat burner supplement. His coach had a long talk with Mickey and his parents and suggested that Mickey visit the family physician to have a checkup. Mickey stopped taking the supplement but gained weight and felt that he was not as competitive at the higher weight. He was convinced he could not maintain a low weight without the supplement and decided to quit the team.

When you finish reading this chapter, you should be able to explain

- what vitamins and minerals your athletes need,
- what other common supplements are available and which are effective,
- the possible dangers of supplement use,
- the pros and cons of steroids and how to prevent their use, and
- how to educate your athletes about supplement use.

The dietary supplement industry makes billions of dollars. Energy drinks, protein powders, bars, and pills line the shelves of supermarkets and health food stores. Many studies have looked at the prevalence of supplement use among adolescents, including one done recently on U.S. adolescents (Castillo and Comstock 2007). Supplement studies show the following usage rates in athletes:

- 3 to 5 percent of athletes in sixth through eighth grades (O'Dea 2003)
- 22 to 58 percent of adolescent athletes (Laos and Metzl, 2006; Scofield and Unruh 2006)
- 42 percent of college freshmen football players (Jonnalagadda et al. 2001)
- 76 percent of collegiate athletes (Froiland et al. 2004)

You and your athletes need to speak the same language when you talk about supplements. Froiland et al. (2004) surveyed athletes and found that they defined supplements in many ways, such as the following:

- Products that increase performance, strength, and muscle mass
- Products that enhance recovery
- Vitamins and minerals
- Products that improve the health of the body
- Anything other than food
- Substances that help athletes gain or lose weight

Your definition of supplements may not be the same as your athletes' definitions. So when you talk to your athletes about supplements, remember the following:

- Be very clear. Give examples; for instance, many athletes do not consider sports drinks, shakes, or bars to be supplements and thus won't tell you about them unless you specifically ask.
- Be in the know about currently popular supplements.
- Ask athletes questions about their supplement use and ask them to show you the products that they use.

Supplements are used to augment or enhance the diet, not as a replacement for food. Athletes don't always realize that consuming a supplement such as a protein powder is not the same as eating a piece of chicken. The chicken provides not just protein but also vitamins, minerals, and fat, whereas the protein powder may contain select vitamins and minerals and is not a source of fat. Many supplements, such as a carbohydrate gel or a branched chain amino acid, contain just one nutrient. Athletes who don't eat well and take a lot of supplements will only end up with a well-supplemented poor diet!

Athletes and parents need to be educated about the potential dangers of supplements. Athletes who have food allergies or food intolerances may know what foods they have to avoid but don't always consider that supplements can contain the same ingredients and could cause an adverse reaction. Athletes who take prescription or over-the-counter medications need to be very careful with supplements, because some can interact with medications. Supplements that increase heart rate, such as caffeine, synephrine, and green tea extract, may not be the best choice before exercise. Exercise itself increases heart rate, so if heart rate is already elevated before one starts practice, the result may be early fatigue and breathlessness. In addition, synephrine can increase blood pressure. Table 7.1 lists some supplements and their side effects.

These dangers can be present even with recommended doses, and not everyone follows the dosing instructions on the label. Sometimes athletes assume that if a little is good, more is better; they don't realize that too much may be quite harmful.

In this area you are asked to be not only a coach but also an educator and sometimes an enforcer. You do not want to discourage the athlete's desire to pursue an advantage or an edge; however, if the means to that end involve an illegal or harmful substance, you must step in.

The majority of supplements have not been tested in young people, so the possible side effects are unknown. You also have liability concerns. If you recommend a supplement and your athletes suffer negative consequences from taking it, you may be held responsible.

Do not simply say no to your athletes when it comes to supplements, because the athletes will find a person or a Web site that will sell supplements to them. The salesperson may not know (or care) whether the product is harmful, helpful, or banned, and a Web site may overstate claims about what the supplements can do. Instead, educate your athletes about the facts versus the claims and about the risks and benefits of supplement use. Start by discussing supplements that are known to enhance performance. Sports drinks can be useful before, during, and after activity to deliver fluid, carbohydrate, and electrolytes to the muscles. Sports gels can be consumed during endurance exercise or during breaks in competition, and they provide a quick, portable, and easily digestible carbohydrate source. A sports shake can serve as an additional calorie source for the athlete trying to gain weight or, in a controlled portion size, as a low-calorie alternative for the athlete looking to shed body fat.

Let's start by looking at a common supplement that most people take—vitamin and mineral supplements.

Vitamins and Minerals

Vitamin and mineral supplements are among the most commonly used supplements. In some cases, athletes take these supplements because they believe that a supplement will compensate for poor eating or

TABLE 7.1

Side Effects of Supplements

Supplement	Side effects
Ginkgo biloba, ginger, garlic, ginseng	Can act as blood thinner and cause bleeding
Ephedra and synephrine	Can lead to high blood pressure, nervousness, insomnia, and headaches
Yohimbe	Can lead to high blood pressure
Senna	Has very potent laxative effects
Cascara sagrada	Can cause severe electrolyte loss (sodium and potassium loss)
Panax ginseng	Can decrease blood sugar, resulting in hypoglycemia
White willow bark	Increases gastrointestinal irritation and ulcers in those who have aspirin sensitivity and can interact with other medications
Nitric oxide stimulators	Act as a vasodilator (dilate blood vessels) and can cause headaches

because their parents think it is a good idea. **Vitamins** are essential, noncaloric organic substances that can be obtained through food sources and supplements. Vitamins are involved in the maintenance and formation of red blood cells, hormones, nervous system chemicals (neurotransmitters), and genetic material (DNA).

Vitamins are divided into fat-soluble or water-soluble vitamins. Fat-soluble vitamins dissolve in fat and are transported through the body attached to fat. The body stores fat-soluble vitamins in adipose (fat) tissue, which is why we don't want to consume excess amounts of fat-soluble vitamins. When vitamin A is consumed in excess quantities, it can cause headaches, dry skin, liver damage, and bone and joint pain. An excess of vitamin D, a problem rarely encountered in athletes, could lead to kidney stones and weakened muscles and bones. Vitamin E and K excesses are also rare, although people who use blood thinners need to be careful with their vitamin E and K intake because both of these vitamins can have blood-thinning effects.

Water-soluble vitamins dissolve in water and are not stored in significant amounts. Although toxicity is less likely with water-soluble vitamins than with fat-soluble vitamins, it is not wise to consume excess quantities of water-soluble vitamins. This is the case for pyridoxine, or vitamin B_6, which can cause nerve damage when consumed in megadose levels. For the most part, what the body doesn't need is excreted, so it is important that water-soluble vitamins be consumed (ideally through food) daily.

Table 7.2 lists the vitamins by categories. Some supplements contain substances that are vitamin-like compounds required for metabolic processes in the body.

Unless an athlete needs to take a particular vitamin to compensate for a deficiency, he or she should take a multivitamin–mineral supplement to get all of the micronutrients. There is no need for a mega-supplement; a supplement that provides between 100 and 250 percent of the Daily Value (% DV), which is based on average nutrient level requirements, is sufficient. The Supplement Facts panel on a product will provide % DV; however, recommendations for vitamin requirements are based on the **Dietary Reference Intakes (DRIs)**, which are nutrition recommendations from the Institute of Medicine of the National Academies of the United States. The DRIs include average requirements and Recommended Dietary Allowances (RDAs; amounts considered adequate for healthy people) or Acceptable Intakes (AIs; amounts considered to pose no significant health risk). These are listed in table 7.3.

TABLE 7.2

Types of Vitamins

VITAMINS	
Fat soluble	**Water soluble**
Vitamin A	Thiamin (B_1)
Vitamin D	Riboflavin (B_2)
Vitamin E	Niacin (B_3)
Vitamin K	Folic acid
	Cobalamin (B_{12})
	Pyridoxine (B_6)
	Pantothenic acid
	Biotin
	Vitamin C
VITAMIN-LIKE COMPOUNDS	
Choline	Alpha-lipoic acid
Ubiquinone (coenzyme Q10)	Pangamic acid

TABLE 7.3

Daily Vitamin Requirements by Age

	A, µg	D, µg	E, mg	K, µg	B$_1$, mg	B$_2$, mg	Ni, mg	B$_6$, mg	Folate, µg	B$_{12}$, µg	B$_3$*, mg	Biotin, µg	Choline, mg	C, mg
MALES														
Ages 9-13	600	5	11	60	0.9	0.9	12	1.0	300	1.8	4	20	375	45
14-18	900	5	15	75	1.2	1.3	16	1.3	400	2.4	5	25	550	75
19-30	900	5	15	120	1.2	1.3	16	1.4	400	2.4	5	30	550	90
FEMALES														
Ages 9-13	600	5	11	60	0.9	0.9	12	1.0	300	1.8	4	20	375	45
14-18	700	5	15	75	1.0	1.0	14	1.2	400	2.4	5	25	400	65
19-30	700	5	15	90	1.1	1.1	14	1.3	400	2.4	5	30	425	75

Note: B$_1$ = thiamin; B$_2$ = riboflavin; Ni = niacin; B$_{12}$ = cobalamin; B$_3$ = pantothenic acid. Vitamin D amount may be given in international units on a Supplement Facts panel. 1 µg = 40 IU, so 5 µg = 200 IU.

Minerals are inorganic compounds and, like vitamins, are not a source of energy for the body. They are part of the molecules that make up tissue, bones, teeth, and other parts of the body and assist in various body processes. Minerals are classified as major minerals, which are needed in amounts of approximately 250 milligrams per day, and trace minerals, which are needed in amounts of 20 milligrams or less per day. These classifications are shown in table 7.4. Table 7.5 shows the daily requirements for each mineral.

What do your athletes need to know about multivitamin and mineral supplements?

- Supplements do not replace food. Vitamins and minerals are not sources of energy for the body and therefore cannot provide fuel for exercising muscles.
- More is not better! There is a Tolerable Upper Intake for supplements. This is the maximum recommended amount of a supplement, beyond which there may be consequences of overuse, such as toxicity.
- Look for products with 100 percent of the Daily Value for vitamins plus vitamin K. Supplements can contain up to 100 percent of the Daily Value for minerals, but many have only around 25 percent of the Daily Value.

TABLE 7.4

Types of Minerals

Major	Trace
Calcium	Iron
Phosphorus	Zinc
Magnesium	Copper
Sulfur*	Selenium
Potassium	Iodide
Sodium	Fluoride
Chloride	Chromium
	Manganese
	Molybdenum*
	Boron
	Vanadium*

*No Dietary Reference Intakes have been established.

TABLE 7.5.

Daily Mineral Requirements

MAJOR MINERAL REQUIREMENTS						
	Calcium, mg	Phosphorus, mg	Magnesium, mg	Potassium, g	Sodium, g	Chloride, g
Males						
Ages 9-13	1,300	1,250	240	4.5	1.5	2.3
14-18	1,300	1,250	410	4.7	1.5	2.3
19-30	1,000	700	400	4.7	1.5	2.3
Females						
Ages 9-13	1,300	1,250	240	4.5	1.5	2.3
14-18	1,300	1,250	360	4.7	1.5	2.3
19-30	1,000	700	310	4.7	1.5	2.3

Note: Potassium, sodium, and chloride values are presented in grams. You may also see milligrams on labels: 1 g = 1,000 mg, so 4.5 g = 4,500 mg.

TRACE MINERAL REQUIREMENTS									
	Fe, mg	Zn, mg	Cu, µg	I, µg	F, µg	Cr, µg	Mn, mg	Mb, µg	Se, µg
Males									
Ages 9-13	8	8	700	120	2	25	1.9	34	40
14-18	11	11	890	150	3	35	2.2	43	55
19-30	8	11	900	150	4	35	2.3	45	55
Females									
Ages 9-13	8	8	700	120	2	21	1.6	34	40
14-18	15	9	890	150	3	24	1.6	43	55
19-30	18	8	900	150	3	25	1.8	45	55

Note: Fe = iron; Zn = zinc; Cu = copper; I = iodine; F = fluoride; Cr = chromium; Mn = manganese; Mb = molybdenum; Se = selenium.

Reprinted with permission from the National Academies Press, Copyright 2005, National Academy of Sciences. Source: *Dietary Reference Intakes for Energy, Carbohydrate, Fiber, Fat, Fatty Acids, Cholesterol, Protein, and Amino Acids (Macronutrients)*, pp. 1322-1323.

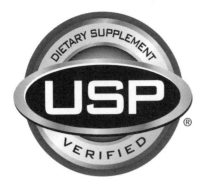

FIGURE 7.1 USP symbol.

© 2009 The United States Pharmacopeial Convention. All rights reserved. Reprinted with permission.

- Products should display the USP symbol (see figure 7.1) and an expiration date. USP stands for United States Pharmacopeia. This symbol indicates that the product has been tested to ensure that it contains the ingredients stated on the label, which will release and dissolve to be absorbed by the body; does not contain harmful levels of contaminants; and was made according to good manufacturing practice regulations (GMPs) promulgated by the US Food and Drug Administration.

- Supplements used past the expiration date do not have their original potency, so the athlete will not receive their full benefit.

- Calcium in supplements is absorbed better if taken in 500-milligram doses (Heaney, Recker, & Hinders 1988).

- Calcium carbonate supplements should be taken with food to help with absorption; calcium citrate is better absorbed on an empty stomach, so it should be taken between meals (Levenson and Bockman 1985).

- Calcium and iron supplements should not be taken together because calcium may interfere with iron absorption (Hallberg, Rossander-Hulten, Brune et al. 1992).

Other Common Supplements

Let's look at some common supplements widely used by athletes. They include creatine, protein powders, amino acids, caffeine, muscle gainers, and fat burners.

Creatine

Some supplements see a surge in popularity and then interest wanes. This has been the case with **creatine**: It is still used, but not to the same extent as a few years ago. This may be in part because there are so many other products on the market that claim to increase muscle mass. Protein powders and bars continue to be popular as well as other substances advertised to increase muscle mass, such as nitric oxide stimulators and fat burners, the latter of which often contain green tea extract, caffeine, and synephrine. (Chapters 5 and 6 address supplements that assist with muscle gain or body fat loss.)

Creatine is obtained in the diet through beef, pork, veal, lamb, poultry, and fish. The amino acids in these foods—glycine, arginine, and methionine—are the building blocks for creatine synthesis. Creatine phosphate is used to produce ATP, as discussed in chapter 1. However, because the amount of creatine in muscles is limited, the phosphagen energy system (ATP and creatine phosphate) is used for short-duration, high-intensity activities. So it would make sense to consume creatine to have more energy to fuel the cells for sport, right?

More than a thousand studies of creatine have been conducted. It is safe, but it is not necessarily effective for every athlete. Some athletes are hyper-responders, who notice that when they take creatine they can push themselves more, lift more, recover more quickly, and see an increase in muscle size. However, some athletes are hyporesponders, who do not notice any changes in their performance or body when taking creatine.

Creatine is a cell volumizer that causes the muscle cells to hold water; therefore, some of the muscle "gain" is caused by increased fluid in the cells, resulting in puffiness. Athletes who experience weight gain as a result of creatine use may notice that the extra weight affects their balance, agility, and speed, thereby negating any performance-enhancing effect. A dose of 3 grams of creatine per day for 30 days is preferred over a loading dose of 20 grams a day for 5 days. The smaller dose may prevent some of the puffiness associated with larger volumes of creatine but can be just as effective, and the athlete will use less total creatine.

Your athletes may ask you what form of creatine to use. Creatine monohydrate is the preferred form, because it seems to be the best absorbed and metabolized and is less expensive than creatine esters or serum.

Let your athletes know that protein foods are sources of creatine. Eight ounces (about 225 g) of pork, fish, or beef will each provide 1 gram of creatine. If your athletes consume a pound (450 g) of meat, poultry, or fish over the course of the day, they don't need creatine supplementation. Once the muscle reaches saturation point with creatine, through either food or supplement, the muscle cannot store more creatine and the rest will be excreted from the body. In addition, meats provide protein and calories, which creatine supplements do not.

Protein Powders

Another very popular type of supplement is **protein powder**, which is used to increase muscle mass. The maximum usable amount of protein is 1 gram per pound (2.2 grams per kg) of body weight per day from all sources, both food and protein powders.

There is much debate about the type of protein to use, and whey protein isolate may be the most effective for maintaining and increasing muscle mass. Whey protein contains high levels of the amino acid leucine, which may play a role in increasing muscle mass.

Remind your athletes to consume protein both before and after lifting in order to receive the maximum benefit. However, a glass of chocolate milk or cup of yogurt can be as effective as a protein powder, because the combination of protein and carbohydrate most effectively increases muscle mass.

Amino Acids

Some athletes believe that amino acid supplements are of benefit, because they are advertised to digest more rapidly than food to provide a quicker increase in muscle size and strength. The truth is that it takes longer for individual **amino acids** to form new proteins than it does for the body to break down a piece of chicken. In addition, amino acid supplements are measured in milligrams, but protein is measured in grams. Athletes can be lured into thinking they are getting a lot of protein through supplements, but because there are 1,000 milligrams in a gram, 7,000 milligrams of amino acids is only 7 grams, the amount of protein in one egg or one thin slice of turkey breast. And the amino acids are much more expensive!

Caffeine

Many athletes believe they cannot get through a day without one or more energy drinks. Most of these products contain **caffeine**, which is a stimulant, not a source of energy. Some of these products can be quite high in calories, whereas others have no calories at all. Caffeine may be listed on the label as caffeine or as guarana, kola nut, or mate. What should you tell your athletes about these products?

Caffeine is not dehydrating to the body, but it may cause someone to need to urinate more frequently. Caffeine may also have the following side effects:

- Rapid heart beat
- Increased blood pressure
- Insomnia
- Nervousness
- Jitters
- Anxiety
- Inability to focus
- Irritability

Although there is not an upper limit for the amount of caffeine that can be safely consumed daily, various organizations and researchers (Council on Scientific Affairs 1984; Nawrot et al. 2003) recommend an upper intake of 400 milligrams of caffeine daily. If one consumes more than that amount, the side effects previously discussed may occur. Table 7.6 lists the amount of caffeine in various products.

Some studies have shown that consuming caffeine before an endurance sport may help delay fatigue. Caffeine causes fatty acids to be released early in exercise to be used as a fuel source, thereby sparing some carbohydrate. Because caffeine pills are more concentrated in caffeine than coffee, tea, or energy drinks, these pills may cause nervousness and restlessness that would not optimize performance. There are no bans on caffeine use in the NCAA, IOC, or professional sport organizations.

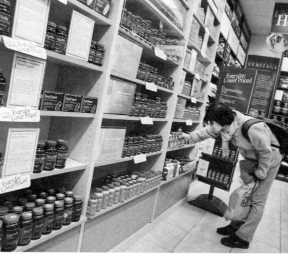

Athletes should shop carefully for supplements and remember that many of the ingredients found in supplements are available through food sources.

© Chris Hondros/Getty Images

Example

Ned was a Division I baseball player who constantly complained of being tired. He was carrying a heavy course load, and with daily practices and workouts he had to stay up late to get his work done. He thought consuming more caffeine would help him focus in class and be more alert during practice, so one day Ned had a large coffee with a shot of espresso mid-afternoon and three energy drinks before practice. When he got to the field he wasn't feeling well and complained to the athletic trainer that his heart was racing and he felt very nervous and jittery. The symptoms became worse and he was not able to take the field; he ended up going to the emergency room for an electrocardiogram. Luckily his heart was fine, but he had to miss a few days of practice, which did not make his coach too happy.

TABLE 7.6

Amount of Caffeine in Various Products

Beverage	Amount, oz (ml)	Caffeine per serving, mg
Espresso	2 (60)	100
Coffee	8 (240)	100
Starbucks Tall	12 (360)	375
Starbucks Grande	20 (600)	555
Starbucks Venti	24 (720)	650
Soft drink	12 (360)	30-50
Black tea	8 (240)	50
Green tea	8 (240)	30
Mountain Dew	12 (360)	55
Red Bull	12 (360)	80
Amp	8 (240)	75
Monster	16 (480)	400
Jolt	12 (360)	70
Bawls	12 (360)	80
Rockstar	16 (480)	275
KMX	12 (360)	38
Adrenaline Rush	12 (360)	79
XS	12 (360)	83

Because excess caffeine use can cause cardiostimulatory effects such as rapid heart rate and increased blood pressure, as well as insomnia, anxiety, and nervousness, it is prudent that athletes limit caffeine intake. In addition, caffeine is considered to be a drug, and there is a potential for addiction with as little as 100 milligrams of caffeine per day. If your athlete misses her daily caffeine fix, she may pay with a headache or other withdrawal symptoms. Explain to your athletes that energy drinks and other caffeine-loaded beverages may make them feel great in the short term but will not necessarily translate to success in sport.

Muscle Gainers

Many of your athletes may be looking for **muscle-mass enhancers**, products to help them put on muscle mass. Several supplements that claim to increase muscle mass are ineffective. Other products are banned by the National Collegiate Athletic Association (NCAA), International Olympic Committee (IOC), and professional sport organizations. Here are some of them:

- Steroid prohormones such as androstenedione, norandrostenedione, and tribulus are advertised to increase muscle mass or strength but have not been shown to do so. They are banned by most sport organizations.

- Dehydroepiandrosterone (DHEA) and human growth hormone are banned in the NCAA, IOC, NFL, and Major League Baseball (MLB) among others. In clinical studies these supplements have not been shown to consistently increase muscle size or strength.

- Boron is a mineral that is advertised to increase muscle mass but doesn't live up to this claim. Taking more than 50 milligrams per day can cause gastrointestinal distress and appetite loss.

- Chromium is another mineral that is supposed to increase muscle mass but doesn't.

- Plant sitosterols such as gamma-oryzanol have no effect on increasing muscle mass, but plant sterols and stanols may help to lower cholesterol levels in people with moderately elevated cholesterol.

- Myostatin inhibitors are very popular with bodybuilders because of the belief that blocking the enzyme that regulates muscle mass will lead to more bulky muscles. The majority of studies that have shown an increase in mass have been done on animals. A human study that combined myostatin inhibitors and strength training demonstrated no effect on muscle strength or mass (Willoughby 2004).

- Beta-hydroxy-beta-methyl butyrate (HMB) may increase muscle mass but is very expensive.

- Nitric oxide stimulators contain the essential amino acid arginine, which is thought to stimulate human growth hormone and insulin secretion, but the research to support this is not strong. Doses greater than 10 grams can cause digestive distress.

- Vanadyl sulfate (a salt of the mineral vanadium) is claimed to increase muscle mass but doesn't. In large doses it can turn the tongue green!

Many of these products are quite costly and don't work. In addition, some of them can cause digestive distress. And supplements that show a benefit in animals may not necessarily be effective in humans. Although your athletes may find it easier to take a pill than eat, they may not achieve gains in muscle because the product may be ineffective. As mentioned in chapter 6, the only way to increase muscle is to strength train and eat enough. Most supplements do not provide sufficient calories or may have no calories.

Fat Burners

For athletes who want to lose body fat, **fat burners** sound very enticing. Ephedra is one: Although this substance is no longer available on the shelves in America, it can still be purchased online under other names. The word *ephedra* may not be on the label but it is in any product that contains or is marketed as ephedrine, ma huang, Mormon's tea, epitonin, or *Sida cordifolia*. This substance is a central nervous system stimulant that can increase heart rate, blood pressure, and rate of breathing and can alter moods.

Synephrine is another fat burner. It's also known as zhi shi, citrus aurantium, or bitter orange, and it is a central nervous system stimulant as well.

Your athletes may not know what ephedra or synephrine is, but they may be familiar with the brand-name products that contain these substances, such as Ripped Fuel, Hydroxycut, Xenadrene, and Red Line.

Both ephedra and synephrine are banned by the NCAA, the IOC, and professional sporting associations. Again, it is possible for your athletes to obtain, knowingly or unknowingly, products with ephedra (online) or synephrine (in stores or online). Advise them to be vigilant about what they put into their bodies.

New Supplements

New supplements come to market all the time that have no effect on performance. Here are some of them:

- Meditropin is advertised as an anabolic but has no effect. It contains the essential amino acid arginine, which has not been proven to increase muscle mass or strength, and glutamine, which may support a healthy immune system but does not increase muscle mass or strength. There are no evidence-based studies or clinical trials that demonstrate the efficacy of meditropin.

- Microhydrin claims to buffer hydrogen ions in the muscle to reduce lactic acid buildup, but there are no clinical trials to demonstrate efficacy.

- GAKIC and Epovar contain the essential amino acid arginine, which is also found in nitric oxide stimulators. When taken as a supplement, arginine is supposed to result in increased muscle mass by increasing growth hormone levels, but this contention has been challenged (Lambert et al. 1993).

- Glutamine is a nonessential amino acid, the levels of which decrease during physical stress. Product makers claim that glutamine supplementation will keep the immune system strong, especially during periods of strenuous and prolonged physical activity. Glutamine supplementation does not increase muscle mass (Candow et al. 2001). Carbohydrate supplementation during and after exercise may be more effective than glutamine supplementation in maintaining the body's glutamine stores. In addition, glutamine is found in foods such as meat, poultry, and milk. Glutamine seems to be more effective when consumed in food rather than as a supplement (Zanker et al. 1997).

Supplement Safety

Your first concern should be that the supplement do no harm. The athlete may be allergic to ingredients in the supplement, or the supplement may interact with medications. Even beyond these possibilities, some supplements are harmful, including the following:

- Gamma hydroxy butryone (GHB), gamma butyrolactone (GBL), or Furanone di-hydro (sold as Rest-Eze), which can result in seizures or coma and can be fatal

- Star Caps, which contain Lasix, a diuretic, in quantities that exceed prescription doses

- Dieter's Tea, which contains senna and cascara, two very potent laxatives

- Yohimbe, which may be toxic to the kidneys and can increase blood pressure

- Aristolochic acid, an ingredient in some over-the-counter weight-loss products that can be toxic to the liver

- Comfrey, chapparal, and germander, which are herbs added to some herbal preparations that can be toxic to the kidneys

- White willow bark, which contains salicylates that are contraindicated in those who cannot tolerate aspirin

Ask your athletes to show you anything they are considering taking *before* they take it so that you, the athletic trainer, the sports dietitian, the school nurse, or the team physician can look at the product before it is used. Have your athletes fill out a supplement form (see figure 7.2) and instruct them to update the form if they add or discontinue the use of any medication or supplement.

Anabolic Steroids

It seems that almost every day we hear another story about an athlete banned from his or her sport for taking banned supplements, which often turn out to be **anabolic steroids.** Anabolic steroids are synthetic substances related to the male sex hormones, or androgens. Anabolic steroids are used to promote the growth of skeletal muscle (the anabolic effect) and the development of male sexual characteristics (the androgenic effect), particularly an increase in strength.

At the beginning of the season, provide to athletes and their parents a written policy banning steroid use and have every athlete fill out a Supplement and Medication Form (figure 7.2). Follow up with athletes as necessary. (Preseason Activities)

Although anabolic steroids can confer an unfair competitive advantage by improving muscle strength, size, and speed, they are banned because they can be harmful to the body. Several studies have looked at the long-term consequences of anabolic steroid use, such as increased risk for heart disease and cancer, and short-term studies have shown that anabolic

Supplement and Medication Form

Name:_____

Please list all medications and supplements you are currently taking.

Supplement or medication	Dose	Frequency of use	Reason for use

From L. Bonci, 2009, *Sport Nutrition for Coaches* (Champaign, IL: Human Kinetics).

FIGURE 7.2 Supplement and medication form.

steroids can have deleterious psychological consequences such as aggressive behavior, depression, and suicidal ideation (Hartgens and Kulpers 2004; Maravelias et al. 2005).

There are two types of anabolic steroids; oral and injectable. Table 7.7 lists them by type. Your athletes may also be familiar with other terms for steroids such as *gym candy, juice, Arnolds, pumpers, stackers,* and *weight gainers.* Many slang terms have grown up around steroid use, including the following:

Shotgunning: cycling with steroids

Stacking: using two or more steroids

Roid rage: unexplained outburst of anger, combativeness, or frustration

Pyramid: schedule of doses in 6- to 12-week cycles, starting with low doses that slowly increase to higher doses during the second half of the cycle and then decrease

The best way to prevent steroid abuse is to have prevention policies in place. Ignoring or allowing steroid use to continue is dangerous for all. Develop a written policy that bans steroid use and specifies consequences for violators. Do this in conjunction with your school's administrators, athletic director, athletic trainer, and student representatives (for high school athletes, include parent representatives). The policy should require coaches to receive training on spotting steroid use and educating athletes about steroids. It should prohibit companies that manufacture muscle-building supplements from sponsoring school sports or events. The policy should also prohibit school staff members or parents from encouraging or distributing muscle-building supplements to students, with penalties for violators. Staff members who violate the policy would put their jobs at risk; parents who do so would be banned from attending sporting events.

If your school or organization does not have a written policy banning steroid use, consider developing one in conjunction with your school or organization's administrators, the athletic staff, and student and parent representatives. (Start-Up Activities)

You have a role to play in preventing steroid abuse. You may not like confrontations, but your athletes are your responsibility. Just as you wouldn't allow them to drive drunk, you shouldn't allow them to experiment with supplements that could harm them. So have the courage to say something. Don't be combative, but do educate your athletes with facts about steroids, and approach athletes if you suspect that they are using steroids. Make sure that you communicate with compassion and know your limits; you may need to refer athletes to a physician or psychologist.

Some of the signs of steroid abuse that you need to watch for are listed in table 7.8.

To create a substance-free environment, implement the following strategies:

- Have an open-door policy so your athletes are comfortable talking to you.

- Require your athletes to tell you if they are considering using supplements and, if so, which supplements.

- Be confident of your expertise, and take a zero-tolerance attitude about steroids.

- Talk about both sides of the issue, performance enhancement as well as the harm to health. Involve student-athletes in the discussion, and invite an athlete who has used steroids to share his or her story with your athletes.

TABLE 7.7

Types of Steroids

Oral	Injectable
Anadrol (oxymetholone)	*Deca-Durabolin* (nandrolone deconoate)
Oxandrin (oxandrolone)	*Duobolin* (nandrolone phenpropionate)
Dianobol (methandrostenolone)	*Depo-testosterone* (testosterone cypionate)
Winstrol (stanozolal)	*Equipoise* (boldenone undecylenate)

Italicized terms are brand names.

TABLE 7.8.

Signs of Steroid Abuse

Physical	Psychological
Sudden increase in strength	Depression
Sudden increase in body weight	Irritability
Sudden increase in lean body mass	Anxiety
Acne	Mood swings
Puffiness	Fatigue
Growth stunting	Insomnia
Growth of body hair in women	Suicidal thoughts
Decreased breast size in women	Obsessive behavior related to conditioning and physique
Oily hair and skin	Restlessness
Enlarged breasts in men (gynecomastia)	Appetite loss
Swelling of feet and ankles	Hallucinations
Bad breath	
Trembling	
Weakened immune system	
Shrunken testicles	

Users of injectable steroids are also at increased risk of contracting or transmitting HIV and hepatitis B and C.

- Take 5 to 10 minutes of practice time monthly to address supplement issues and nutrition.
- Do not use scare tactics; they don't work.

Educate your athletes on the consequences of steroid abuse. Also let them know that steroids can interact with prescription or over-the-counter medications.

Do not allow athletes who use steroids to be part of your team. In collegiate athletics, steroid use results in a 1-year suspension. In professional sports, athletes who use steroids are fined, suspended for a number of games, or both.

Some educational programs have been extremely effective in preventing steroid abuse. The most well-known and most successful one is ATLAS, which stands for Athletes Training and Learning to Avoid Steroids. This program has resulted in a 50 percent decrease in new use of anabolic steroids in high school athletes, a decrease in the use of alcohol and other drugs, and a decrease in other risky behaviors. You can learn more about this program at http://www.ohsu.cc/hpsm/atlas.html.

Another great resource is Drug Free Sport. This organization's Web site, www.drugfreesport.org, provides information on preventing substance abuse and educating athletes, and your athletes can use this site to anonymously ask questions about supplements.

Supplement Legality

Sometimes athletes are shocked to learn that they can fail a drug test because they take an over-the-counter medication. A legal product can be banned within a sport. You need to know which products are allowed

Become familiar with your sport's list of banned substances. (Start-Up Activities)

or banned in your sports. The NCAA and other sport governing bodies provide regularly updated lists of banned substances. Here are some online sources for these lists:

Baseball: http://mlbplayers.mlb.com/pa/pdf/jda .pdf

Football: http://www.prostaronline.com/ banned_subs2.html

NCAA: www.ncaa.org/health-safety

IOC: www.wada-ama.org/en/

Supplement Education

Foods should be considered before supplements. Encourage your athletes to improve their diets and gauge the results before considering a supplement. Remind your athletes that their edge may come from something in the refrigerator rather than the medi-

 Discuss supplement and steroid use with athletes during the season and encourage them to talk with you about supplements before beginning to use them. (Season-Long Activities)

cine cabinet. There are also some supplements that are fine to use, which are listed in table 7.9.

Talk to your athletes not only about the supplements but also about why the athletes want to take supplements and what they notice as a result of taking supplements. Explain that *natural* and *safe* are not the same thing. For instance, mushrooms are natural, but some mushrooms are poisonous and therefore unsafe to eat. Many supplement products state that they are made of natural ingredients, such as plants, but certain plants and other natural substances can have toxic side effects. Supplements are not inexpensive, so you may want to have your athletes price these items and compare them with food. Some cost comparisons for sources of protein are listed in table 7.10.

Athletes learn through their stomachs, so have them taste the protein powders, bars, and gels to determine whether they like them or find them hard to get down. Supplements always have the same taste and mouth feel, and that gets boring quickly; there is much more variety in the look and the taste of food.

Have athletes compare the cost of supplements with the cost of foods with similar nutrients. (Season-Long Activities)

TABLE 7.9

Acceptable Sport Nutrition Supplements

Product	Nutrient	Purpose
Sports drinks	Fluid, carbohydrate, electrolytes	Hydrate and fuel during exercise
High-carbohydrate sports bars	Carbohydrate, protein, fat, vitamins, minerals	Provide a convenient, portable source of energy before or after exercise
Gels or honey*	Carbohydrate	Provide an easily digestible fuel source for use during activity or between events
Sports beans* (jelly beans with electrolytes added)	Carbohydrate and electrolytes	Provide fuel during activity or events
Protein isolates	Typically whey or soy protein	Provide concentrated protein source to augment dietary protein intake to help to increase muscle mass
Electrolytes	Sodium, potassium, and chloride	Improve fluid balance
Multivitamin–mineral supplements	Vitamins and minerals	Augment the diet

*Gels, honey, and sports beans are concentrated carbohydrate sources, so athletes who use these products should consume them with water to expedite absorption.

TABLE 7.10

Comparisons of Costs for Protein Sources

Mega protein, 1 scoop + 8 oz (240 ml) skim milk	**Chunk tuna,** packed in water, 6 oz (170 g)	
Protein: 31 g	Protein: 40 g	
Cost: US$1.34	Cost: US$1.29	
	OR	
	Cottage cheese, 1 cup (225 g)	
	Protein: 26 g	
	Cost: US$0.90	
	OR	
	Three eggs, scrambled	
	with 1/4 cup (120 ml) milk and1/4 cup (25 g) shredded cheddar cheese	
	Protein: 32 g	
	Cost: US$0.67	
Weight Gainer, two scoops + water	**Skim milk,** 8 oz (240 ml)	
Protein: 10 g	Protein: 8 g	
Cost: US$0.87	Cost: US$1.19	
MetRx Bar	**Cheese and crackers**	
Protein: 32 g	Four slices of muenster cheese and 20 crackers	
Cost: US$2.49	Protein: 37 g	
	Cost: US$1.76	
Power Bar	**Roasted soybeans** (1/2 cup)	
Protein: 24 g	Protein: 14 g	
Cost: US$1.99	Cost: US$0.53	
	OR	
	Turkey sandwich	
	Four slices of turkey breast on a roll	
	Protein: 33 g	
	Cost: US$1.53	
Amino acid supplements	**1 egg**	
Protein: 5.3 g	Protein: 7 g	
Cost: US$1.33	Cost: US$0.10	

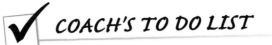

COACH'S TO DO LIST

☐ Advise athletes to talk with you, the athletic trainer, and their physician before taking any supplements.

☐ Ask athletes to tell you and the athletic trainer about any medications or over-the-counter substances that they take regularly.

☐ Teach athletes to read the ingredient list before taking anything, especially if they have food allergies or take medication.

☐ Be sure that athletes know that they should stop taking a supplement if they notice any side effects such as a headache, nausea, vomiting, or changes in bowel movements.

☐ Counsel athletes not to believe everything they read about supplements.

☐ Remind athletes that not all supplements have the same effects in all people; what works for one player may not work for another.

☐ Work with athletes to improve their diet rather than take supplements.

SUMMARY

- Dietary supplements are used by child, adolescent, and adult athletes.
- Athletes are always looking for an edge, and many of them think that supplements will provide that edge.
- Supplements can be harmful as well as helpful.
- Some supplements impair performance.
- Vitamins and minerals may be useful but not in excess quantities.
- The supplements most commonly used by athletes do not have the same efficacy in everyone who uses them.
- Athletes need to understand the consequences of supplement use.
- Some supplements are banned by sport governing bodies.
- Anabolic steroids can have adverse long-term physical effects and short-term psychological effects.
- It is important to establish a supplement-informed policy.
- Education of athletes and parents is key.

KEY TERMS

amino acids
anabolic steroids
creatine
caffeine

Dietary Reference
 Intakes (DRIs)
fat burners
minerals

muscle-mass enhancers
protein powders
vitamins

GAME PLAN QUESTIONS

1. Why are athletes attracted to supplements?

2. What should an athlete look for in a vitamin–mineral supplement?

3. Why should you establish a supplement policy?

4. What are some of the adverse effects of caffeine overuse?

5. What are some of the problems with anabolic steroids?

PART II

Special Situations

The four chapters in this second section explain how you can deal with some common nutrition-related problems you may encounter in coaching. In chapter 8, Preventing Common Complaints, you learn how to prevent three physical problems that often keep athletes from performing at their best: muscle cramps, gastrointestinal distress, and "hitting the wall." You may also run into a problem if some of your athletes have diets that are different from the rest of the team, whether for religious or medical reasons. To accommodate these athletes and help them perform at their best, you can use the information in chapter 9, Coping With Special Diets. This chapter covers vegetarian and vegan diets; diets for those who have diabetes or hypoglycemia, food allergies or intolerances; and fasts. As you work with your athletes during the season, you may suspect a few of them have eating disorders. Chapter 10, Dealing With Disordered Eating, explains what signs to look for, how you can encourage healthy eating, and what you can do if one of your athletes does have an eating disorder. Finally, you may struggle with the issue of alcohol use if you work with athletes in middle school, high school, or college settings. In chapter 11, Dealing With Alcohol Use, you get the facts on alcohol's short- and long-term effects on the body and learn how to talk to your athletes about alcohol and how to set team policies for alcohol use.

Preventing Common
Complaints

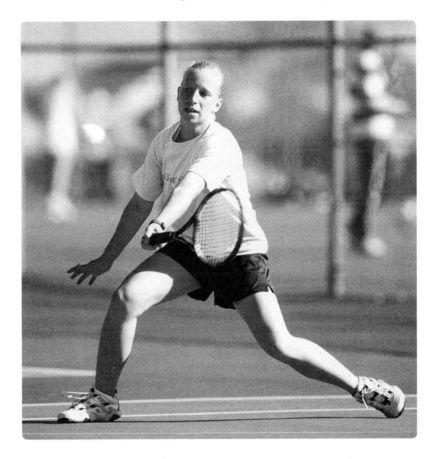

Jen is a high school tennis player who has always brought sports drinks and water to practice and games and hydrated during the day. She started her senior year playing well, but one month into the season, she started complaining of severe leg cramps during matches. She also noticed that her hands and ankles were puffy after practices or matches, a problem she had never had before. The cramps often were bad enough that she had to forfeit.

Her father was recently diagnosed with high blood pressure and was told that salt was bad. Her mom started cooking without salt, and Jen tried to help her father become an astute label reader. When she looked at her sports drink and saw that it contained sodium, she decided to quit using it and just drink water.

Jen was told that foods high in potassium would help with muscle cramps, and she started drinking a large glass of orange juice every day as well as eating two or three bananas daily, but the cramps didn't go away.

Jen is a salty sweater (see chapter 4), who notices that her skin feels gritty after practice. She can see white streaks on her arms and sometimes inside her visor, and she says her sweat stings her eyes.

I recommended that she put sodium back into her diet. She started to use more sports drinks during practice and games, used salt on her foods, and added some salty foods to her diet such as pickles, pretzels, and crackers. She started to feel better and noticed less swelling and no more muscle cramps. She finished the season strong and is looking forward to playing in college.

When you finish reading this chapter, you should be able to explain how your athletes can avoid

- muscle cramps,
- gastrointestinal distress, and
- running out of fuel for their muscles ("hitting the wall" or "bonking").

Muscle cramps and digestive distress can take the athlete out of the game. Not only can cramps and stomach upset be uncomfortable or painful, but they are also extremely distracting. The athlete with muscle cramps or an upset stomach will not be able to focus on practice or competition. The good news is that with proper hydration and electrolyte intake, the frequency of muscle cramps can decrease. Athletes can learn to monitor food intake to discover which foods and beverages, as well as what kind of timing of fueling and hydration and what quantities, cause digestive problems. In addition, your endurance athletes need to know how to avoid running out of fuel for their muscles so they can finish strong.

This chapter offers ways to deal with common, preventable physical problems that can occur during activity. Each solution is related to eating or drinking the right foods or liquids at the right times, so that if you educate your athletes about possible problems and make sure they follow through with solutions, you can prevent these problems from interfering with your athletes' performance.

Identify which common complaints are most widely seen in your sport. (Start-Up Activities)

Muscle Cramps

Nothing can sideline an athlete faster than muscle cramps. Whether the athlete has a leg cramp or a whole-body cramp, it is almost impossible to push through and keep playing with a cramp. The goal is education and prevention, because once the athlete has a cramp, little can be done except to let the cramp subside.

There are a lot of misconceptions about the cause and treatment of muscle cramps. Certainly skeletal muscle fatigue and overload attributable to overuse or inadequate conditioning can result in muscle cramps in muscles that are overworked (Bentley 1996; Jung et al. 2005; Schwellnus et al. 1997). Extensive sweat losses and **sodium** losses can also lead to muscle cramping even when the muscles are not overworked. Although you may think that this second type of cramping occurs only in hot or humid conditions, athletes can experience muscle cramps even when the weather is cool. Some athletes may sweat more than others because of genetics, adults sweat more than children, and men sweat more than women. Athletes who are acclimatized to heat will lose less sodium in their sweat.

You should have a cramp prevention game plan. Such plans are common in sports like football, but given that muscle cramps can occur in all sports, you must make a plan for all of your athletes.

There are two priority items for managing cramps. One is to have the athlete consume adequate amounts of fluid (refer to chapter 4). The second is to make sure your athletes consume enough sodium.

Why don't athletes consume enough sodium? Some athletes don't like the taste, some have sweat sodium losses that far outpace their sodium intake, and others don't have easy access to salty foods. But many athletes believe that sodium is bad. Remind them that because they sweat, they need to consume more sodium than does a friend or family member who is not physically active. The USDA Dietary Guidelines Tolerable Upper Intake for sodium is 2,300 milligrams per day (Food and Nutrition Board 2004), which is equal to 1 teaspoon of salt. Most athletes will require more sodium. Sodium is the key electrolyte that helps to reduce the risk of whole-body muscle and heat cramps during practice and competition (Bergeron 2003). Sodium is important to

- replace sweat losses,
- enhance rehydration, and
- speed fluid absorption.

Sodium and fluid losses during exercise can be huge. Many athletes lose between 1 and 1.5 quarts (roughly equal to the same number of liters) of fluid and 1 to 1.5 grams, or 1,000 to 1,500 milligrams, of sodium per hour. A teaspoon of salt contains 2,300 milligrams of sodium, so basically we are talking about 1/2 teaspoon of salt loss per hour. For athletes who have back-to-back competitions, or two practices per day, sodium losses can be enormous.

Sweat rates, fluid losses, and sodium losses will vary. Some athletes sweat a lot but lose relatively little sodium, whereas others may not be heavy sweaters but may be **salty sweaters** (see chapter 4) who lose a great deal of sodium. The longer athletes practice or compete, the more they sweat and thus the higher their fluid and sodium losses. Your athletes must plan their fluid and sodium intake before, during, and after exercise.

Educate your athletes on the need to consume sodium, especially for salty sweaters. Your sodium "losers" can be identified by the following signs:

- Frequent cramping
- Sweat that stings the eyes
- Sweat that tastes salty
- Caked sweat on uniform
- Gritty skin
- White streaks on face or clothes
- Drinking water to the exclusion of any other beverage, especially during exercise

Taking in sodium stimulates thirst, which will help athletes increase voluntary fluid consumption and thus maintain fluid balance (Casa et al. 2000).

Potassium: Not the Key to Halting Cramps

Many athletes mistakenly believe that **potassium** is the key electrolyte to help prevent muscle and whole-body heat cramps. Potassium loss during exercise occurs but is minimal, and sodium losses will always outpace potassium losses. However, potassium is important to help regulate fluid balance within and out of the cells and also helps muscles to contract.

Good sources of potassium include the following:

- Bananas
- Citrus fruits and juices
- Tomatoes
- Yogurt
- Milk
- Beans
- Potatoes

This is why a sports drink is preferable to water, especially for salty sweaters. The recommendation for sodium is 70 to 200 milligrams of sodium per 8-ounce (240 ml) serving of beverage. Athletes can determine sodium content by looking at the Nutrition Facts panel on the label of a beverage. Most sports drinks contain approximately 100 milligrams of sodium per 8 ounces. If you have salty sweaters on your team, suggest that they add 1/2 teaspoon of salt to 32 ounces (~1 L) of sports drink.

Establish a game plan to keep your athletes cramp free and on the field:

- Make sure your athletes acclimatize to heat well in advance of their sport season.

- Encourage salty sweaters to drink sports drinks instead of water during practice and competitions.

- Have high-sodium foods available after practice, such as Chex mix, crackers, pretzels, or pickles, or encourage your athletes to bring salty foods to practice.

- Remind your salty sweaters to add salt or salty foods or beverages to every meal. They can salt their food, flavor food with soy or Worcestershire sauce, eat pickles, eat soup, drink tomato or vegetable juices, and snack on salty baked chips, pretzels, and crackers.

- Remember the acronym SALT—Sodium Advances the Level of Training.

Identify athletes who are salty sweaters and teach them how to consume more salt. (Beginning-of-Season Activities)

Gastrointestinal Distress

Digestive distress can bring even the strongest athlete to his knees. If the gut doesn't work well, the athlete won't be able to focus on practice or the game and won't play well. Heartburn, nausea, vomiting, constipation, diarrhea, and abdominal cramps can all sideline the athlete, and these conditions are fairly common. Thirty to fifty percent of endurance athletes, particularly runners, may be affected by digestive disorders (Moses 1990; Peters et al. 2001). Digestive problems occur less frequently in sports where the body is more stable, such as cycling and pool swimming, although swimming in rough waters can result in digestive distress.

Your athletes lead busy lives. They work, train, and travel and as a result may need to eat under less than optimal conditions. Depending on the sport, athletes may have to eat on their way to practice, training, or competition or during breaks between contests or events. When we eat, blood is diverted from our limbs to the gut to help with digestion, and that doesn't always feel comfortable during activity; athletes need to learn not only what to eat but when and how much to eat to prevent digestive distress.

One of the most common causes of digestive distress is food-borne illness. We have all heard about cases of food poisoning caused by improperly cooked meats, but many other things can cause illness. Remind athletes to rinse their blenders well, to keep cold foods cold and hot foods hot, and to not share water bottles. I have known athletes who tried to keep food cold by placing it on top of the air-conditioning vent. Some of my professional football players have been known to keep their unwashed blenders, used to mix protein shakes, in their lockers. High school athletes who keep meat-containing sandwiches in their lockers all morning increase their risk of food-borne illness.

Here are some suggestions to reduce the risk of food-borne illness:

- Make sure that your athletes don't share water bottles, and warn them not to reuse bottles from water they've purchased. The bottles can be a breeding ground for bacteria and should be discarded after the first use.

- Remind athletes not to bring perishable foods such as milk, yogurt, eggs, meat, or cheese to games unless coolers and ice are available to keep them cold.

- Insist that your athletes clean their water bottles and blenders after every use.

- Inspect athletes' sports bags, or remind your athletes to clean out their bags regularly to get rid of food that may not be safe to eat.

- Bring disposable wipes or a hand sanitizer for your athletes to use before they refuel after practices or games.

Educate athletes on ways to prevent food-borne illness. (Beginning-of-Season Activities)

Some of the other frequent causes of digestive distress in athletes occur in the upper gastrointestinal tract. Upper gastrointestinal (GI) complaints include heartburn, nausea, vomiting, bloating, stomach pain, and feelings of food heaviness. The major concern with vomiting is dehydration caused by fluid and electrolyte loss. If your athletes are nauseated, chances are they are not optimally hydrating and are not taking in enough fuel.

The most frequent lower GI complaints are of gas, abdominal cramping, the urge to defecate, and diarrhea. The athlete who has diarrhea is at increased risk of dehydration attributable to fluid and electrolyte loss.

The type of sport athletes play can affect the gut. Sports with more jostling tend to result in greater digestive distress. The more intense the exercise, the greater the likelihood that the athlete will experience GI distress. Athletes who are well trained have less digestive distress than untrained individuals. Extremes of temperature and altitude can affect the gut, which is why athletes who are able to acclimate usually experience fewer gut issues.

Athletes can control digestive distress, but they need to experiment with foods, fluids, timing, and volume during training. Remind your athletes to bring familiar foods to training and competition and to practice with the foods and fluids they intend to

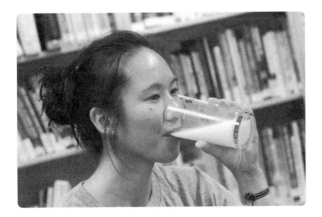

To prevent digestive upsets that can jeopardize performance, teach athletes to monitor what they put into their bodies and when.

use for events. Although athletes cannot control the weather, the competition, and travel issues, athletes can control food choices and eating habits.

Help your athletes avoid GI distress by guiding them to eat the right foods at the right times, supervising their use of supplements, and giving them tips for eating right while on the road.

Eating the Right Foods at the Right Times

Although some gastrointestinal conditions require pharmacological intervention, often the problem and its solution are related to food choices and eating habits. The rate at which food leaves the stomach (gastric emptying) may contribute to an upset stomach or distention. The longer food stays in the stomach, the higher the risk of an upset stomach. Athletes need to think about the timing of food relative to exercise as well as the consistency of the food (solid or liquid). Foods with a high liquid content, such as yogurt, soup, and gelatin, as well as fluids will empty from the stomach more rapidly than solid foods.

Athletes also need to understand that quantity matters. Taking in too much food or fluid at any given time will result in a feeling of fullness that can be quite uncomfortable.

Although fiber is important for health, eating too much fiber at one time can result in bloating and possibly diarrhea. Carbohydrate is an important fuel for exercise, but athletes need to know how much carbohydrate to consume to ensure rapid stomach emptying, especially before and during exercise.

Eating a lot of fatty foods such as fried foods and fatty lunchmeats can also increase the risk of indigestion. Both fiber- and fat-containing foods take longer to empty from the stomach.

Example

Beth is a high school soccer midfielder who routinely finishes games exhausted. She doesn't like to eat or drink much before she plays and often needs to be replaced in the latter part of the game because of fatigue. She recently decided to try eating a large meal and drinking more fluid before the start of the game. Before her last game, she ate a peanut butter sandwich and drank 12 ounces (360 ml) of chocolate milk and 20 ounces (600 ml) of sports drink. Within the first 10 minutes of the game she had to leave the field and vomited on the sideline. Although her intentions were good, she tried too much too soon!

One of the hallmarks of digestive disorder management is establishing some degree of consistency in the timing and size of meals. To decrease the likelihood of experiencing gut issues during practice or competition, your athletes should time eating to activity. Table 8.1 shows recommendations for the size of the meal and the amount of time before activity.

An athlete who plans an intense workout or interval training should allow an additional hour before exercising to decrease the chance for GI upset.

Consuming too little or too much fluid can cause GI discomfort. Dehydration can result in nausea, vomiting, and delayed gastric emptying so that even though the athlete needs more fluid, she is so uncomfortable that the urge to drink is not present. If the athlete experiences hyponatremia (low blood sodium) attributable to inadequate sodium intake or water overload, she may also feel nauseous and bloated because of the fluid load.

A carbohydrate-containing beverage that is too concentrated can take a while to leave the stomach, which is why energy drinks or fruit juice are not preferred before exercise. Carbonated beverages also may take longer to empty from the stomach and cause the athlete to feel uncomfortably full.

Your athletes should always choose noncarbonated beverages, which empty more quickly from the stomach than the carbonated variety. Beverages with a 6 percent carbohydrate solution empty from the stomach more rapidly than more concentrated carbohydrate beverages such as juices and energy drinks. Athletes should not consume more than 40 ounces (1.2 L) of fluids per hour of exercise, and they should try to gulp instead of sip fluid during practices or games to expedite gastric emptying.

Athletes need to test what feels comfortable during activity. Some prefer consuming liquids rather than solids so they do not experience the sensation of food heaviness. Athletes may need to experiment with several different foods and fluids to find out what works best. For example, an athlete with a sensitive stomach may want to try 20 ounces (600 ml) of sports drink in the hour before practice. If this volume seems too large, she can start with 10 ounces (300 ml) and build up gradually. If food is preferred, recommend something like a 6-ounce (172 g) container of yogurt or 8 ounces (240 ml) of chocolate milk, flavored soy milk, or smoothie. For the athlete who doesn't want something creamy, a small bowl of oatmeal or a slice of toast with a thin spread of jam or honey may be more appealing.

Athletes who complain of gas or bloating may be causing the problem by eating too fast. The "grab, gulp, and go" method of eating may cause more discomfort than taking the time to sit and eat. Eating quickly can cause the athlete to take in extra air, which can lead to abdominal distention and gas.

 Have athletes identify when and what to eat before and during exercise. (Beginning-of-Season Activities)

Taking Supplements

Athletes who take supplements don't always realize that their digestive distress may be caused by the product that they are taking. For example, these vitamins and minerals can cause problems:

- Megadoses of vitamin C may cause an upset stomach.
- Potassium supplements may cause nausea.
- Calcium carbonate may cause bloating and constipation.
- Iron supplements may cause nausea and constipation.
- Large doses of magnesium may cause nausea and vomiting.

TABLE 8.1

Meal Size and Waiting Time Before Activity

Meal size	Number of hours before activity
Large meal	3-4
Small meal (e.g., cereal, sandwich)	1-2
Shake or smoothie	1-2
Small snack (e.g., sports drink, granola, cereal bar)	<1

Some energy drinks are very concentrated in carbohydrate and may lead to an upset stomach when consumed before exercise. Athletes who have food sensitivities or food intolerances may experience digestive distress when they consume sports bars or protein powders if those products contain bothersome ingredients. Athletes who use dieter's tea for weight loss do not always realize that this product contains senna and cascara, two very potent laxatives. Some of the "low-carbohydrate" or sugar-free products contain sugar alcohols such as sorbitol, mannitol, lactitol, xylitol, and erythritol, which can cause bloating and diarrhea in athletes who are sensitive to these ingredients or when they are consumed in large quantities.

Some supplements may enhance performance but may also adversely affect the gut. For example, sodium bicarbonate may serve as a lactic acid buffer, preventing the buildup of lactic acid that could lead to earlier onset of fatigue. Sodium bicarbonate also can cause bloating, nausea, and, in some cases, explosive diarrhea. Amino acid supplementation during exercise can result in nausea and vomiting. Some athletes experience digestive distress with creatine. Some athletes take fish oil supplements for the anti-inflammatory benefit but may complain of heartburn. Athletes who take ginger to help prevent nausea or motion sickness may experience heartburn if they take this supplement on an empty stomach.

> *Educate athletes about how supplements can contribute to digestive distress. (Season-Long Activities)*

Eating on the Road

Travel is a way of life for many athletes. Although travel cannot be avoided, athletes who don't plan may find that their digestive tract pays the price. To decrease the chance for digestive distress when traveling, your athletes should try to travel with "security" foods, foods that they have tried before and have felt comfortable eating. When traveling abroad, check to see whether there are restrictions or regulations about bringing food into the country or countries to which you will be traveling. Also check the Centers for Disease Control and Prevention Web site, www.cdc.gov, to see whether there are any outbreaks or food concerns in the region. When athletes travel to countries where their language is not the native tongue, it is worthwhile for them to bring a list of food concerns translated into the languages of the destination countries. Encourage your athletes to travel with hand sanitizer or hand wipes and to wash their hands frequently.

Have your athletes bring familiar, nonperishable, nonliquid foods whenever they travel, especially when traveling by air. Remind your athletes that these foods must be sealed before they can be carried onto the plane. Travel foods may include the following:

Oatmeal

Dried soups

Dried fruit

Nuts

Peanut butter

Crackers

Pouches of tuna, salmon, chicken

Trail mix

Cereal

Hot cocoa mix

Nonfat dry milk powder

The athlete should always request bottled water during air travel or purchase fluid once through security.

Have your athletes carry a Good Gut Travel Kit, which could contain the following:

- Sports drink powder and salt, to replace electrolytes if athletes have vomiting or diarrhea.
- Candied gingerroot, which can be helpful for nausea. Some of your athletes may tell you that they would prefer ginger ale, but oftentimes the sweetness and the carbonation of ginger ale can make nausea worse.
- Chamomile tea, which can help to alleviate abdominal spasms because it relaxes the gut.
- Fig bars and dried plums, to help with constipation.
- Raspberry leaf or blackberry root bark tea, which can reduce diarrhea.
- Sure Jel or Certo, sources of pectin which, when mixed in a little water or juice, can help with diarrhea.

> *Encourage athletes to bring familiar foods and a Good Gut Travel Kit on road trips. (Season-Long Activities)*

Hitting the Wall or Bonking

Have you had an endurance athlete start a race feeling strong and perform well during the event only to drop out near the end, saying she can't push any farther? This phenomenon, often known as **hitting the wall** or **bonking,** happens when glycogen use outpaces intake. The body has limited stores of glycogen for fuel, and once those stores have been used, there is no more fuel for the muscles. If the muscles don't have any more glycogen, they can no longer contract, and the muscle fibers become fatigued. If this occurs before the end of a race or practice, then the athlete is done or may struggle to finish but at a much slower pace.

Why can't the body just use stored fat as a fuel source? It does, but it takes a while for the body to break down fatty acids and convert them to usable energy during exercise, and in the meantime, fatigue sets in.

In chapter 1 we discussed the energy systems used during exercise. The exercising body uses carbohydrate from the blood, or blood glucose, as well as muscle and liver glycogen. But the brain, which needs to be fueled 24 hours a day, also needs carbohydrate, so not all stored carbohydrate can be earmarked to fuel exercise. Thus, if your athlete starts practice or competition without adequate carbohydrate stores and exercises for a long duration, she is probably going to experience suboptimal performance.

For activity lasting less than 1 hour, athletes typically have enough stored carbohydrate available, but for longer-duration or back-to-back events without carbohydrate repletion, the liver cannot keep up with the demand to release enough glucose to fuel the brain and the muscles. In addition to experiencing muscle fatigue, athletes may become dizzy or disoriented. They may even become combative when their blood sugar level drops. They lose concentration and focus and may injure themselves or someone else. These symptoms, seen in athletes who experience hypoglycemia or low blood sugar, need to be addressed right away.

This is why being prepared is so important. You need to help your athletes establish a fueling plan to prevent them from running out of gas. To help keep your athletes stay strong while on the course or in the game, encourage them to fuel regularly during exercise lasting longer than 1 hour. The rule is 30 to 60 grams of carbohydrate per hour. That amount of carbohydrate translates to relatively small amounts of food. There is no need for athletes to overconsume carbohydrates, because they likely will end up with an upset stomach. Here are some 30-gram carbohydrate fueling choices:

One sports gel

Two tablespoons of honey

Six honey sticks

32 ounces (1 L) of sports drink

Six sugar cubes

1 cup (270 g) flavored gelatin

10 gumdrops or gummi-type candy

10 large jelly beans

Have your athletes practice with foods and fluids so that they learn what does and does not affect their gut. Some athletes may prefer gels, honey, or sports drinks. Some may use sugar cubes, gumdrops, or jelly beans, and others may prefer gelatin. The goal is to have your athletes be proactive about fueling. Once they bonk, it becomes more difficult to replete. If they have a fueling plan in place, they will be more likely to finish strong.

Make 30-gram carbohydrate snacks available to athletes during exercise or encourage athletes to bring their own snacks. Another option is to designate one player, each practice, to provide a snack for the team. (Beginning-of-Season Activities)

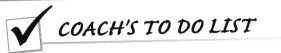

COACH'S TO DO LIST

- Make sure your players get used to the heat one month before the start of their season.
- Educate your athletes on the importance of consuming enough fluid and sodium to prevent muscle cramps.
- Remind salty sweaters to increase their sodium intake.
- Encourage salty sweaters to drink sports drink instead of water during practice and competition.
- Have salty snacks available after practice.
- Do not let athletes share water bottles.
- Provide coolers for perishable foods or remind athletes to leave them at home.
- Have disposable wipes and hand sanitizers available for your athletes to decrease the spread of germs.
- Educate your athletes about preventing digestive distress through the selection, amount, and timing of their food and drink.
- Remind athletes to stick with familiar foods before competition.
- Tell your athletes that certain supplements may cause digestive distress.
- Pack nonperishable foods for travel to competitions.
- Encourage your athletes to travel with a Good Gut Travel Kit.
- Make sure your athletes fuel during events that last longer than one hour to prevent bonking.
- Have easily digestible and absorbed carbohydrate sources on hand during prolonged events.

SUMMARY

- Muscle cramps can be caused by skeletal muscle fatigue and muscle overload.
- Extensive sweat and sodium losses can contribute to muscle cramps.
- Consuming adequate fluid and sodium is a key factor in preventing muscle cramps.
- Some athletes are salty sweaters, and you need to teach them how to replace sodium.
- Food-borne illness is a major cause of digestive distress; athletes must take care to ensure that they eat foods at the proper temperature and do not share water bottles.
- Use of hand sanitizer or disposable wipes can help to decrease the spread of germs.
- The type of food, volume consumed, and timing of eating can all adversely affect the gut.
- A ban on new food or drink before exercise can cut down on digestive distress.
- Supplements as well as foods can contribute to digestive distress.
- Athletes should travel with familiar, nonperishable foods.
- To prevent hitting the wall or bonking, athletes need to consume enough carbohydrate before and during exercise.
- Athletes need to practice consuming carbohydrate during exercise to discover which items are best tolerated.

KEY TERMS

hitting the wall
or bonking

potassium

salty sweater

sodium

GAME PLAN QUESTIONS

1. What are the main reasons that muscle cramps occur?

2. What are some of the main causes of digestive distress in athletes?

3. How can you help to prevent your athletes from bonking?

Coping With
Special Diets

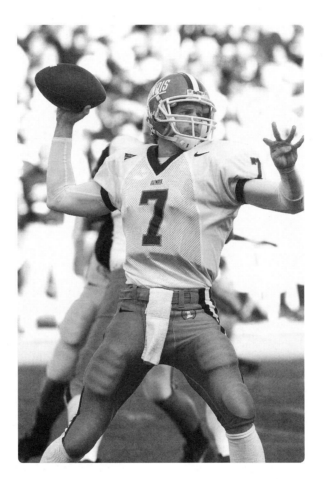

John is a freshman quarterback at a Division I university. He has had diabetes since age 12 and has multiple daily injections of insulin. Prior to starting college, he had good blood glucose control, mostly because his mother and the high school nurse made sure that he ate regularly and monitored his blood glucose consistently. His high school coach had a child with diabetes, so the coach was very familiar with symptoms and kept a close eye on John.

Once John arrived at college, he dove right into classwork, practice, and other activities that the school offered. As a result his schedule started to vary, his eating was not as consistent, and he didn't monitor his blood glucose as often as before. Although his football coach and the team physician were aware of his diabetes, they weren't with John 24 hours a day. After the starting quarterback was injured early in a game, John had to step in. He started out fine, and then his play became erratic before the half. When he came to the sideline, a blood glucose check revealed that his levels were low. He drank a sports drink and ate half of a cereal bar, and when he checked his blood glucose again, the reading was very high. He didn't play in the second half because his glucose readings were fluctuating widely. After the game, his coach called me and I met with John to map out a plan.

We devised a daily eating schedule and I provided a list of snack options to have available on the sideline. John realized that he needed to take responsibility for good blood glucose control and was able to finish the season well. He became the starting quarterback for his four years at college and went on to play in the NFL.

When you finish reading this chapter, you should be able to explain how to manage

- vegetarian and vegan diets,
- diets for those with diabetes or hypoglycemia,
- diets for those with food allergies or intolerances, and
- religious diets or fasts.

Although all of your athletes need to consume adequate amounts of calories, carbohydrate, protein, and fat, food choices are going to vary based on personal preferences as well as religious reasons, moral or ethical concerns, and health issues. For instance, you may have athletes on your teams who are vegetarian, so it is not reasonable or fair to go to a fast food restaurant that only serves hamburgers and provides no viable options for those who don't eat meat. It is likely that you will have athletes on your team who have diabetes. No one expects you to be the team physician, but you must be the watchdog for your athletes with diabetes and ensure that they are comfortable talking to you about their physical well-being during practice and competition. If your athletes need more help than you can give them, you must enlist the help of other medical professionals. There are also athletes who have food intolerances or food allergies. If you normally provide chocolate milk for your team after practice and games and have athletes with a milk allergy or lactose intolerance,

you must have a back-up option for them such as chocolate soy milk or rice milk. If you have athletes who observe Ramadan and who do not consume liquids or food from sunrise to sunset, yet still want to practice and compete, you must know how to handle this situation.

Identify any athletes on your team who need special diets. (Preseason Activities)

Vegetarian and Vegan Diets

Many athletes choose to eat **vegetarian** or **vegan** diets for moral, ethical, performance, weight management, or health reasons. Several professional and Olympic athletes are vegetarians and are able to compete well on plant-based diets. Many people believe that vegetarian diets are deficient in protein. Although this can be true in some cases, vegetarians can meet their protein needs by replacing animal protein with

plant protein. Here are some mistakes that vegetarians tend to make:

- They eliminate meat without considering their body's needs.
- They fail to include plant-based protein sources.
- They forget to replace the micronutrients that animal-based protein provides, such as zinc, iron, calcium, and B$_{12}$.
- They fail to take in enough calories.
- They become too restrictive with eating.
- They strive to combine plant proteins to consume a complete protein at every meal.

Most plant proteins (except for soy protein) are incomplete, meaning they do not contain all of the essential amino acids (discussed in chapter 2 in the section on protein). Rice by itself does not contain all of the essential amino acids; however, combining rice with beans would provide all of these nutrients. To meet their protein needs, athletes don't have to combine foods to get all of the essential amino acids at every meal; they just need to do this throughout the course of the day. More on this topic is provided in the section titled Protein Sources.

The biggest obstacle for vegetarian athletes who say they don't like beans, tofu, or vegetables is meeting their protein needs. Grains and fruits cannot provide all the protein an active body needs. However, dairy foods and eggs are complete protein sources and are good substitutes for meat.

There are several different types of vegetarians. Table 9.1 lists the categories of vegetarianism.

Let's look at some of the ways that your vegetarian athletes can get enough protein and the necessary vitamins and minerals. They also may have to do some planning and preparation when your team is going to be on the road.

Protein Sources

Although it is possible for athletes to meet protein requirements by consuming a plant-based diet, one of the challenges is that they have to consume larger amounts of plant-based food to get the same amount of protein as they would by consuming a smaller amount of animal-based food. For example, 3 ounces (85 g) of chicken breast (about the size of a deck of cards) contains 21 grams of protein. An athlete would have to eat 1 1/2 cups of beans to get 21 grams of protein. Beans are an excellent source of protein but are also high in fiber and can contribute to a feeling of fullness, which could be a problem for an athlete who needs to gain weight. Bean dips such as hummus often contain some fat and seem less dense, so an athlete can eat more of this for a larger number of calories than beans alone.

Soy foods are a great source of protein and are the only plant foods that contain all of the essential amino acids. Soy foods such as tofu, soy milk, and edamame (raw soybeans) and meat analogs such as texturized vegetable protein, veggie burgers, and soy hot dogs can be used to help an athlete meet her needs.

Soy foods, nuts, nut butter, seeds, all grains, and all vegetables contain some protein. Fruits; fats such as oil, mayonnaise, butter, margarine, and salad dressings; and sweets such as candies, jams, jellies, honey, and syrup contain little or no protein.

Table 9.2 on page 133 lists the protein content of some popular vegetarian foods.

Athletes may ask about combining protein or complementary protein. Because none of the plant-based proteins, with the exception of soy, contain all of the amino acids, plant-based proteins are considered to be **incomplete proteins.** Combining two incomplete proteins can make a **complete protein,** which has all of the essential amino acids. It is not

Example

Susan is a high school softball pitcher who saw a documentary in health class about meat processing. She decided at that moment to stop eating meat, chicken, and fish. She would have a granola bar for breakfast, grab a peanut butter sandwich or salad for lunch, and eat pasta with marinara sauce for dinner. After a few weeks, she began to notice that she didn't feel as strong during practice or games and wasn't throwing as well. She felt strongly about not wanting to eat meat but needed to know how to meet her protein needs. After meeting with a sports dietitian, Susan was able to increase her protein intake through milk, yogurt, vegetarian meatballs, and beans, and within a short period of time she was back to her previous level of play.

TABLE 9.1

Types of Vegetarians

Term	Description
Semivegetarian	Includes some but not all animal products—such as meat, poultry, seafood, eggs, milk and milk products—but may not eat animal products daily
Lacto-vegetarian	Includes milk and milk products but does not consume eggs, fish, seafood, poultry, or meat
Lacto-ovo vegetarian	Includes only milk and milk products and eggs as protein sources; does not consume meat, poultry, fish, and shellfish
Ovo-vegetarian	Includes only eggs as an animal protein source; no dairy, meat, poultry, fish, or shellfish
Vegan	Excludes all animal products: eggs, milk and milk products, meat, poultry, fish, and shellfish
Fruitarian	Eats only nuts, fruit, honey, and olive oil
Macrobiotic vegetarian	Does not include many animal foods but does eat some fish; foods need to be consumed in certain combinations to balance food choices, which, for an athlete, can be overly restrictive

necessary to combine incomplete proteins at each meal; the body can synthesize amino acids to create new protein in a 24-hour period, provided all of the essential amino acids are consumed. So if an athlete decides to just have a spoonful of peanut butter for breakfast and crackers for lunch, his body will be able to synthesize new protein by the time the day is done. Here are some examples of complementary protein combinations:

Grains + nuts: peanut butter sandwich

Beans + seeds: hummus, which is garbanzo beans and tahini (sesame seed paste)

Beans + grains: red beans and rice

To meet their nutritional needs, vegetarian athletes should try to eat the following foods daily:

Milk and milk alternatives (six to eight servings per day)

1/2 cup (120 ml) milk, yogurt, fortified soy milk, or soy yogurt

1 ounce (28 g) cheese

1/2 cup (110 g) cottage cheese

1/4 cup (55 g) tofu

1/4 cup (35 g) almonds

3 tbsp sesame or almond butter

Dry beans, nuts, seeds, eggs, and meat substitutes (two to three servings per day)

1 cup cooked dry beans, lentils, or peas

2 cups (480 ml) soy milk

1/2 cup (110 g) tofu

2 ounces (56 g) veggie meat or soy cheese

Two eggs or four egg whites

1/4 cup (35 g) nuts or seeds

3 tbsp peanut butter

Vegetables (three to four servings per day)

1/2 cup cooked or chopped raw vegetables

1 cup raw, leafy vegetables

3/4 cup (180 ml) vegetable juice

Fruit (two to four servings daily)

3/4 cup (180 ml) fruit juice

1/4 cup dried fruit

1/2 cup chopped, raw fruit

1/2 cup canned fruit

One piece of fruit

TABLE 9.2

Protein Content of Vegetarian Foods

Food	Protein, g
Egg, one large	7
Egg whites, four	7
Milk, 1 cup (240 ml)	8
Cottage cheese, 1/2 cup (110 g)	13
Beans, 1/2 cup	7
Tofu, 1/2 cup (110 g)	10
Yogurt, 8 oz (230 g)	10
Cheese, 1 oz (28 g)	7
Soy cheese, 1 oz (28 g)	7
Pasta, 1 cup cooked	6
Textured vegetable protein, 1/4 cup	12
Soy veggie burger	7-10
Nuts or seeds, 1/4 cup (35 g)	7
Peanut butter, 2 tbsp	7
Rice, 1/2 cup (100 g)	3
Bread, one slice	2-3
Protein-fortified cereal, 1 cup (30 g)	5
Hummus, 1/4 cup (60 g)	4
Quorn*, one cutlet	11

*Quorn is made from a mushroom-based protein, also known as a mycoprotein.

***Bread, cereal, rice, and pasta
(6-11 servings per day)***

One slice of bread

Half of a bagel, English muffin, or bun

1 ounce (30 g) ready-to-eat-cereal

1/2 cup (120 g) cooked cereal

1/2 cup pasta or rice

Vitamin, Mineral, and Fatty Acid Sources

In addition to meeting their calorie and protein needs, your vegetarian athletes also need to consume adequate amounts of micronutrients (vitamins and minerals) and certain fatty acids (which are found in some animal foods as well as in nuts, seeds, oils, and margarines). Many vegans do not consume enough vitamin B_{12} because it is only found naturally in animal foods and Brewer's yeast; however, many cereals available on the market are fortified with vitamin B_{12}. Vitamin D is important for bones and muscles and is found in milk, some cheeses, and egg yolks. Athletes who do not consume dairy foods or eggs can take a calcium supplement with vitamin D to meet daily needs. Zinc can be found in whole-grain breads and cereals as well as nuts and seeds.

Consuming enough iron is always a challenge for athletes, but it is even more tricky if they don't eat meat. Iron is not as well absorbed from plant sources

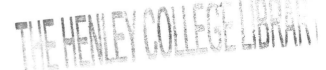

as it is from animal sources. The best way to increase iron intake, aside from taking a multivitamin–mineral supplement, is to consume iron-fortified cold or hot cereals. Remind your athletes to consume a vitamin C source such as citrus juice or fruit with these cereals or with other iron-fortified foods, because vitamin C helps to improve the iron absorption from plant-based foods. Suggest that athletes wait a few hours after eating before consuming coffee or tea, which contain phytonutrients, plant nutrients (tannins in coffee and tea and polyphenols in coffee) that prevent iron from being fully absorbed.

If your athletes do not consume dairy foods, they can meet their calcium needs through calcium-fortified soy milk or through juices, cereals, and calcium supplements. The calcium recommendation for males and females ages 13 to 18 is 1,300 milligrams per day. Table 9.3 lists plant sources for vitamins and minerals that are hard to obtain in a vegetarian diet.

TABLE 9.3

Vegetarian Food Sources of Vitamins and Minerals

VITAMIN B (DRI 1.2-2.4 µg)		
Food	**Amount**	**Vitamin B$_{12}$, µg**
Egg	One	.6
Yogurt	1 cup (230 g)	.6
Milk	1 cup (240 ml)	.9
Cheese	1 oz (28 g)	.2
Cereal, fortified	1 oz (30 g)	6
Soy milk, fortified	1 cup (240 ml)	.2
Veggie burger	One	2
Red Star Yeast 6635+		
Powder	1 tsp	1
Flakes	2 tsp	1
VITAMIN D (DRI 400 IU)		
Food	**Amount**	**Vitamin D, IU**
Orange juice	1 cup (240 ml)	100
Milk	1 cup (240 ml)	98
Egg yolk	1	25
Soy milk, fortified	1 cup (240 ml)	100
Rice milk, fortified	1 cup (240 ml)	100
Some cereals	1 oz (30 g)	40
IRON (DRI 8 MG FOR MALES, 18 MG FOR FEMALES)		
Food	**Amount**	**Iron, mg**
Blackstrap molasses	1 tbsp	3.6
Soybeans	1 cup	8.8

IRON (DRI 8 MG FOR MALES, 18 MG FOR FEMALES), *continued*		
Food	**Amount**	**Iron, mg**
Tofu, firm	1/2 cup (110 g)	3.4
Tofu, soft	1/2 cup (110 g)	6.7
Lentils	1 cup	6.6
Beans	1 cup	2.2-3.6
Chickpeas	1 cup	4.7
Enriched cereals	1 cup	4.5-18
Pumpkin seeds	1 oz (28 g)	4.2
CALCIUM (DRI 1,300 MG/DAY FOR AGES 13-18; 1,000 MG/DAY FOR AGES 19-50)		
Food	**Amount**	**Calcium, mg**
Cow's milk	1 cup (240 ml)	300
Yogurt	1 cup (230 g)	450-490
Cheese	1 oz (28 g)	200
Soy milk, calcium-fortified	1 cup (240 ml)	250-350
Soy yogurt	1 cup (230 g)	300
Tofu, calcium set	1/2 cup (110 g)	435
Orange juice, calcium-fortified	3/4 cup (180 ml)	260
Cereal, calcium-fortified	1 oz (30 g)	125-1,000
Greens (collard, mustard, kale)	1 cup	94-264
ZINC (DRI 8 MG FOR FEMALES, 11 MG FOR MALES)		
Food	**Amount**	**Zinc, mg**
Black beans	1 cup	1.9
Kidney beans	1 cup	1.9
Pinto beans	1 cup	1.7
Black-eyed peas	1 cup	2.2
Tofu, firm	1/2 cup (110 g)	2.0
Pumpkin seeds	1 oz (28 g)	2.1
Cashews	1 oz (28 g)	1.6
Veggie burger	One	.88
Cereal, fortified	1 oz (30 g)	1.2-3.8
Peas	1 cup	1.9

DRI = Dietary Reference Intake.

U.S. Department of Agriculture, Agricultural Research Service. 1998. USDA National Nutrient Database for Standard Reference, Release 12. Nutrient Data Laboratory Home Page, http://www.ars.usda.gov/nutrientdata.

Omega-3 fatty acids are important as anti-inflammatory agents and also for cardiovascular health. Fish is a good source of omega-3 fatty acids, but if your athletes do not eat fish, they can get omega-3 fatty acids in enriched eggs, flaxseed, walnuts, and canola and soybean oils.

Although it would be easier for a vegetarian athlete to take a supplement rather than worry about food sources of vitamins and minerals, foods also contribute calories and other important nutrients. Encourage your athletes to eat a variety of foods, and if you or they notice increased fatigue, decreased performance, or weight changes, it may be necessary to reevaluate their eating to make sure their needs are being met.

> *Educate vegetarian athletes about non-meat sources of protein and vitamins. (Season-Long Activities)*

Vegetarians on the Road

Although there are more vegetarian choices in restaurants today than ever before, travel can still be a challenge for vegetarians. Make sure that when the team is on the road you stop at places that have choices for your vegetarian athletes. Here are some vegetarian options that are available at most restaurants:

- Vegetable hoagies or wraps
- Baked potatoes, plain or with broccoli and cheese
- Salads
- Egg sandwiches with or without cheese
- Veggie burgers
- Pizza (for the vegan, no cheese)
- Bean burritos
- Rice and beans
- Corn
- Veggie stir-fry
- Bagels
- Pasta
- Cereals
- Pancakes and waffles
- Salad bars

If you are going to be on an extended road trip, encourage your vegetarian athletes to travel with nonperishable protein foods such as peanut butter, trail mix, roasted soybeans, and soy milk (which is sold in aseptic packages so it does not need to be refrigerated). Packaged vegetarian soups just require hot water, and instant hot cereals are also very easy to pack and are lightweight as well. Several brands of sports bars provide protein. The other option is to bring a protein powder or a ready-to-drink protein shake if there are no acceptable food choices.

There are several quick and easy ways for athletes to prepare vegetarian dishes. Here are some examples of easy, nutritious vegetarian meals:

- Oatmeal with walnuts, raisins, and soy or cow's milk
- Lentil soup with rice or pasta added
- Vegetarian refried beans in corn tortillas
- Peanut butter sandwich
- Chili with texturized vegetable protein, tomato sauce, and kidney beans
- Veggie burgers
- Stir-fry with vegetables and beans over rice
- Pizza with cheese or soy cheese
- Pasta with vegetables and olive oil
- Pasta with marinara sauce and texturized vegetable protein
- Cheese ravioli
- Cheese-filled manicotti
- Vegetable omelet
- Rice and beans (several combinations are commercially available)
- Hummus in a pita bread, add feta cheese for additional protein
- Vegetarian vegetable soup and a bagel with melted cheese or soy cheese
- Vegetable, tomato, or bean soups

Diets for Athletes With Diabetes or Hypoglycemia

With increasing rates of diabetes in the United States, it's likely that you will work with athletes who have diabetes. You also may have players who have a problem with hypoglycemia, or low blood sugar. If your players are educated about how to take care of themselves, these conditions shouldn't keep them off the field or court. With your help and supervision, these athletes can perform well.

Diabetes

Diabetes is a chronic disease in which **blood glucose** (blood sugar) stays higher than normal. This happens because the pancreas does not produce enough insulin, the hormone that regulates blood glucose levels, or because the receptors that work to remove glucose from the blood for use by the cells don't function as efficiently as they should. When blood glucose levels are too high, there can be several complications including excess thirst, frequent urination, blurry vision, and kidney, cardiovascular, and nervous system complications. Diabetes is detected through blood tests, as fasting blood glucose measured in milligrams per deciliter (mg/dl), or through a more sensitive blood test called HgbA1C. High blood glucose can also be detected in the urine.

The two types of diabetes are referred to as **type 1** and **type 2**. Type 1 is seen most often in young people, who need to take insulin daily through injections or an insulin pump because the pancreas does not produce insulin. Type 2 diabetes is more common. In this form of the disease, even though the pancreas produces insulin, it does not produce enough or the receptors don't work well, so blood glucose levels are higher than normal. Some people with type 2 diabetes can control their blood glucose through diet, and others use a combination of diet and medication.

The most important issue with diabetes is regulating blood glucose levels so they are neither too high **(hyperglycemia)** nor too low **(hypoglycemia)**. With high blood glucose levels, the risk of dehydration increases the risk for **ketosis,** which is the appearance of ketone bodies (free fatty acids released from storage to be used as fuel). It is possible to tell whether someone is in ketosis, or is ketotic, by measuring urinary ketone levels. Increased amounts of ketone bodies can make the blood more acidic and can result in a condition known as metabolic or diabetic ketoacidosis, which can lead to coma and possibly death. Low blood glucose or hypoglycemia can increase the likelihood of dizziness, fainting, and **hypothermia** (lowered core body temperature).

The incidence of type 2 diabetes is on the rise, although you may encounter both type 2 and type 1 diabetes on your team. If you have athletes with diabetes, sit down with them, their parents or caregivers, and preferably with their physician and the athletic trainer so you can map out a plan of action. Although it is not your job to be these athletes' physician, you need to be aware of symptoms and have an open-door policy so they are comfortable telling you when they don't feel good. There is no reason that athletes with diabetes cannot compete provided they have good blood glucose control.

Your diabetic athletes face challenges that other athletes do not, because they need to deal with

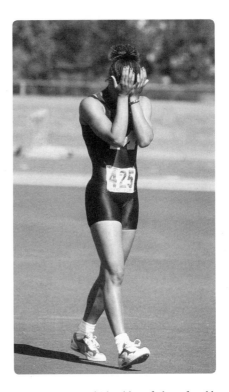

Create an environment in which athletes feel comfortable speaking up about illness and health conditions. Symptoms of high or low blood sugar must be addressed immediately.

medicine, glucometers, and dietary adjustments to stabilize and control blood glucose. Diabetes is a disease that requires patients to take care of themselves daily. Some athletes who have diabetes try to give their sports precedence over their diabetes management, but this can result in adverse health consequences and impaired performance. Reassure these athletes that they will be able to participate and compete provided their blood glucose is within acceptable ranges.

Although many diabetic athletes are vigilant about monitoring themselves and their food choices, others take too relaxed an approach and may do the following:

- Exercise without checking their blood glucose
- Mismanage high or low blood glucose
- Eat too much to compensate for low blood glucose readings
- Wait too long to eat after exercise
- Fail to hydrate adequately (described later in this section)
- Cut their carbohydrate intake to a level too low to fuel their muscles in the hope of having better blood glucose control

Exercise can affect blood glucose. Endurance or stop-and-go sports typically lower blood glucose levels. High-intensity, short-duration exercise such as powerlifting, sprints, pitching, 800-meter track events, or 200-meter swim events typically do not lower blood glucose. However, athletes with diabetes must monitor their blood glucose before, during, and after exercise so they can respond appropriately with medications and carbohydrate intake.

You need to know your diabetic athlete's blood glucose numbers before every practice and competition. If you think that you are going to be too occupied with other athletes, then make sure that your diabetic athlete reports to someone, such as an assistant coach or athletic trainer, before every practice and competition for a blood glucose check.

 Assign someone on your staff to do blood glucose checks on diabetic athletes. (Beginning-of-Season Activities)

The following glucose levels are contraindications to practice or competition, according to the American Diabetes Association position statement on diabetes mellitus and exercise (2002):

Type 1 diabetes

Blood glucose less than 100 or more than 250 milligrams per deciliter and the presence of urinary ketones

OR

Blood glucose greater than 300 milligrams per deciliter with no urinary ketones

Type 2 diabetes

Blood glucose greater than 400 milligrams per deciliter and no urinary ketones

Hyperglycemia (high blood sugar) is defined as abnormally high blood glucose levels. If circulating insulin levels are low, it is difficult for glucose to enter the exercising muscle cells, resulting in hyperglycemia. The main concern with hyperglycemia is dehydration and the presence of urinary ketones; therefore, exercise is contraindicated until the blood glucose levels decrease.

One of the other major concerns with diabetic athletes is hypoglycemia (low blood sugar), which is a blood glucose reading of less than 70 milligrams per deciliter. Elevated circulating insulin levels cause glucose to enter the exercising muscle cells rapidly, which can lead to hypoglycemia during exercise. This phenomenon can occur several hours after exercise or when the athlete is asleep. Hypoglycemia can cause symptoms including shakiness, fatigue, weakness, sweats or clamminess, pallor, loss of concentration, irritability, hunger, and impaired coordination, all of which can impair performance and curtail participation in athletic events. Hypoglycemia also can impair temperature regulation, making the hypoglycemic athlete more susceptible to hypothermia and hyperthermia.

The goal is to be proactive, not reactive. To prevent hypoglycemia, your athletes must do the following:

- Check blood glucose levels before, during, and after exercise.
- Keep records of the time of day, duration, and intensity of exercise.
- Keep track of the time between exercise and the last meal ingested.
- Monitor carbohydrate intake.

Figure 9.1 shows a sample day of blood glucose monitoring.

Figure 9.2 is a blank monitoring form for your diabetic athletes to use.

 Ask diabetic athletes to track their eating and exercise using the blood glucose monitoring form. (Beginning-of-Season Activities)

Your role is to know the signs and symptoms of hypoglycemia and know how to treat it. You may also want to educate one or more of your athletes about how to respond as well. The best way to treat a hypoglycemic episode is to administer 15 grams of quickly absorbed carbohydrate until stable blood glucose is achieved. Although an athlete who has diabetes should always carry sources of easily absorbed carohydrate, it is a good idea for you to have them available as well. Table 9.4 lists foods that would supply 15 grams of fast-acting carbohydrate.

Have 15-gram carbohydrate foods available at all times to treat hypoglycemia. Have a glucagon injection and someone who knows how to administer it on hand. (Beginning-of-Season Activities)

Sample Blood Glucose Monitoring Form

Time of meals, snacks, and exercise	Food eaten	Carbohydrate intake, g	Blood glucose before exercise, mg/dl	Blood glucose during exercise, mg/dl	Blood glucose after exercise, mg/dl
7 a.m.—breakfast	2 Eggs Toast, two slices Orange juice, 8 oz (240 ml)	60			
8 a.m.—lifting			100		110
9 a.m.—snack	Protein shake	10			
11 a.m.—lunch	Sandwich: Turkey breast, three slices Cheese, two slices Whole-wheat bread, two slices Mayonnaise, 1 tbsp An apple Small bag of baked potato chips Skim milk, 12 oz (360 ml)	72			
2 p.m.—snack	A low-sugar granola bar	20			
3-5 p.m.—soccer practice			150	130	120
5:15 p.m.—snack	Trail mix, two handfuls: pretzels, raisins, nuts	50			
7 p.m.—dinner	Chicken breasts, two Mashed potatoes, two scoops (1.5 cups) Green beans, 1 cup Whole-wheat bread, one slice Crystal Light, 12 oz (360 ml)	70			
9 p.m.—snack	Sugar-free ice cream, 1 1/2 cups (200 g)	30			

FIGURE 9.1 Sample blood glucose monitoring form.

Blood Glucose Monitoring Form

Time of meals, snacks, and exercise	Food eaten	Carbohydrate intake, g	Blood glucose before exercise, mg/dl	Blood glucose during exercise, mg/dl	Blood glucose after exercise, mg/dl

From L. Bonci, 2009, *Sport Nutrition for Coaches* (Champaign, IL: Human Kinetics).

FIGURE 9.2 Blood glucose monitoring form.

TABLE 9.4

15-Gram Carbohydrate Food Equivalents

4 oz (120 ml) apple or orange juice*
4 oz (120 ml) carbonated beverage (not sugar free)
One half of a candy bar **
Five gummy-type candies
Eight jelly beans
1/2 cup (135 g) gelatin (not sugar free)
Five hard candies (Lifesaver size)
1 tbsp honey *
8 oz (240 ml) skim milk
2 tbsp raisins *
6 1/2 in. (1.3 cm) sugar cubes
8 oz (240 ml) sports drink
Three glucose tablets

*These foods are higher in fructose, which is slower and less effective in elevating blood glucose levels than other types of carbohydrate.

**This food can be higher in fat content which can slow digestion, thereby delaying the effectiveness of the carbohydrate.

You may also want to carry a food kit stocked with the following items:

Dextrose or glucose tabs	Sports drink powder
Sugar cubes	Gelatin
Cake icing	Peanut butter crackers
Honey or honey sticks	Jerky
Lifesavers	Pretzels
Sports gels	Trail mix
	Granola bars

If the athlete is not feeling better after 15 to 20 minutes, someone needs to test the athlete's blood glucose level and, if the reading is still less than 70 milligrams per deciliter, feed the athlete another 15 grams of carbohydrate. If the athlete is unconscious, do not give the athlete food or beverages. An option is to place a small amount of glucose gel or cake decorating gel between the athlete's cheek and gums and rub the cheek from the outside until the gel dissolves. If this does not work, it may be necessary for a trained individual—the athletic trainer, you, or a teammate—to give the athlete a glucagon injection if blood glucose levels do not start to improve. Glucagon is a hormone that allows glycogen to convert to glucose to restore normal blood glucose levels.

In addition to monitoring their blood glucose prior to exercise and adjusting carbohydrate intake, athletes with diabetes must consume some carbohydrate during practice and competition. Your job is to remind those athletes that they need to fuel their body during activity. Table 9.5 shows some examples of sports and the amount and timing of carbohydrate required.

Achieving optimal hydration is especially critical for athletes with diabetes, because higher blood glucose levels increase the risk of dehydration. These athletes can use sports drinks but must account for the carbohydrate in these drinks as part of their overall daily carbohydrate intake. Some new products provide less sugar but the same amount of electrolytes as regular sports drinks.

Remind your athletes with diabetes to take in fluid and carbohydrate-containing foods during exercise. (Season-Long Activities)

TABLE 9.5

Amount of Carbohydrate Needed to Fuel Activity

Sport	Amount of carbohydrate, g	When to consume
Soccer	15-20	Every 60 min of play
Swimming	15-30	Every 60 min of swimming
Running	15-20	Every 30-45 min of running
Basketball	15-30	Every 60 min of play

Alcohol is a potent inhibitor of hepatic (liver) glucose production, which can result in late and severe hypoglycemia in athletes with type 1 diabetes. Alcohol could also precipitate hyperglycemia depending on the type of mixer used, such as carbonated beverages or juice, and the types and amount of alcohol consumed. Educate your athletes about the adverse consequences of alcohol on blood glucose, and remind all athletes to optimally rehydrate and to refuel after exercise.

Reactive Hypoglycemia

Any athlete, not only those with diabetes, can experience **reactive hypoglycemia,** a rapid decrease in blood glucose that occurs one to four hours after eating a carbohydrate-rich food. Symptoms can include these:

Weakness	Perspiration
Faintness	Anxiety
Palpitations	Hunger

Maintaining adequate blood glucose levels during activity can be a challenge for any athlete. Dietary carbohydrate is stored as glycogen in the liver and muscles. Adequate carbohydrate intake is the only way to ensure optimal glycogen stores. If liver glycogen stores are low because of exercise and decreased carbohydrate intake, the liver is unable to maintain circulating glucose concentrations, which can lead to hypoglycemia. Fatigue during prolonged exercise can be associated with hypoglycemia. Those who are participating in prolonged exercise following several hours without food, such as morning events, or who have been restricting carbohydrate intake for the purpose of losing weight will be more likely to experience problems such as fatigue.

Although the actual number of athletes with diagnosed hypoglycemia is low, all athletes should modify their diet to decrease the likelihood of hypoglycemic symptoms. Diets that advocate protein intake to the exclusion of all else, and those that severely curtail carbohydrates, are never recommended for an athlete. Consuming carbohydrate-containing food at every meal and snack can be an easy way to meet athletes' needs.

Consuming carbohydrate-containing food during exercise can help prevent hypoglycemia by supplementing the liver's ability to maintain blood glucose levels. In addition, it can delay the rate of muscle glycogen depletion and therefore delay fatigue. The body can effectively use solid or liquid carbohydrate sources during exercise. Your athletes should experiment to find what is most comfortable and palatable.

Controlling Glucose Levels

Frequent meals provide athletes with an opportunity to ingest carbohydrate throughout the day, stabilizing blood glucose. For those with reactive hypoglycemia, larger meals can increase the likelihood of a reaction, so remind these athletes to establish an eating schedule. Educate your athletes about some of the fads concerning carbohydrate intake that may exacerbate symptoms. For example, there is no reason for an athlete with hypoglycemia, or any athlete for that matter, to consume carbohydrates early in the day and restrict carbohydrate intake at night. Eating an evening meal of only protein and vegetables may precipitate a hypoglycemic reaction during the night. It is much better to consume a mixed-nutrient meal, such as pasta with meat sauce, that includes protein and fat in addition to carbohydrate. Eating soluble-fiber foods (oats, barley, fruits, vegetables, and dried beans and peas such as kidney, pinto, navy, split peas, and lentils) may help to stabilize blood glucose, and these foods should be eaten throughout the day as part of overall carbohydrate consumption.

You may have athletes who are sensitive to caffeine and may need to restrict intake to prevent fluctuations in blood glucose. Energy drinks, and even some sports drinks and waters, can have caffeine added, so athletes may be better off choosing noncaffeinated versions of these products.

An athlete who has fasted, or who has not eaten for several hours, such as during and after an endurance event, is more likely to experience hypoglycemia when drinking alcohol after exercise. Therefore, alcohol should never be consumed on an empty stomach.

Dietary recommendations for athletes with hypoglycemia and reactive hypoglycemia are as follows:

- Frequent feedings, every three to four hours
- Moderate caffeine consumption, less than 200 milligrams per day
- Alcohol with meals only, not on an empty stomach

Spend some time with your athletes with diabetes or hypoglycemia in advance of the season to lay down the ground rules:

- Insist that they eat before practice or competition; if they show up without having eaten, they will not be permitted to participate.
- You can choose to provide food for athletes before they are permitted to exercise, but this should only be in cases of emergency. You need to instill a sense of responsibility in your athletes.
- Recommend that your athletes (if they have not already done so) meet with a registered dietitian to develop meal plans.
- Remind these athletes that they need to consume some carbohydrate during exercise.
- Ask your athletes with diabetes about their blood glucose readings before exercise, and provide breaks so that they can test blood glucose during exercise.
- Keep a survival kit on hand that contains fast-acting carbohydrate foods that don't spoil:
  - A box of sugar cubes
  - Cake decorating gel
  - Glucose tablets
  - Gummy candies or jelly beans
  - A roll of Lifesavers
  - Powdered sports drink

Food Allergies and Food Intolerances

Although the incidence of food allergies is relatively small, there are few things scarier than witnessing someone having a dangerous allergic reaction. It can start as extreme itching, sweating, rapid or irregular heartbeat, and low blood pressure and progress to **anaphylaxis,** where the person's throat can swell, resulting in breathing difficulty, loss of consciousness, cardiac arrest, and shock.

If an athlete has a **food allergy,** he is allergic to the protein in foods. Although any food could be the cause of an allergic reaction, some foods are more likely to be the culprit, such as the following:

Milk	Fish
Eggs	Peanuts
Wheat	Tree nuts
Soy	Corn (not as common)

Keep in mind that an athlete may be allergic to more than one type of food.

Athletes with food allergies need to let you know what they are allergic to so you can inform the team and prevent problems. The team mom who makes brownies with walnuts could endanger the athlete who has a tree nut allergy. An athlete with a peanut allergy who touches a knife that has trace amounts of peanut butter could have an allergic reaction. If you provide pregame meals and team snacks, either make provisions for the athlete with food allergies or ask the athlete to bring along safe foods to eat. Insist that the athlete with food allergies bring epinephrine or an Epi-pen (an injector with adrenaline, which is used to counter the allergen to prevent symptoms from occurring; instructions for use are included in the packaging) so that someone can administer the medication if an allergic reaction occurs. Epinephrine can only be obtained by prescription, and it is given as an injection so it can be administered quickly.

Some athletes cannot tolerate **lactose,** the sugar in milk, or **gluten,** the protein in wheat, rye, barley, and oats. Often the symptoms are gastrointestinal such as diarrhea, nausea, vomiting, and abdominal distention. Athletes with **food intolerances** typically know what foods cause them problems, although unlike athletes with food allergies, those with food intolerances may be able to ingest small amounts of foods to which they react. Request that athletes on your team let you know whether they have any food intolerances.

Make a list of all your athletes' food allergies and food intolerances. Keep these in mind when providing food before, during, or after practice and on the road. (Beginning-of-Season Activities)

Religious Diets and Fasts

You may have athletes who observe fasts for religious reasons. This does not have to be a reason for excluding any athlete from participation in sports. Certainly the lack of food or fluid prior to and during exercise can present challenges, but as long as you and your athletes are educated on how to handle these situations, and the athlete does not experience any adverse side effects, he or she should be able to participate.

Athletes who observe the month of Ramadan do not eat or drink anything, including water, from sunrise to sunset. This creates some logistical challenges for optimal fueling and hydration. However, even cross country runners and football players are able to practice and compete during Ramadan without a significant decrease in performance.

Because these athletes are going to be without food or fluid for most of the day, the goal is to concentrate fueling and hydration into two times of the day, before sunrise and after sunset. Advise your athletes to consume one third of their daily calories and one half of their daily fluid requirements before sunrise.

Because this can be quite a volume to ingest at one time, advise your athletes to get up one to one and a half hours before sunrise so that they can take their time to eat and hydrate.

Recommend that your athletes choose fluids that contain calories to provide both hydration and fuel, such as juice, milk, lemonade, sweetened tea, or sports drinks. Because a person can consume only so much food at one sitting, it is a good idea to maximize the calories by including nutrient-dense foods such as granola, oatmeal, bagels, yogurt, cheese, and eggs.

Encourage your athletes to break the fast as soon as they can. If practice is still going on past sunset, give your athletes who fast permission to stop and fuel. Encourage them to have a sports drink right away to elevate blood glucose levels and then allow them to eat something such as a bagel, crackers, trail mix, or a sports bar. Remind them to let you know if they feel dizzy or lightheaded during practice or competition and that they are allowed to break the fast for illness or heat exhaustion (and make up the fasting when they have recovered).

Make sure these athletes eat again as soon as practice is done, and watch them eat to make sure they have done so. If you remind your athletes to replete and rehydrate, they will be more likely to do so. Remind them that over the course of the evening they must focus on eating to ingest two thirds of their daily calories as well as the remaining one half of their fluid intake.

Example

Joseph is a collegiate cross country athlete who wanted me to help him devise an eating plan for Ramadan. He told me that his high school cross country performance had always suffered during this time and that he typically lost several pounds. He thought that by modifying his diet he would have a better outcome.

Per our plan, he set his alarm clock for one hour before sunrise and consumed his first meal of the day, a bagel with honey, oatmeal, a handful of nuts, and three glasses of fluid: milk, juice, and water. He brought trail mix and sports drink to consume as soon as practice was over around 7 p.m. so that he could start to rehydrate and refuel right away. He had dinner at the dining hall and consumed an evening snack with more fluids. He made it through the month without losing a pound and thought that his running was better as well.

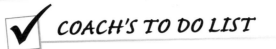

COACH'S TO DO LIST

- Ask every athlete to inform you of any food or diet issues prior to their participation in sport.
- Become familiar with these issues and attempt to make your athletes comfortable talking to you about their concerns.
- Make special provisions for snack items and precompetition meals for athletes with special diet requirements or restrictions.
- Have foods available for athletes with diabetes or hypoglycemia.
- Be aware and understanding of the food and beverage restrictions for athletes who observe Ramadan or other religious fasts or restrictions.
- Designate an athlete and the athletic trainer—and perhaps a team parent—to help athletes with medical issues.

RESOURCES

American Dietetic Association: www.eatright.org

Vegetarian Resource Group: www.vrg.org

American Diabetes Association: www.diabetes.org

Diabetes Exercise and Sports Association: www.diabetes-exercise.org

Food Allergy & Anaphylaxis Network: www.foodallergy.org

SUMMARY

- Health, moral, ethical, and religious concerns will affect athletes' food choices.
- Vegetarian athletes must fulfill their caloric, protein, fat, and micronutrient needs.
- Offer appropriate options for food on the road for athletes with special dietary needs.
- There is no reason why athletes with diabetes or hypoglycemia cannot participate in sports.
- Attaining optimal blood glucose levels can keep athletes with diabetes in the game.
- The coach must know the symptoms of hyperglycemia or hypoglycemia and what to do should this occur.
- A food kit should be available at practices and competition.
- Athletes with hypoglycemia need to eat at regular intervals and limit caffeine and alcohol use.
- Athletes with food allergies need to inform the coach of their food allergens and carry epinephrine.
- Athletes who observe fasts for religious reasons need to plan their hydration and fueling around allowed eating times so that performance is not impaired.

KEY TERMS

anaphylaxis	gluten	ketosis
blood glucose	hyperglycemia	lactose
complete proteins	hypoglycemia	reactive hypoglycemia
diabetes (types 1 and 2)	hypothermia	vegan
food allergy	incomplete proteins	vegetarian
food intolerance		

GAME PLAN QUESTIONS

1. How would you handle eating on the road with your vegetarian athletes?

2. Why do athletes with diabetes need to monitor blood glucose levels?

3. What types of foods should you have available for your athletes with diabetes?

4. How should you handle a low blood glucose episode in your athlete?

5. What nutrition advice should you give an athlete who is observing Ramadan?

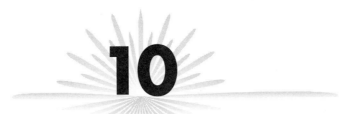

Dealing With Disordered Eating

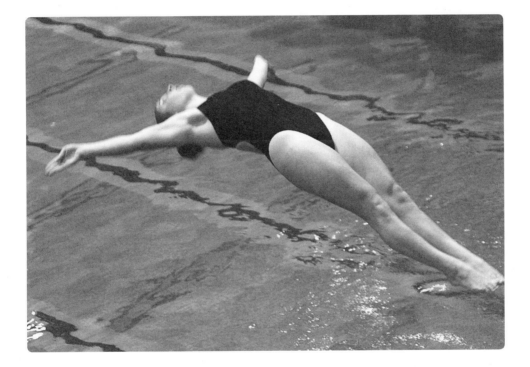

Carolyn is a high school diver who thought she was heavier than all of the other girls on her team. She worried that, on the basis of the weight problem she felt she had, the judges would lower her score. She started to change her eating by cutting back on junk food and also decided to add two hours of exercise to her day by running, biking, and using the elliptical machine at her parents' gym. Her weight started to drop but still she thought that she had loads more weight to lose; she would pinch her thighs and call herself a fat pig. She cut out all snacks and began to skip meals, eliminating breakfast and rarely eating lunch. At the same time, she started to make herself vomit when she did eat, claiming that if she ate anything, she would gain weight. A friend gave her a box of laxatives and told Carolyn that if she took them, she would lose even more weight.

During one practice, Carolyn was at the end of the diving board and started to get dizzy. She complained of blurred vision and felt very lightheaded. She slowly made her way back to the end of board and climbed down the ladder. When her coach asked her what was wrong, she burst into tears and told the coach she needed to quit the team. The athletic trainer had observed the change in Carolyn's appearance and had also heard from her teammates that Carolyn was very moody and always excused herself right after meals to go to the bathroom. On more than one occasion her teammates noticed that when she returned to the table, her eyes were red and her nose was runny.

Carolyn's coach sat down with her and her parents to express his concern. He told Carolyn that he only wanted her to focus on taking care of herself, and if she decided she no longer wanted to be part of the team, it was her choice, but he still wanted her to get help. The athletic trainer suggested that Carolyn see a treatment team consisting of a physician, therapist, and dietitian. She ended up missing the season but used her treatment team to get well. Ultimately she decided to quit diving, but she is still quite active and is now healthy and much happier.

When you finish reading this chapter, you should be able to explain

- the types of eating disorders,
- how to recognize eating disorders,
- the female athlete triad,
- how to foster a positive eating environment,
- how to get help for athletes with eating disorders, and
- how to include parents in treatment.

We think of athletes as people who are healthy and fit, yet many athletes engage in **disordered eating**, regularly either eating too much or starving themselves. In female athletes, disordered eating can occur in all sports, at estimates of up to 62% of female athletes. In male athletes, disordered eating is more common in weight-class sports (wrestling, crew, horse racing) and aesthetic sports (bodybuilding, gymnastics, swimming, diving) and affects about 33% of male athletes (Byrne et al. 2001; Sundot-Borgen & Torstviet 2004).

Although body image concerns and eating issues may be more prevalent in women, men can have them, too. Men can become anorexic or spend hours lifting in order to gain muscle mass. A recent study in the *International Journal of Eating Disorders* found that there was a significant increase in the prevalence of eating disorders from 1995 to 2005 among teenage American boys (Chao et al. 2007). Harrison Pope, the lead author of *The Adonis Complex: The Secret Crisis of Male Body Obsession* (2000), talks about the increase in compulsive exercise, dieting, bulimic behaviors, and supplement abuse among young men.

Why might athletes be at risk for developing disordered eating? Here are some reasons:

- *Desire to improve performance by dropping weight.* Some athletes believe that if they are lighter and have less body fat, they will be faster or better able to delay fatigue. However, if the athlete loses too much muscle through inadequate calorie consumption, the end result is performance impairment.

- *Imbalance between energy intake and energy output that results in weight loss.* This is especially true in athletes with considerable energy expenditure in their sport such as distance runners, who may expend 7,000 or more calories per week while training and competing but fail to replace them and so lose weight.

- *Fear of failure.* Athletes who are not performing to what they perceive to be their optimum may believe that altering their body composition will improve performance. If they do not see a marked difference, they may believe that they didn't lose enough weight or body fat and may continue to try to alter their physique until they are successful in sport or receive attention or praise from teammates or the coach.

Let's now look at some of the types of eating disorders you may encounter with the athletes you coach.

Eating Disorders

When you hear the words *eating disorders*, you may immediately think of anorexia or bulimia, and we discuss those in this section. We also discuss a number of other less severe disorders, which are grouped under the term *eating disorders not otherwise specified* (EDNOS). Some signs of disordered eating you can watch for are shown in table 10.1 on pages 150 and 151.

Anorexia

Anorexia is defined as a disorder of self-starvation, either through restricting calories or excessive exercise or both. Anorexics are very thin for their height and often appear underweight. The criteria for anorexia, taken from the *Diagnostic and Statistical Manual of Mental Disorders, Fourth Edition* (*DSM-IV*, APA 1994), are as follows:

- Failure to maintain body weight at or above a minimally normal weight for age and height
- Intense fear of becoming fat
- Body image distortion
- Loss of three consecutive menstrual cycles

Bulimia

Bulimia is a disorder of binging and purging. Binging is defined as overconsumption of food, and the purging can occur through self-induced vomiting, enemas, laxative or diuretic abuse, excessive exercise (above and beyond that required for sport), or fasting. Bulimics may or may not be underweight; more often they are of normal weight and sometimes they are overweight. The criteria for bulimia, taken from *DSM-IV* (APA 1994), are as follows:

- Recurrent episodes of binge eating characterized by
    -large volume of food consumed or
    -lack of control over eating during a binge
- Recurrent harmful behaviors to prevent weight gain, such as self-induced vomiting, excessive exercise, fasting, laxative or diuretic abuse, and enemas

- Binge and purge episodes that occur at least two times a week over a three-month period
- Body image distortion

Eating Disorders Not Otherwise Specified (EDNOS)

Although you may have athletes with anorexia or bulimia, you may have many more athletes with disordered eating behaviors. Disordered eating is characterized by attitudes about weight, food, and body size and shape that cause the person to follow very rigid eating and exercise habits—used to attain and maintain a low or unhealthy body weight and body fat—that jeopardize their health, happiness, and safety (Otis et al. 1997). These behaviors can occur along a continuum from clinical eating disorders to occasional binge-and-purge episodes (Thompson and Sherman 1993). **Eating disorders not otherwise specified (EDNOS)** include

- binge eating disorder,
- orthorexia, and
- seasonal eating issues such as restricted eating in athletes in weight-class sports.

Binge Eating Disorder

An athlete may binge or overeat for many reasons:

- Stress management
- Injury
- Emotional reasons
- Self-esteem
- Comfort
- Relationship difficulties with a coach, teammates, significant other, or parents

Compulsive overeating or **binge eating disorder** can be as big a problem as restricting or binge–purge behaviors. The individual who is a binge eater eats in secret, typically consuming large volumes of food, but does not purge. The caloric intake can be quite large, resulting in increased body fat as well as shame, isolation, and in some cases depression. Athletes with binge eating disorder, like athletes with any disordered eating behavior, may be embarrassed by the quantity of food consumed as well as the feelings of eating being out of control and may not readily admit to a problem.

Orthorexia

Although not a true eating disorder, **orthorexia** can lead to severe health consequences. It is defined

TABLE 10.1

Signs of Disordered Eating

PHYSICAL SIGNS		
	Athlete who restricts eating	**Athlete who purges**
Hair loss	✗	✗
Dry skin and hair	✗	✗
Brittle nails	✗	✗
Weight fluctuations	✗	✗
Calluses on the palms of the hand		✗
Dental enamel erosion		✗
Increased risk of stress fractures	✗	✗
Dehydration	✗	✗
Swelling of the parotid glands*		✗
Facial swelling (edema)		✗
Jaundice	✗	
Lanugo**	✗	
Hypotension (low blood pressure)	✗	✗
Hypothermia (low core body temperature)	✗	
Constipation or diarrhea	✗	✗
Upset stomach	✗	✗
Delayed wound healing	✗	✗

*Parotid glands are salivary glands located toward the back of the jaw. Their function is to secrete saliva and aid digestion, and they can swell in response to self-induced vomiting.

**Lanugo is a layer of fine downy hair that grows on the arms and chest in response to lack of body fat as a way to insulate the body.

MEDICAL ABNORMALITIES		
Anemia*	✗	✗
Musculoskeletal injuries	✗	✗
Bradycardia (slowed heartbeat)	✗	✗
Amenorrhea**	✗	✗

MEDICAL ABNORMALITIES, *continued*		
	Athlete who restricts eating	**Athlete who purges**
Esophageal irritation		✗
Sore throat		✗
Hypokalemia***	✗	✗

*Anemia is characterized by low levels of hemoglobin in the blood attributable to iron deficiency.

**Amenorrhea is lack of a menstrual cycle.

***Hypokalemia is a low serum potassium level. Potassium levels can decrease because of vomiting or laxative or diuretic abuse. Low potassium levels can be harmful to the heart and can impair muscle function.

EATING HABIT CHANGES		
Large amounts of foods consumed by a very thin person		✗
Eating in private	✗	✗
Refusal to eat with others	✗	
Excessive use of condiments	✗	
Pushing foods around the plate	✗	✗
Leaving the table immediately after or during meals to go to the restroom		✗
Subpar caloric intake or macronutrient intake	✗	✗
Binge eating		✗

BEHAVIOR ISSUES		
Asking whether he or she is fat	✗	✗
Constantly comparing his or her body to others	✗	✗
Alcohol or substance abuse		✗
Compulsive exercise beyond that required for sport	✗	✗
Purging		✗
Laxative, diet pill, or diuretic abuse	✗	✗

INDICATORS OF ANXIETY		
Social isolation	✗	✗
Mood changes	✗	✗
Personality changes	✗	✗

as disordered eating characterized by a fixation on eating healthy food. Individuals with orthorexia may obsess about eating a healthy diet and will not allow themselves to deviate from select food items they allow themselves. They tend to avoid processed foods, and this can become problematic when the team is on the road and fast food or snacks are the only choices available. The athlete who won't eat these foods may not eat at all. Also, people with orthorexia often consume insufficient calories to support body weight, which may compromise their sport performance.

Seasonal Eating Disorders

Athletes in weight-class sports may participate in unhealthy behaviors to make weight, but only during their competitive season. Their disordered eating behaviors, called **seasonal eating disorders,** occur in spurts rather than continuously. However, even a short period of weight cutting typically results in a decrease in water weight, which can leave the athlete dehydrated. In addition, if weight goals are met by restricting carbohydrate intake, the athlete may notice a decline in strength, speed, or stamina. Thus, restricting eating to make weight or dehydrating to lose a few more ounces does not optimize performance or health and should be considered as harmful as any other eating disorder.

Now that you know the types of disordered eating possible, we can discuss some of the signs to watch for in your athletes.

Signs of Disordered Eating

Be alert for clues that your athletes may have eating disorders. Your athletes may tell you that they like to feel light and that food weighs them down. An athlete who doesn't eat at a team meal may give excuses such as "I ate earlier," "I'm not hungry," or "My stomach hurts." Skipping a meal once or twice is understandable, but when this becomes a pattern, it is time to worry. A female athlete who doesn't have a period may be thrilled about this, but lack of menstruation may be a sign of insufficient caloric intake. The same physiological markers are not present in males, but you may be able to detect heightened anxiety, mood changes, or weight changes and muscle loss as well as performance deficits in male athletes with eating problems.

Sometimes it is easy to detect weight changes, such as in the case of an athlete who returns from summer break and is markedly thinner. But if your athletes wear baggy clothes, you may not notice a weight change. You will be able to see changes in

sport performance, however, and more often than not those changes are negative.

Another condition closely related to disordered eating is the female athlete triad.

Female Athlete Triad

The **female athlete triad** refers to three interrelated health issues that are seen in female athletes:

- Insufficient calorie intake
- Menstrual disorders (missed periods and irregular menstrual cycles)
- Low bone mineral density

Each component of the triad may develop separately along a spectrum of severity. In the most severe cases, the athlete with the triad may develop these problems:

- Eating disorders
- Lack of menstrual periods for three consecutive months
- Increased risk of fractures

Every one of the components of the triad is distinct, but they are interrelated. Although all three components of the triad are not present in every affected female athlete, if she is identified to have one component of the triad, she needs to be evaluated for the presence of the other two.

The precipitating factor of the triad is an energy (caloric) imbalance created by insufficient intake of energy (calories) to meet or sustain the energy demands (calories expended) of exercise. Insufficient caloric intake affects all body processes, including growth, thermoregulation, and reproduction. Low energy availability can result in menstrual disturbances, and the resulting decrease in estrogen can cause a decrease in bone mass, increasing the risk of fractures.

Energy availability is the key to whether a female athlete will progress to the triad. Energy availability is defined as the amount of energy remaining for body functions in addition to exercise-related energy expenditure:

Dietary energy intake > Exercise expenditure = Energy availability

Dietary energy intake < Exercise expenditure = Energy drain or energy imbalance

Example

Beth is a high school field hockey player who is entering her senior year. She decided to add running to her routine in the spring, averaging 30 or more miles per week in addition to conditioning, practice, and tournaments for field hockey. Even though her exercise increased, she did not increase her caloric intake. By the start of the fall season she had been amenorrheic for five months and also had developed a stress fracture.

Her primary care physician prescribed a prolonged period of rest (for the stress fracture) and oral contraceptives (for the amenorrhea) but did not talk about the need to increase calories. Consequently, it took a long time for her to heal, and her period was still irregular. It was not until Beth sat down with a sports dietitian to work out an eating plan to achieve positive energy balance that she was able to optimize her health and performance.

Next let's discuss how you can recognize the female athlete triad and what you can do to encourage female athletes to eat an optimal diet.

Recognizing Signs

In many cases, the female athlete is not intentionally restricting calories but rather is overexercising. However, some female athletes do restrict eating and exercise excessively to deliberately lose weight to improve performance or alter their appearance.

You need to be on the lookout for some of the warning signs of the triad:

- Prolonged or additional training above and beyond that required for sport
- A decrease in caloric intake during training or a noticeable decrease in eating during team meal times
- Weight loss
- Personality changes
- Cold hands and feet
- Dry skin
- Increased injury occurrences
- Delayed healing

One of the ways to identify female athletes who may be at risk for the triad is to screen using the acronym TRIAD:

Training excess—The cross country athlete who is running 60 to 70 miles per week during the season and decides to supplement her running with biking and extra running may be training excessively.

Repetitive injuries—The soccer player who has recurrent stress injuries and whose weight has steadily declined from preseason to the end of the season might need help.

Initial menstrual cycle age—An athlete who is not menstruating by age 16 may be at risk for the triad.

Amenorrhea—Any female athlete who is not presently menstruating also can be at risk.

Dieting—Female athletes who diet regularly, even during the sport season, when energy output can be great, should be monitored.

If you suspect that any of your female athletes are at risk, you need to ask questions about each of these elements and obtain information from the athlete, her parents, the athletic trainer, and the athlete's physician.

Encouraging Female Athletes to Eat

One of the nutrition issues that is more applicable to female athletes than males is consuming enough calories to train optimally. Many female athletes significantly undercut calories, demanding that their bodies survive on the minimum number of calories rather than fueling the body adequately. Although many high-level athletes seem to survive on the minimum while expending the maximum, this type of eating pattern is certainly not conducive to optimal health, especially in young athletes, who need energy to grow as well as train. The challenge is to encourage the athlete to eat without drastically altering current eating patterns.

A distance runner weighing 110 pounds (50 kg) might require a minimum of 2,200 calories per day, which could increase as training intensifies. If she is currently consuming 1,200 calories per day, she will be very reluctant to add an additional 1,000 calories to her daily intake. A compromise is a better approach. Starting with a 200-calorie increase through a food or beverage and gradually increasing calories over time may be more acceptable to her.

Consuming enough meals is an issue for all athletes, but women are more likely to skip meals for weight loss. Women may also be more concerned that eating at night will add more fat to their bodies. The athlete who eats only once a day is not going to be willing to try five small meals immediately but may try two meals instead of one. Small, gradual changes in eating behaviors tend to work better, so start with a small change and then ask the athlete what results she notices, such as less hunger or more energy.

Female athletes also are more likely than males to skimp on protein and fat intake, assuming that these foods can lead to weight gain. The athlete who does not meet protein requirements may suppress her immune system function, resulting in nagging upper–respiratory tract infections. These can prevent the athlete from competing at an optimal level, causing her to cut back even more on eating in response to decreased energy output. In addition to supporting a healthy immune system, protein-containing foods can confer a greater sense of satiety, helping to curb appetite between meals. Encourage athletes to eat some type of protein at each meal, whether an animal or a vegetable source. For the athlete who does not like red meat, point out that poultry, fish, eggs, low-fat dairy products, dried beans, and soy are all excellent protein sources. Recommend to your athletes that they eat protein at every meal and snack so they develop the habit of eating multinutrient meals. The athlete who does not consume any animal products and is a very picky eater should try a protein-containing sports bar or sports beverage to meet protein requirements.

If your athletes strive to maintain a minimal fat intake, gently remind them that fat is used as a fuel substrate during any exercise with the exception of an all-out sprint and that restricting fat intake may result in earlier fatigue, negatively affecting performance. Recommend that they increase fat intake gradually, perhaps only 5 grams at a time. This would be equal to the following:

One thumbnail-sized serving of oil, margarine, peanut butter, or mayonnaise

One thumbnail-sized serving of salad dressing or cream cheese

One ounce of part-skim mozzarella cheese or one serving of string cheese

When you work with female athletes, do not lose sight of the fact that they are women as well as athletes. One of your jobs is to help them successfully balance their athleticism and feminism. Your female athletes are not immune to the concept of the "ideal" feminine body, which is probably of someone who does not engage in regular physical activity. We tread in dangerous waters when we put too much emphasis on weight and performance, and such an emphasis always has deleterious consequences for athletes. Although males can be affected as well, females are more likely to try to alter body composition and weight, not just to optimize performance but to improve their self-image.

You can help your female athletes have a better sense of themselves by focusing on improvements in these areas:

- Agility
- Power
- Motor control
- Speed
- Strength
- Stamina

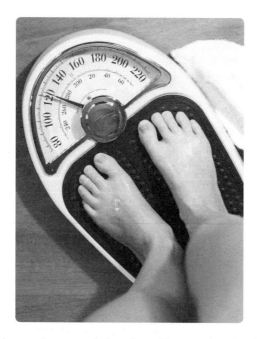

Athletes can become overly focused on arbitrary numbers that don't take into account the demands of their sport.

Praise your female athletes for achieving and excelling in these areas of performance. Fostering a sense of satisfaction in your athletes for what their bodies allow them to do may help protect them from body dissatisfaction. If your athletes have a strong sense of self or feel comfortable in their skin, they will be better able to focus on performance and less likely to jeopardize their health. The effort put forth in fostering healthy and positive body images may keep your female athletes from developing the female athlete triad.

Fostering a Positive Eating Environment

Set the tone by making good nutrition a priority for your entire team. Administer a preseason nutrition screening form to all athletes that includes questions such as number of meals consumed per day, food preferences, fluid intake, weight history, and differences between in-season and off-season eating. A sample form in appendix C asks questions about food choices, eating habits, and diet history. In addition, ask all athletes to complete a three-day food diary and bring it to a preseason meeting so you have a chance to review the information before the start of the season.

Include brief discussions about nutrition in your regular team meetings. Encourage your athletes to submit various questions, anonymously if desired, and if possible have a sports dietitian talk to the team. If that resource is not available, assign a question to two or three team members, steer them toward appropriate resources, let them research the answer, and have each group present their findings at the next training session. This approach can be quite eye opening. It also gets everyone involved, and the information reaches the entire team at one time.

You can take other steps to keep your team focused on eating well and to help team members who have eating disorders: Educate athletes about the consequences of poor nutrition, help them to develop positive body images, and talk openly about eating disorders.

> *Before the season begins, have your athletes fill out a preseason nutrition screening form. In addition, ask your athletes to complete a three-day food diary. Review the results and discuss any food issues with the athletes individually. (Preseason Activities)*

Education

You may find that your athletes harbor misconceptions about food and eating habits. Unfortunately, these are usually negative statements that categorize foods as good or bad. You may have athletes who regularly use the words *can't*, *won't*, or *shouldn't* when describing their food choices. They may believe that they can only eat reduced-calorie, fat-free, or sugar-free items and are often very rigid about the amount of foods consumed and the time of day they eat.

It is your job to educate your athletes to keep them healthy. You can challenge their distorted thinking about food by presenting facts about calories and nutrients.

Start by discussing the role of food as it relates to performance. This can be an informative and non-threatening segue into a very touchy subject. Try these sample statements:

- If you eliminate carbohydrate, your mental and physical performance suffer.
- If you restrict protein, the risks for muscle wasting, weakness, and injury increase.
- If you restrict fat, the body cannot efficiently absorb fat-soluble vitamins, essential fatty acid stores diminish, and fatigue increases, compromising performance.
- If your vitamin and mineral needs are unmet, energy production is compromised, muscle tissue synthesis and repair are jeopardized, the immune system is suppressed, and bone health is at risk.
- If nutritional intake is inadequate, it will take longer for you to bounce back from injuries.

When you talk to your athletes about foods, try to keep your discussions neutral and inclusive, rather than exclusive. Do not label foods as good, bad, or fattening. Focus on the role of food for performance, not just for health. Remind your athletes that they have to eat well to perform at the highest level. Reiterate the importance of fuel to provide both the mental and physical edge.

Your athletes need to understand the consequences of eating calories insufficient for good nutrition and the impact doing so will have on performance:

- Glycogen depletion results in muscle fatigue, psychological fatigue, and reduced mental capacity.
- Increased lactate production attributable to insufficient carbohydrate intake results in premature muscle fatigue.

- Dehydration impairs regulation of body temperature (thermoregulation), oxygen transport, and nutrient exchange, leading to premature muscular fatigue.
- Loss of lean body mass results in reduced muscular strength and endurance and decreased anaerobic performance.
- Restriction of calories may reduce cardiac output. The heart is a muscle that can become depleted after long-term caloric restriction, which results in decreased aerobic capacity, affecting endurance.

As athletes lose more weight, training becomes ineffective and performance suffers. Inadequate caloric intake, especially when carbohydrates are restricted, will limit training efficiency. Table 10.2 shows how insufficient caloric intake can affect your athletes.

Body Image

When dealing with issues of body size and appearance, be careful about what you say to athletes:

- Never give improper weight-loss advice. Don't tell your athletes to lose or gain weight and pick a number just because it sounds good to you. Do not put time limits on weight changes, such as mandating a 20-pound (9 kg) weight loss in a two-month period.
- Unless their sport demands that athletes make weight, do not conduct mandatory weigh-ins,

Locate a sports dietitian in your area and have her discuss with your team the role of food in sport performance. (Season-Long Activities)

especially group weigh-ins. The only reason to monitor weight in other sports is to check hydration status.

- Do not set a weight but rather a weight range for your athletes. There is not one best weight, and only your athlete can determine where he or she feels and performs best.
- Do not pressure or use scare tactics or humiliate your athletes into losing weight.
- Do not threaten the athlete with being kicked off the team because of weight or eating issues.
- Do not ignore the weight discussion; if you are not comfortable talking with your athletes about weight, then find someone who is.

To create a body-friendly environment, ban scales from the public areas. There is no need to have a scale where it is visible to everyone; if a scale is truly necessary, put it in a private place.

Have photographs of athletes of all shapes, sizes, and colors in your office and on the walls of your training facility. Refer to your athletes' bodies with only positive descriptors, and encourage them to do the same. It's hard to be self-critical when you're smiling!

TABLE 10.2

Effects of Insufficient Intake of Calories

Decreases in	Increases in
Strength	Preoccupation with food and body
Endurance	Anxiety
Speed	Agitation and irritability
Coordination	Fear
Motivation	Risk of injury
Confidence and self-esteem	Risk of upper–respiratory tract infections
Growth and development	Fractures
Reproductive function	Impaired bone health in later life
Achievement of performance goals	

Openness

For athletes with eating issues, it is critically important to address eating behaviors. Eating disorders need to be destigmatized and discussed openly, truthfully, and factually in a comfortable environment.

Athletes who restrict fluid, make themselves vomit, or abuse laxatives or diuretics need to understand the effects of these practices on the body. Dehydration caused by a binge–purge episode can affect the body for a week and can result in the following:

- Fatigue
- Irritability
- Muscle spasms
- Dizziness
- Bloating
- Swelling of hands and feet
- Impaired coordination
- Impaired thermoregulation
- Increased risk of hypothermia
- Increased risk of injury attributable to loss of protective body fat

Many athletes with eating disorders need direction regarding weight goals and eating habits. Talk with them about the need to control their behavior instead of allowing themselves to be controlled by food. These athletes need to learn how to set realistic and sustainable nutrition goals, and they need to understand that eating is influenced by emotions and stress.

Have a zero-tolerance policy for unhealthy eating behaviors. For example, if athletes come to a training session without having eaten all day, don't allow them to practice until they eat something. This lets them know that you care and are concerned about their well-being.

Most of all, be a role model for healthy eating through your own food choices and eating habits. Better yet, eat with your athletes on a regular basis or let them see you eat. Your actions may convey a message more effectively than your words.

Getting Help for Your Athletes With Eating Disorders

In most cases, athletes with eating disorders are not going to come into your office and admit to a problem. You may observe physical and performance changes in your athletes, or perhaps a teammate or the athletic trainer will make you aware of her concerns regarding an affected athlete. How you approach the athlete is extremely important. Consider the following strategies before you address the athlete (Rosen et al. 1988):

- Have the authority figure (certified athletic trainer, teacher, coach) who has the best rapport with the athlete arrange a private meeting.
- Express support for the athlete and concern for his best interests. Stress that health and happiness transcend the athletic arena. Be empathetic and caring. Let the athlete know that you are aware that the demands of the sport may have played a role in the development of the problem.
- In an objective and nonpunitive way, list what you have seen and what you have heard that have led you to be concerned. Let the athlete respond fully. Expect denial and rationalization.
- Emphasize that the athlete's place on the team or in the program will not be endangered by an admission that she has an eating disorder unless the eating disorder has compromised the athlete's health or increased her injury risk potential. If that is the case, consult with a physician to decide the wisest course of action.
- Let the athlete know that eating disorders are treatable and that people do recover from them. Almost always, though, professional help is necessary. Needing help should not be regarded as a sign of weakness, inadequacy, or lack of effort. Remind your athletes that most people with eating disorders have tried, and failed, to correct the problem on their own. Failure is especially demoralizing to athletes, who are constantly oriented toward success. Focus on winning the battle and gaining control over the eating disorder.
- If the athlete is working with a physician or counselor, ask that resource person how you can help. Then do it.

It takes a treatment team to help an athlete with an eating disorder. Medical treatment, psychological treatment, and nutritional management are the priorities to get the athlete to a state of health. The treatment team should consist of the athlete's physician, sports dietitian, therapist, and athletic trainer. The goal is to treat the athlete and allow him to continue to participate in sport. This requires total commitment on the part of the athlete as well as open communication with all members of the team.

There must be a point person on the team to make sure that the athlete keeps appointments with the health care providers. A sports dietitian who is also an eating disorder specialist is best qualified to work with these athletes. If such a person is not available, enlist the help of a dietitian in the student health services department or a local hospital. If a dietitian is not available, the athletic trainer should step in. If appropriate, the athletic trainer can call upon an athlete who is recovering from an eating disorder, who may have better rapport with the affected athlete, to be an effective peer leader and to assist the point person in providing support.

The athlete must trust the point person and connect with her. This individual should be the one who does body composition measurements and sets weight and body composition goals for the athlete. (Rockwell 2002). She will be the resource for you as well as for the athletes and should provide appropriate education materials for you, your athletes, and your staff. The point person will also provide the input necessary for determining return to play (Beals 2004).

Although important people in the affected athlete's life—friends, teammates, roommates, boyfriend or girlfriend—are not part of the treatment team, they should be involved in the athlete's care. For instance, a roommate or close teammate can accompany the athlete to counseling appointments or have dinner with an athlete who is struggling at mealtimes.

You probably won't be directly involved in the day-to-day treatment of the athlete. However, the point person should keep you informed of the athlete's progress toward recovery and what you can do to help.

Several universities have developed performance teams and performance protocols to deal with athletes with eating disorders. Figure 10.1 is an example of a performance team protocol. Note that there are consequences if the athlete does not keep appointments and that the end result may be that the athlete is not allowed to return to sport. Figure 10.2 highlights the rationale behind the protocol as well as the objectives and the plan for implementation.

Including Parents in Treatment

The athlete's family is a critical component of treatment. Even though family dynamics may have contributed to the development of the athlete's eating disorder, when dealing with players of high school age or younger the athlete's family must be involved in treatment. Insist that parents attend your preseason team meetings, talk about how eating disorders will be managed, and let parents know that you have an open-door policy. Tell them that if they suspect that their child may have an eating problem, they can talk to you. You may have a parent who pleads with you to let her child finish the season even though he is clearly underweight. Don't forget that you are responsible for the health and well-being of your athletes, and allowing an underfed athlete to compete is a liability to you and your institution. At the college level, NCAA guidelines would hold the institution liable for improper treatment of athletes with eating disorders.

Suggest appropriate resources for parents if they raise concerns about their child's eating. Maintain a list of dietitians and therapists in your area who specialize in treating eating disorders. You can locate dietitians through the American Dietetic Association at www.scandpg.org (select About Scan, then Search for a Dietitian) or through www.eatright.org (select Find a Nutrition Professional). The school nurse or student health services may have a list of qualified health professionals. If you are a collegiate coach, find out whether the student health service on campus has a counseling center. It is very important that the athlete be seen by someone who is an expert in sports as well as in treating eating disorders. Not all dietitians and therapists have expertise in both areas.

Remind parents that the treatment of an eating disorder always takes precedence over sports; reassure them that their child will not lose his or her place on the team but that you will only allow the athlete to participate in sports if all members of the treatment team are in agreement. You may have to deal with irate parents who want their child to continue playing no matter what, but ultimately you have to advocate for your athletes. Your goal as a coach is to safeguard your athlete's health, and if you believe that the eating disorder is jeopardizing your athlete's well-being, or the safety of his or her teammates, that is reason enough to withhold participation in practice or competition.

> *If you suspect that any of your athletes have an eating disorder, talk with them individually. Make it clear that they will retain their place on the team but that their health comes before participation in sports. Form a treatment team for each athlete, and include parents in the treatment. (Season-Long Activities)*

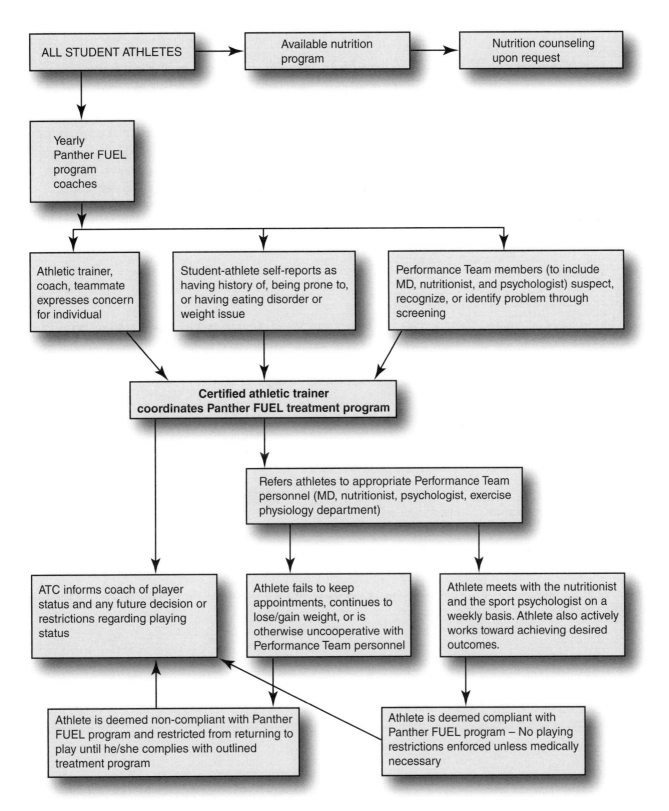

FIGURE 10.1 **University of Pittsburgh Fostering Useful Eating Lessons (FUEL) protocol for dealing with eating disorders among student-athletes.**

Panther FUEL: Fostering Useful Eating Lessons

Mission Statement

The University of Pittsburgh Department of Athletics and the Performance Team are committed to the health and welfare of the student-athlete. With this in mind, we seek to establish this policy by means of a twofold approach. It is our mission to identify nutritional, weight, and body image–related concerns that affect both the health and the performance of the student-athlete. Both overall physical health and the ability to perform are essential ingredients in successful competitive athletics. Thus, it is our goal to assess and maintain health and performance in student-athletes at the University of Pittsburgh.

Objective

Bring about prevention through education

Increase awareness of eating disorders and disordered eating among coaches and student-athletes

Establish a protocol to effectively identify, treat, and follow up all potential cases

Use a multidisciplinary approach to recognition and treatment including consultation from a primary medical physician, nutritionist, psychologist, and athletic trainer

Educational Exposure

Implement yearly nutrition in-services for all coaches and student-athletes early in the fall semester:

> To be conducted by performance team staff
>
> To include physical and psychological characteristics of eating disorders
>
> To conduct preseason screening on all athletes
>
> To inform and outline regarding eating disorder protocol
>
> To encourage coaches and athletes to refer and seek help if needed

FIGURE 10.2 Mission statement and overview of the University of Pittsburgh's Fostering Useful Eating Lessons (FUEL) protocol.

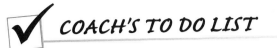

COACH'S TO DO LIST

- ▣ Establish eating policies before the season begins. Insist that athletes eat sufficiently before working out or playing. Do not allow them to participate if they haven't eaten.
- ▣ Tell your athletes to let you know if they are worried about the eating habits of someone on the team.
- ▣ Tell your athletes that they can come to you if they have an eating disorder and that it won't necessarily prevent them from playing.
- ▣ Observe your athletes eat after practice.
- ▣ Promote the idea that athletes come in all sizes and shapes and there is not one ideal body image.
- ▣ Insist that the athlete with an eating disorder seek help. Refer the athlete to professionals who can help.
- ▣ Do your own body checklist:
  - ⬦ Are you comfortable with your body?
  - ⬦ Do you have good food attitudes?
  - ⬦ Do you talk about losing weight in front of your athletes?
  - ⬦ Do you describe foods as good or bad?

RESOURCES

Academy of Eating Disorders (AED) (www.aedweb.org)

Bloomington Center for Counseling and Human Development (www.bloomington-eating-disorders.com)

International Association of Eating Disorder Professionals (IAEDP) (www.iaedp.com)

National Eating Disorder Association (NEDA) (www.nationaleatingdisorders.org)

National Association of Anorexia Nervosa and Associated Disorders (www.iaedp.com)

NCAA Web site on Nutrition and Performance (www.ncaa.org/membership/ed_outreach/nutrition-performance/index.html)

Sports, Cardiovascular, and Wellness Nutrition (www.scandpg.org)

POSITION STANDS

American Academy of Pediatrics (AAP) (www.aap.org) (aappolicy.aappublications.org/cgi/content/full/pediatrics;111/1/204)

American College of Sports Medicine (ACSM) (www.acsm.org)

American Dietetic Association (ADA) (www.eatright.org)

American Psychiatric Association (APA) (www.psych.org) (www.psychiatryonline.com/pracGuide/pracGuideHome.aspx)

Female Athlete Triad (www.femaleathletetriad.org)

International Olympic Committee Position Stand on the Female Athlete Triad (http://multimedia.olympic.org/pdf/en_report_917.pdf)

National Athletic Trainers' Association (www.nata.org)

National Athletic Trainers' Association Position Statement: Preventing, Detecting, and Managing Disordered Eating in Athletes. *J Ath Train.* 2008;43:80-108.

SUMMARY

- Disordered eating behavior and eating disorders can occur in both male and female athletes in a variety of sports.
- The three types of eating disorders are anorexia, bulimia, and eating disorders not otherwise specified (EDNOS).
- Eating disorders are characterized by physical signs, medical abnormalities, behavior issues, and eating habit changes.
- Athletes need to be educated on the physical, psychological, and performance consequences of disordered eating behaviors.
- The female athlete triad consists of insufficient caloric intake, menstrual disorders, and low bone mineral density and can put the athlete at risk for adverse health consequences and impaired performance.
- Athletes need to eat an optimal amount of calories to fuel sport.
- Athletes who consume an inadequate amount of calories will experience negative effects on performance and training.
- Creating a body-friendly environment and an open-door policy establishes a better comfort level for athletes with eating issues.
- Athletes with eating disorders need to be followed by a treatment team.
- Parents need to understand that eating disorders always take precedence over sport.

KEY TERMS

amenorrhea	disordered eating	female athlete triad
anorexia	eating disorders not otherwise specified (EDNOS)	orthorexia
binge eating disorder		seasonal eating disorders
bulimia		

GAME PLAN QUESTIONS

1. Why are athletes at risk of developing eating disorders?

2. What are three health consequences of an eating disorder?

3. How can an eating disorder adversely affect performance?

4. What should you say to an athlete who has an eating disorder?

5. What are some strategies you can adopt to create a positive food environment for your athletes?

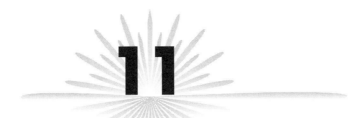

Dealing With Alcohol Use

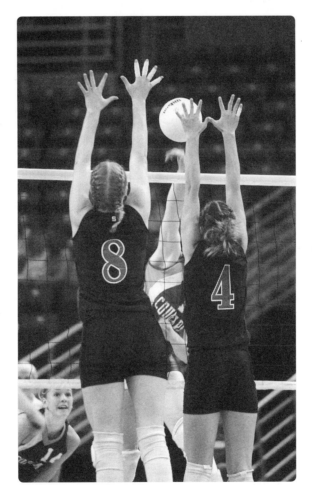

Nikki was a volleyball standout in high school. She received many scholarship offers to big-name universities and finally decided to attend a Big Ten university. She fit in well with her team, did very well in her classes, and had a lot of friends on campus. One of her teammates encouraged Nikki to pledge a sorority that many of the athletes belonged to. She was very excited about this opportunity and loved being part of yet another aspect of college life. Towards the middle of the fall semester, she attended a party and had too much to drink. She wasn't feeling well and decided to find a place to lie down.

When she woke up, her clothes were on the floor and she realized she had been raped. Even though she pressed charges and ultimately won the case, the damage had been done. Nikki became withdrawn, quit the sorority, quit the team, and left school before finishing her first semester.

When you finish reading this chapter, you should be able to explain

- the short-term effects of drinking alcohol on the body and on athletic performance,
- the long-term effects of drinking alcohol on the body,
- how to talk to your athletes about the effects of alcohol, and
- how to set team policies on alcohol.

You have probably dealt with at least one athlete who missed practice, had an accident, or did something he or she regretted because of **alcohol.** Although we all know that alcohol has some health-promoting effects, the bottom line is that it can impair performance, affect health, and get your athletes into a lot of trouble. Many universities have cracked down on hazing because of the number of deaths associated with alcohol intoxication. Yet it seems that drinking is a rite of passage and is considered cool by many young people—all the more reason for you to be the voice of reason, even though this may make you unpopular with your athletes.

If you coach middle school or high school athletes, you may think that you don't need to have this discussion with them, but here are some sobering statistics from the 2006 National Survey on Drug Use and Health and Monitoring the Future conducted by the Substance Abuse and Mental Health Services Administration of the United States Department of Health and Human Services. (Johnston et al. 2008)

- Almost 20 percent of 8th graders and 41 percent of 10th graders have been drunk at least once.
- Approximately 11 percent of 8th graders, 22 percent of 10th graders, and 27 percent of 12th graders report binge drinking (five drinks in a row) in the previous two weeks.
- In 2005, almost 36 percent of 8th graders and 58 percent of 10th graders reported trying flavored alcoholic beverages at least once.
- Adolescents who abuse alcohol may have cognitive deficits; they may only be able to recall 90 percent of what they have learned compared with classmates who do not drink.

Even though the legal drinking age is 21 in the United States, you are going to have athletes who drink. The advertisements for alcohol make it nearly irresistible, and your underage athletes may feel pressure from friends and teammates to drink. Remember, and remind them, that they are committing a crime if they drink.

If you work with underage athletes, you need to take some responsibility for protecting and educating your athletes and enforcing consequences if they break the law by drinking. It is not always easy to be the enforcer, but nothing could be worse than getting a call from the police or distraught parents that something catastrophic has happened to an athlete because he or she was drinking.

As a coach, you need to educate your athletes about the effects of alcohol on performance, weight, and health. You also need to develop an alcohol policy for your team and have each of your athletes—and at the middle school or high school level, their parents or guardians—sign a form that spells out the rules and consequences. Your athletes need to know that you adhere to a zero-tolerance policy for alcohol use during the entire season. This is essential to protect all the athletes who are your responsibility.

The advertisements for alcohol portray glamour and fun, but your athletes also need to see the ugly side of alcohol. Emphasize the performance aspect rather than health. There are very few 18-year-olds who are going to lose sleep worrying about cirrhosis of the liver. But if they are benched or suspended because of alcohol use, then the message starts to resonate.

What Alcohol Does in the Short Term

There is no doubt that alcohol can wreak havoc on performance. The athlete who drinks may notice delayed reaction time, decreased coordination, poor concentration, and impaired visual perception; athletes who participate in team sports are a detriment and risk to their teammates as well as to themselves. Your athletes may not understand the magnitude of the effects of alcohol on their body and their ability to participate in their sport.

Teach your athletes about the downside of alcohol and sports. They see commercials and advertisements that show active people drinking, but they probably don't know what alcohol actually does to an active body.

First, they need to know that drinking alcohol will affect how well they perform athletically:

- Common unpleasant side effects of drinking alcohol may include dry or cotton mouth, nausea, vomiting, heartburn, and headaches. The athlete with these symptoms will not be able to focus fully or perform to the best of his ability.

- Athletes who drink before a practice or competition will have delayed reaction time and possibly lessened motor skills.

- Alcohol is the only fluid that can dehydrate the body. If athletes do not optimally hydrate during exercise or rehydrate after exercise and consume alcohol as well, they are going to end up dehydrated, which can impair subsequent performance.

- If your athletes become injured and drink alcohol in the 24 hours after the injury, it may take them longer to heal. Alcohol opens the blood vessels so that there may be more swelling around the injured area.

- Alcohol can decrease sensitivity to pain, which may offer a false sense of security to an athlete with a nagging injury. If an athlete drinks to deaden pain and then participates in sport, he may end up with a more serious injury as a result of playing through the pain.

- Athletes who play in cold-weather sports need to know that the vasodilating (blood vessel–opening) effects of alcohol can speed heat loss from the skin, putting them at risk for hypothermia, or a lowered core body temperature.

- Endurance athletes need to know that if they consume alcohol prior to practice or competition, they may be at increased risk for hypoglycemia, or lowered blood glucose. Alcohol inhibits liver glycogen release, increasing the risk of lowered blood glucose during exercise. A hypoglycemic athlete is also at risk for hypothermia and certainly is not going to be able to perform at her optimum.

Second, athletes need to know the effects of drinking on their bodies:

- Athletes who train intensely for several hours and drink afterward are not replacing the calories or energy that the body lost during physical activity, because alcohol is not a significant source of carbohydrate. Athletes who drink a lot may not have an appetite to eat, therefore delaying muscle glycogen resynthesis. Athletes who drink beer, which is carbonated, may also feel full or bloated and probably won't want to eat well.

- Alcoholic beverages are not a source of sodium, and alcohol itself may increase urinary sodium losses, so salty sweaters need to be very careful with alcohol consumption.

- Alcohol is fairly high in calories. It contains 7 calories per gram, slightly less than fat (9 calories per gram) but more than both carbohydrate and protein (each 4 calories per gram). In addition, alcohol can be an appetite stimulant, and typically if your athletes are drinking and eating, they aren't eating vegetables! More likely they are eating high-calorie snack foods such as chips or bar foods such as pizza, wings, or ribs.

- Alcohol can affect sleep quality. Most athletes are sleep deprived anyway because of academics, athletics, and jobs. Alcohol prevents your athletes from getting adequate REM sleep so they wake up tired instead of well rested.

- Alcohol can affect athletes' ability to learn and achieve in the classroom.

Even though you don't want to encourage your athletes to drink, you need to tell them that how they drink will affect them:

- If they drink quickly, alcohol will leave the stomach more rapidly and the effects will be felt earlier.

Example

Barry is a freshman pole vaulter whose starting weight in the fall was 175 pounds (79 kg). By November he was 190 (86 kg) and had difficulty clearing the bar. His grades had slipped as well because he had trouble staying awake in class. The coach asked him to meet with me. Barry told me that he didn't understand why his weight was up because he didn't like the food on campus. But he said he went to frat parties every week and was drinking with his friends a few nights per week followed by late-night trips for fast food. He said he never felt rested and was tired in class and during practice. I explained to him that the alcohol was adding a lot of calories to his diet as well as increasing his appetite and disrupting his sleep. He agreed to cut back on his drinking and before the end of the fall semester had totally quit alcohol. His grades went up, his weight went down, and he was soaring once again!

- Women tend to feel the effects of alcohol faster than do men because of a smaller body mass. In addition, women have a lower concentration of total body water than men, so for the same amount of alcohol, a woman will have a higher blood alcohol concentration. And alcohol leaves the gut faster in women than men, so blood alcohol levels are higher in women than in men.

- Athletes who drink on an empty stomach are more likely to get drunk than those who eat before or while drinking.

- If your athletes consume alcohol mixed with carbonated beverages they will feel the effects of the alcohol faster than drinking a beverage that is mixed with juice. The reason is that carbonated beverages are absorbed by the small intestine more quickly, increasing the alcohol concentration in blood more rapidly.

- If athletes have not eaten much on the day of competition and end the day underfueled and dehydrated, they will feel the effects of alcohol much more rapidly.

Many athletes combine alcohol and **energy drinks,** which have caffeine. Alcohol is a depressant, whereas caffeine is a stimulant. When alcohol is mixed with caffeine, athletes may feel the stimulant effects and end up drinking more than they usually would. However, even if they don't feel the effects of the alcohol as much, their motor skills, judgment, coordination, and reaction time are still adversely affected.

You will also have athletes on your team who require medication. Alcohol and medication can be a dangerous combination. In some cases, alcohol can decrease the effectiveness or enhance the toxicity of medications. There are also medications that can increase blood alcohol levels. Here are medications that can have adverse reactions in combination with alcohol used:

- Pain medications
- Allergy medications
- Cough and cold preparations
- Diabetes medications
- Blood pressure medications
- Cholesterol medications
- Antibiotics
- Antidepressants
- Anti-seizure medications

The National Institute of Alcohol Abuse and Alcoholism has a detailed list of alcohol and drug interactions (see its Web site at www.niaaa.nih.gov).

Finally, keep in mind that if your athletes go out to drink after a victory and the opposing team is in the same bar, and someone gets carried away boasting and bragging, a fight may break out. There could be very serious consequences—you don't want to receive a phone call asking you to bail an athlete out of jail.

What Alcohol Does in the Long Term

Even though some of the health consequences of alcohol abuse are not likely to be of immediate concern to your athletes, it is important for them to understand the long-term and the short-term effects of alcohol. The physical harm associated with alcohol may take a while to develop, but the psychological consequences often occur more rapidly. Your athletes need to understand how their actions can affect their health as well as their academic and athletic performance, now and in the future. For example, in small amounts, alcohol may lower the risk of heart disease, but in larger amounts it can elevate triglycerides (blood fats), therefore increasing the risk for cardiovascular disease, high blood pressure, and stroke.

More than 2 million Americans suffer from **alcohol-related liver disease,** according to a survey by the National Institute for Alcohol Abuse and Alcoholism (Grant 2006). Because the liver is the filter for alcohol, regular long-term consumption can result in hepatitis, or inflammation of the liver. Approximately 10 to 20 percent of alcohol abusers will develop alcoholic cirrhosis, or scarring of the liver, which affects liver functioning and, if drinking continues, can lead to death (Grant 2006).

Some people who abuse alcohol will develop pancreatitis, an inflammation of the pancreas, which is painful and causes serious symptoms such as poor absorption of nutrients, weight loss, bleeding, tissue damage, and infection. Pancreatitis attributable to alcohol abuse may develop between the ages of 30 and 40. In addition, regular heavy alcohol use can increase the risk for cancer of the liver, mouth, throat, larynx, and esophagus.

Individuals who abuse alcohol are typically malnourished, even though they may be at normal weight or even overweight. This happens because alcohol does not provide all of the nutrients the body requires and can also cause vitamin deficiencies, particularly of the B vitamins. Some individuals who abuse alcohol develop dementia attributable to deficiencies in thiamin, one of the B vitamins.

Alcohol abuse can result in heartburn and can even be a risk factor for developing stomach ulcers. Gastritis, or irritation of the stomach, can also occur. Symptoms include abdominal pain, nausea, vomiting, and in some cases a feeling of fullness or burning in the stomach. If gastritis is present, the body cannot maximally absorb nutrients, and the condition is very painful as well.

There is a higher rate (44 percent) of psychological disorders including depression and anxiety in those who abuse alcohol compared with those who do not (Grant 2006). Individuals who abuse alcohol have a higher risk of accidents and a higher risk of suicide.

Men who drink excessively may become sexually impotent. Pregnant women who drink to excess are at increased risk of having a baby with fetal alcohol syndrome. Infants with fetal alcohol syndrome may have birth defects, retarded growth, mental impairment, and physical malformations.

Talking to Your Athletes About Alcohol

If all the problems related to alcohol use sound scary, it's because they *are* scary. You cannot sugarcoat the facts! Your athletes need to know what can happen to their performance, and they need to know that if they are found to be drinking, they won't play. No exceptions! Although you may not want to have this discussion with your athletes, you must. You should address this issue several times over the course of the year, and parents of younger athletes should be included in one or more of the discussions.

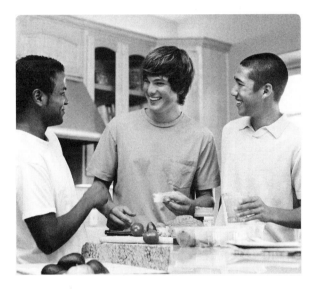

The more information athletes have, the better armed they are to make safe and healthful choices about alcohol in social situations.

Ask your athletes to fill out a questionnaire that asks about alcohol use. You may think that they will not answer truthfully, but don't let that deter you. Ask the questions, get their answers, and then have an alcohol talk with your entire team so no one feels singled out. The following questions are part of the DISCUS tool kit created by the Distilled Spirits Council of the United States:

- Do you drink alcohol?
- How many days a week do you drink?
- How many drinks do you have when you drink?

- What types of alcohol do you drink?
- What do you consider a drink to be?
- Did you use to drink more or less than you do now?
- Has anyone ever said anything to you about your drinking?
- Has anyone in your family ever had a problem with drinking?

The DISCUS tool kit is an excellent resource that includes lesson plans, charts, and online programs for students and parents. It will give you an idea of what your athletes think and do with regard to alcohol.

Have your athletes complete the alcohol questionnaire from the DISCUS tool kit (http://www.alcoholtoolkit.org/discusOnline.html). After you review the answers, invite a guest speaker to address the performance and health consequences of alcohol use. (Season-Long Activities)

During your discussions with athletes, it is also important to dispel some of the myths surrounding alcohol. Your athletes may have heard or believe some or all of the myths in table 11.1.

As far as the body is concerned, the effects of alcohol are going to be the same no matter what the source. Explain this to your athletes and show them alcohol equivalents. The DISCUS tool kit has a great chart that will show your athletes the serving size of an alcoholic beverage. Each of the beverages shown in figure 11.1 is considered to be the equivalent of one drink.

Educate your athletes on the calorie cost of alcohol as well. They may believe that liquids are not high in calories, but depending on the size of the drink, the amount of alcohol, or the mixers, the calorie cost can be staggering.

- 12 ounces (360 ml) beer: 90 to 150 calories
- 5 ounces (150 ml) wine (people often pour 6 to 10 oz): 100 calories
- 1.5 ounces (15 ml) liquor: 100 calories
- Mixed drinks: 200 to 800 calories per drink

TABLE 11.1

Myths About Alcohol

Myth	Reality
One drink won't hurt.	Even 1 oz (30 ml) of alcohol—12 oz (360 ml) of beer, 5 oz (150 ml) of wine, or 1.5 oz (15 ml) (a shot) of liquor—may be enough to affect motor skills.
Beer has less alcohol than wine or liquor.	A 12-oz beer, 12-oz wine cooler, 5-oz glass of wine, or 1.5-oz shot of liquor all have the same amount of alcohol.
Light-colored beverages have less alcohol than darker colored beverages.	Beer can vary in the amount of alcohol, with malt liquor having a higher alcohol content than most other brewed beverages.
Sweet drinks are lower in alcohol.	A sweet wine or wine cooler has as much alcohol as a beverage that is not sweet.
Wine coolers have less alcohol.	A 12-oz wine cooler and a 5-oz glass of wine have the same amount of alcohol.
Low-carbohydrate beer is lower in alcohol.	Low-carbohydrate beer may have less carbohydrate but the alcohol content is the same as regular beer.
Mixing an energy drink with alcohol will prevent you from getting drunk.	The caffeine in the energy drink acts as a stimulant so you may not feel drunk as quickly, but your motor skills and judgment skills are affected. And if you do not feel the effects of alcohol, you may be likely to drink more than you usually would.

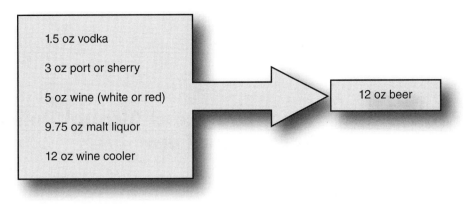

FIGURE 11.1 Equivalents of one drink.

Setting Team Policies on Alcohol

Develop an alcohol policy that you are willing to enforce. Check with your school or other supporting institution to see what policies are already in place, and make sure that your athletes are aware of the policies and the consequences of violating them. In addition to setting a team policy, if you believe that the existing institutional policies are not strict enough, meet with your administrator and work together to toughen them in order to safeguard your athletes.

Use education and awareness to convince your athletes and their support systems to buy in. Stress the importance of being a team. If one member of the team drinks, the whole team will be affected. Your athletes need to know that there will be consequences for drinking and that every athlete on your team must inform you if someone breaks the rules.

Your team policy should prohibit the selling or consumption of alcohol at school or tournament venues. For example, the State of Iowa prohibits the possession or consumption of any type of alcohol on school property (public or private) or while attending a school function.

In addition, you can develop a contract for athletes and their parents or guardians to sign (see figure 11.2). The contract should clearly state that the athlete will not possess or use alcohol, narcotics, or other illegal substances. Have the athlete and a parent sign the contract and make sure you keep a copy on file.

You may want to draft a separate agreement form or letter for parents that explains the alcohol policy in greater detail.

Emphasize that this policy will be in place for the entire school year, not just during the season, and that it applies to any school-related functions. Work with your administrators to determine the consequences of policy violation. For example, the first offense might involve a conference with the athletic director, coach, and player; a six- to eight-week suspension from athletics; and at least one meeting a week with a student assistance counselor. A second violation might involve another conference, permanent suspension from athletics, and mandatory participation in a drug and alcohol rehabilitation program.

There is no time or place for alcohol during the playing season. If your goal is to have a zero-tolerance policy for alcohol, you must spell this out to your athletes before the season begins. They need to know your policy and what the consequences will be. Don't just say it—enforce it. If your star athlete is caught drinking during the season, you will have to bench him even though it may put your team at a competitive disadvantage. If you let any of your athletes off

Learn about your school's or organization's policy on student-athlete alcohol use. If no policy exists or you believe the existing policy should be changed, meet with administrators to develop a more appropriate policy. (Start-Up Activities)

During the preseason parent meeting, describe the school's or organization's alcohol policy. Have students and their parents sign a contract stating that they understand and will follow the policy. (Preseason Activities)

Player Name _____

Athlete and Parent Drug and Alcohol Policy Agreement Form

Athlete's Pledge and Responsibility

As a participant in my school's athletic program, I have read and understand the Drug, Alcohol, and Tobacco Policy for Student-Athletes. I understand that this pledge is for the entire school year, not just the sport season. I agree to honor all the rules regarding the use of drugs, alcohol, and tobacco.

I will not smoke or use tobacco products.

I will not possess or use alcohol.

I will not possess or use unauthorized drugs or substances.

If I use, possess, or am found to be under the influence of any of these substances, I agree to accept the consequences for my behavior.

_____   _____

Student Signature   Date

Parent's Pledge and Responsibility

I have received a copy of the Drug, Alcohol, and Tobacco Policy for Student-Athletes. I have read and understand the policy. I understand that this pledge is for the entire school year, not just the current sport season.

I will not allow my child to use drugs or alcohol.

I will not provide drugs or alcohol to my child.

I will not provide drugs or alcohol to any minor.

I will not be on the school campus or attend any school athletic event, home or away, while under the influence of drugs or alcohol.

I agree to attend an annual player and parent drug and alcohol prevention meeting.

I understand that failure to abide by this policy could lead to my child's losing his or her playing privileges and that I could be banned from attending school athletic events.

_____   _____

Parent's Signature   Date

From L. Bonci, 2009, *Sport Nutrition for Coaches* (Champaign, IL: Human Kinetics).

FIGURE 11.2 Sample Athlete and Parent Drug and Alcohol Policy Agreement Form.

the hook, you lose credibility. Remember, a drunk athlete is a liability to himself or herself, to teammates, to you, and to your institution.

Your athletes need to know that if they drink before practice or competition, they may be unable to finish, they may become injured, and they definitely will perform at a subpar level. The goal is for your athletes to take care of their bodies so they can push themselves to be their best. Most of your athletes would not wear ill-fitting shoes or play with defective equipment; they need to realize that in similar but potentially more serious ways alcohol will jeopardize their performance and, worse, their health.

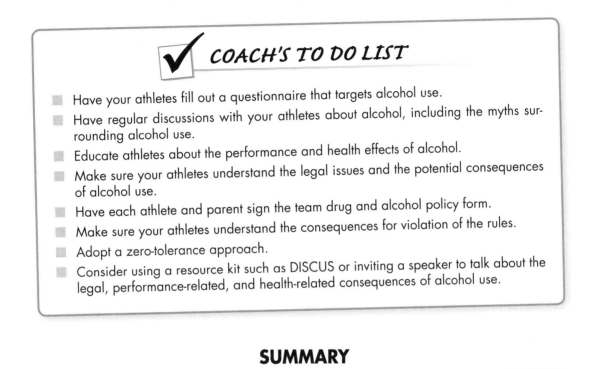

✔ COACH'S TO DO LIST

- Have your athletes fill out a questionnaire that targets alcohol use.
- Have regular discussions with your athletes about alcohol, including the myths surrounding alcohol use.
- Educate athletes about the performance and health effects of alcohol.
- Make sure your athletes understand the legal issues and the potential consequences of alcohol use.
- Have each athlete and parent sign the team drug and alcohol policy form.
- Make sure your athletes understand the consequences for violation of the rules.
- Adopt a zero-tolerance approach.
- Consider using a resource kit such as DISCUS or inviting a speaker to talk about the legal, performance-related, and health-related consequences of alcohol use.

SUMMARY

- Alcohol can adversely affect health and performance and may have serious consequences for athletes.
- Athletes need to be educated about the effects of alcohol.
- Athletes need to be educated on the short-term and long-term consequences of alcohol use in terms of mental and physical health.
- Alcohol use can cause digestive distress and headaches.
- Alcohol can delay reaction time, dehydrate the body, delay recovery from injury, and increase the risk of hypothermia.
- Alcohol can delay recovery from exercise and affect sleep quality.
- The excess calories consumed from alcohol can contribute to weight gain.
- Drinking a large volume of alcohol quickly can affect the body more rapidly.
- Consuming alcohol and energy drinks or alcohol and medications can have adverse health consequences.
- It is important to know whether and what your athletes drink, as well as how much, and to explain some of the myths of alcohol.
- It is imperative to develop and enforce an alcohol policy for students and parents.

KEY TERMS

alcohol   alcohol-related liver disease   energy drinks

GAME PLAN QUESTIONS

1. Why discuss alcohol with your middle and high school athletes?

2. What are some of the performance consequences of alcohol consumption?

3. What strategies can you use to help educate your athletes about alcohol?

PART III

Planning Tools

This final section will help you take what you've learned in the first two sections and make it work in your particular situation. Finding ways to deliver good nutrition to athletes, despite time and travel constraints, is the topic of chapter 12, Facing Logistic Challenges. Finding ways to provide your athletes with the food they need without breaking the bank is covered in chapter 13, Budgeting Good Nutrition. And chapter 14, Implementing a Sport Nutrition Plan, offers you guidelines on setting up a year-long nutrition plan for your team and getting your athletes (and their parents) to buy into it so you can ensure that they stay healthy and fit for play.

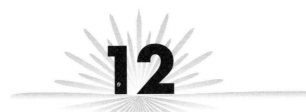

Facing Logistic Challenges

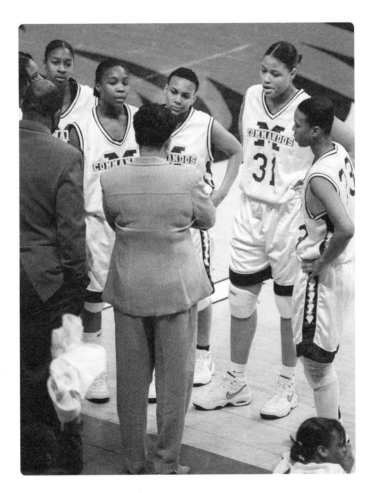

One of the girls' AAU teams had a very successful season and was playing in an out-of-state tournament. The team was traveling by bus and competing in a small town where there was only one diner, a convenience store, and a fast food restaurant. Because of some mechanical problems with the bus, the team left late and didn't have time to stop to eat before the game. Because all of the girls needed to be at the bus by 5 a.m., few of them were awake enough to eat anything before they left home, and most of them fell asleep once they got on the bus.

After a five-hour bus ride, the team arrived late at the tournament venue and had just enough time to change clothes and shoot around before the game started. They played two games and made it to the finals, to be played the next day. The girls were tired, famished, and ready to eat. The diner was packed and the fast food restaurant wasn't appealing to everyone, so they ended up going to the convenience store to get some snack items. Needless to say, no one repleted optimally from their games. The team had breakfast at the hotel the next morning, but it was continental style and only offered sweet rolls, doughnuts, milk, and juice.

The girls were excited about being in the finals, but their bodies were tired and they didn't play well. The game was close throughout but in the final minutes the opposition went on a run; the team couldn't catch up and lost the game.

On the bus ride home the girls talked about what went wrong and decided that they needed to plan better for fueling when they traveled by bringing food with them and looking into their restaurant options ahead of time so that they would have enough energy to finish strong.

When you finish reading this chapter, you should be able to explain how to

- use the off-season to get your athletes into good nutrition habits before the season starts,
- help your athletes work eating into their busy schedules,
- work with your institution's food service to improve access to nutritious foods and encourage athletes to eat them, and
- ensure that your athletes eat a healthy diet while on the road.

It may seem to you that sometimes practice is the least stressful time of the day. Your players show up, go through the workout, and leave. But each player brings with him or her an agenda above and beyond athletic responsibilities. Your athletes may be students, may have jobs, or both, and sports need to fit into an overly busy schedule. You may be a teacher or have another career as well as coaching, and yet you need to prepare and show up for practice and competition.

You can make your life a little less difficult by developing a plan for feeding your athletes. It would be nice if they would remember to pack food for travel, bring money to buy food, or both, but the reality is that they don't always do this. You can hope for the best but you need to prepare for the worst by having a contingency plan. This will require you or someone on your staff to work with the food service staff at your school, university, or camp or the restaurant manager on the road. All of this needs to be coordinated before the team travels; the less left to chance, the better off you and your athletes will be.

Off-Season Nutrition

A good way to ensure that your athletes follow good nutrition habits throughout the playing season is to get them started with those habits during the off-season. Even though your athletes may not be involved in their sport all year long, they still need to fuel and hydrate daily. Often an athlete who is out of season will develop bad eating habits such as skipping meals or eating a lot of high-fat, high-sugar foods. An athlete who eats poorly during the off-season will not be as prepared to play as one who fuels well all year long, so remind your athletes of the importance of continuing their in-season eating habits during the off-season.

You may also have athletes who are trying to increase mass, decrease body fat, or both during the off-season. They need to have a plan to accomplish these goals without compromising health or performance. An athlete who is rehabilitating from injury needs to eat well to heal.

Provide all your athletes with a fueling and hydration plan for the off-season (see figure 12.1 for a sample summer plan). If you have athletes with particular weight goals, make sure that they are working with a health professional and encourage them to start on their plan as soon as the season is over so they have the maximum amount of time to see results.

For the off-season, do the following for your athletes:

- Call a team meeting one week before the end of the season. Ask your players to list the nutrition goals they want to work on during the off-season.

- Provide them with guidelines for off-season fueling and hydrating.

- Encourage those who have weight issues to work on their goals in the off-season under the supervision of a health professional. Meet or talk with these athletes halfway through the off-season to assess their progress and again a month before the start of preseason. Remind them that they may not start if they have not been following their plan.

- Contact all athletes one month before the start of the preseason to see whether they have been following your guidelines on daily fueling and hydrating. For team members who are just entering high school, send a letter on how to hydrate and fuel for preseason and provide them with a sample menu that they can start to follow one month before the preseason.

- Send all athletes a letter one week before the start of preseason reminding them to eat before practice and to bring snacks and fluid to practice.

- Have your athletes calculate their sweat rate for a few days prior to the start of preseason so they know how much fluid they are going to need during practice.

Athletes' Busy Schedules

You need to be the master juggler and timekeeper to make sure your athletes not only come to practice but also make it to class, study halls, and work. Your athletes may stay up late and struggle to wake up early so that they arrive at practice at the last minute. As a result, they may skip breakfast because it takes too much time. If your athletes are late or miss practice for an unexcused reason, you may need to sit them rather than start them for the next competition. They will learn quickly that being on time is one of the responsibilities of being an athlete.

Help your athletes plan their eating schedule around their other obligations. They can plan to eat something within the first hour of waking up and then go to practice or class. If they carry portable

---

Sample Summer Fueling and Hydration Game Plan

- Drink 16 to 20 ounces (480-600 ml) of water when you wake up.
- Eat something within one hour of waking up, such as a bowl of cereal, yogurt and fruit, or a peanut butter sandwich, and have 16 to 20 ounces of water, juice, or milk.
- Try to eat something again within four hours, such as a piece of fruit and some cheese, two handfuls of trail mix, or a sandwich and fruit, and have 16 to 20 ounces of fluid.
- Make sure you eat something one hour before any activity and again within 15 minutes after activity.
- If you are a salty sweater, choose sports drinks when you play, add salt to your foods, and eat salty foods such as pickles, pretzels, and crackers.
- Make sure you eat dinner, and include some kind of protein such as chicken, fish, meat, or veggie burgers; a starch of some kind such as rice, pasta, or potato; and fruit and vegetables. Have 16 to 20 ounces of fluid with dinner.
- If you are going to be up late or have early-morning court time or conditioning, eat something before you go to bed, such as a smoothie, yogurt, or a bowl of cereal.

FIGURE 12.1 Fueling and hydration plan for the off-season.

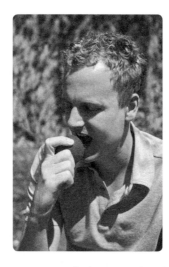

When athletes eat nutritious foods on a regular schedule, they are less tempted to fill up on empty calories.

snacks with them, they can eat something between classes or right after practice to tide them over until the next meal. If your athletes have practice or class or need to work during the lunch hour, they can eat something small, like trail mix and a sports drink, a peanut butter sandwich, or a sports bar rather than go without food.

For high school athletes who have early lunch, remind them to bring a snack to have mid-afternoon. If they have the last lunch period, they should eat a snack midmorning so they aren't starved by lunchtime. This will help them be better energized mentally and physically for practice and competition.

Your team may have to practice during a mealtime because that is the only time that the field, court, or rink is available. These athletes need to have a contingency plan. If they have practice from noon until 2 p.m., they may need to eat at 10 a.m. If practice is 5 to 7 p.m., they should either have dinner before practice or have a light snack before and a light dinner after practice.

Athletes may not have the luxury of sitting down to an evening meal if they have night classes or night practice or need to work. For these athletes, a late-afternoon snack such as yogurt and fruit, a bowl of cereal, or bean dip and crackers can provide enough fuel that they won't be starved the rest of the day.

Remind your athletes that they can have their largest meal of the day after practice, even if that means 9 p.m., if that is the only time they have to eat a relaxed, nutritious meal. I prefer that my athletes sit down to a bowl of pasta or stir-fry and have the luxury of 30 minutes to eat rather than try to wolf down a burger on their way to the next event of the day.

Institutional Food

With the exception of those who have training tables, most of the athletes you work with will probably eat their meals with nonathletes. Many student-athletes don't want to eat at their school cafeteria or dining hall because they don't like the food or because it takes too much time to get a meal; instead, they may go without food or just eat snacks. For athletes who have after-school practice, missing a meal is not going to improve performance in class or in sports.

You may need to work with the food service staff to come up with some appropriate solutions for feeding your athletes. Perhaps the food service can provide breakfast bags to feed athletes who have early-morning practice. This could contain yogurt, a muffin and fruit, or a breakfast sandwich and juice. (The concept of grab-and-go meals also may be helpful for athletes who have practice at lunchtime, are work-study students, or have to go to study hall.) You can schedule mandatory early-morning meetings once or twice a week for your team and have food there. The food service staff may be able to provide cereal, fruit, and juice or a hot breakfast with eggs, pancakes or waffles, and fruit.

Suggest to the food service manager that certain foods in the cafeteria or dining hall be labeled as performance foods. Who doesn't want to perform better? This has appeal for the athletes as well as the nonathletes. The cafeteria manager also may have some ideas about how to make the food more appealing or how to move the kids more efficiently through the line at lunch so they have time to eat.

A performance menu might include foods that strengthen the immune system, help the body recover optimally from training, and help athletes achieve their body composition goals.

Foods that strengthen the immune system include the following:

- Carbohydrate-containing foods with anti-oxidants such as fruits, vegetables, a salad bar, juice

- Omega-3-containing foods such as fish and omega-3-enriched eggs

- Monounsaturated fatty acid–containing foods such as nuts, seeds, nut butters, and olive oil (for cooking and on the salad bar)

- Lean protein such as ground turkey burgers; very lean ground meat for chili, tacos, and meatballs; lean lunch meats

Example

Coach Brown couldn't understand why the girls' basketball players were always so tired early in practice. He scheduled rest periods and fluid breaks, but his players weren't able to do what he wanted them to. After sitting down with his athletes, he found out that most of them weren't eating lunch because they only had 15 minutes and by the time they got through the line, it was time to go to class. Those who had time to get to the cafeteria didn't like what was offered there. He decided to have a meeting with the cafeteria manager and one of his athletes to come up with some strategies. Food service was able to provide grab-and-go lunch bags for the team, and with more fuel in their bodies, the girls were able to make it through practice feeling great!

Foods that help the body recover optimally from training by restoring glycogen and rehydrating contain carbohydrate. Choices include pasta, pasta salad, potatoes, rice, breads, cereals, and fruits and vegetables. Figure 12.2 lists recovery foods that may be made available in the dining hall, in your office, in the training room, or at a sports camp.

Foods to help your athletes achieve body composition goals include the following:

- High-fiber items such as beans, whole-grain breads, whole-grain pasta, brown rice, fruits, and vegetables
- Low-fat protein such as grilled or baked meats instead of fried
- Carbohydrate-rich foods prepared using a low-fat cooking method, such as oven-baked fries

You can provide suggestions rather than just rely on the food service staff or cafeteria manager to come up with ideas. Certainly the menu modifications should be available to all students as well as faculty and staff. Suggest that the following food items be considered:

- Low-fat chocolate milk
- Light salad dressings
- Shredded reduced-fat cheese for pizza or tacos
- Cut-up fruit instead of whole
- Foods prepared with less fat and salt added, so those who need or want more salt can add to taste
- Whole-grain pasta and brown rice

Recovery Foods

To be kept in the refrigerator
Smoothies
Fruit
Soy milk
Low-fat cow's milk or chocolate milk
Yogurt
V8 or tomato juice

Nonperishable items
Cereal
Granola or cereal bars
Trail mix
Crackers

Beverages
Water
Sports drinks
Fitness water
Ready-to-drink shakes such as Instant Breakfast, Ensure, Boost
Sports bars (except those that are high protein, low carbohydrate)

FIGURE 12.2 Recovery foods.

Meet with food service staff and a team member to plan what healthy foods to offer and how to present them. (Beginning-of-Season Activities)

Get feedback from your athletes about what foods they like and don't like, as well as some of the perceived barriers to eating, such as time and cost. If you involve your athletes in the discussion, or even appoint one of your athletes to the food committee, you will get better buy-in. The goal is to balance what your athletes need to eat with what they want to eat.

Work with the food service staff to determine how to handle plate waste. If the food isn't being eaten, changes must be made to the item or how it is prepared. The goal is to get your athletes to eat at school or on campus so that they are better fueled to make it through classes and workouts.

Consider the way foods are positioned. What are the first items your athletes see when they walk into the dining hall? Ideally they should see fruits and vegetables first along with beverages so they can start to hydrate and fill with higher-nutrient density, lower-calorie items.

Take advantage of the expertise of the food service staff to plan cooking lessons for your athletes, to be held during a team meeting or after practice. Bring in a chef to teach your athletes how to cook fast and on the go with low-cost items. Educate your athletes on how to feed themselves whether they are at school, on the road, or at home. Here are some examples of simple meals that your athletes can learn how to prepare:

- Enchiladas made with tortillas, beans, shredded cheese, and salsa
- Stir-fry with 90-second rice, chicken, vegetables
- Potato with chili and cheese
- Baked beans with low-fat hot dogs
- Pasta with meatballs (frozen) and sauce
- Tortellini or ravioli with sauce and salad
- Oatmeal with milk and fruit
- Oatmeal with peanut butter and added soy protein or whey protein powder
- Flavored noodles with added chicken
- Flavored Asian-style rice with tofu and peanut butter
- Spanish-style rice with salmon and tuna or baby shrimp
- Tortilla soup with chicken
- Stuffing with mixed vegetables and turkey

Here are examples of some simple recipes:

Protein-boosted oatmeal: Make a packet of instant oatmeal with skim milk. Stir in 1 tbsp peanut butter and maple syrup to taste.

Baked potato: Top a baked potato with 1/2 cup beans, 2 tbsp salsa, and 1/4 cup (60 ml) melted cheese.

Rice bowl: Put 1 cup (200 g) rice in the bottom of a large salad bowl. Top with 2 cups lettuce, and top the lettuce with a 1 cup of cooked, chopped chicken breast, steak, or shrimp. Flavor with soy sauce or ginger teriyaki sauce.

Spanish rice: Brown one medium onion, chopped, in 2 tsp olive oil. Add 1 pound (450 g) ground turkey breast and cook until meat is done (no longer pink). Add a small jar of salsa and salt and pepper to taste. Serve over rice or in tortilla shells.

Chicken and vegetables: Cook a package of flavored pasta according to package directions. Add a pouch of chicken breast and 1/2 cup of frozen mixed vegetables or peas.

Peanut noodles with chicken: Cook noodles according to package directions. Add 2 tbsp of peanut butter and sliced chicken breast. Add soy sauce to taste.

A great resource for recipes is *Nancy Clark's Sports Nutrition Guidebook, Fourth Edition.*

Consider using other resources. There may be a parent on your team who is a chef, or if you have a culinary school in your area, one of their students may be willing to demonstrate some quick recipes for your team. If you have found a sports dietitian to work with your team, ask him to help you with meal planning or to serve as the liaison between you and the food service staff.

Select a few easy-to-prepare, healthy food recipes. You or a parent, chef, or dietitian can teach athletes how to prepare the recipes. (Season-Long Activities)

Nutrition on the Road

Travel is never easy. It may cause problems that impair your athletes' performance, such as altered sleep schedules, skipped meals, dehydration (especially with air travel), food safety issues, and, if you're traveling abroad, the availability and accessibility of familiar foods. Your athletes need to think about packing food as a priority, not an afterthought.

Make a travel food plan. Encourage your athletes to pack food, and if you are traveling by air remind them that they cannot bring liquids onto the plane. However, athletes can bring many food items that will be allowed through security, and they can pack other items in their checked luggage.

Give your athletes and their parents a list of appropriate snack items, like the one shown in figure 12.3. Explain to your athletes that you want them to think about performance foods, which means foods that provide carbohydrate, protein, and fat. It is certainly fine to have a few cookies or a handful of chips, but if your athletes gorge on candy, soda, chips, and doughnuts, they probably will not to be ready to play.

Make sure that each of your athletes receives this list and packs some of the food items on the list. Suggest that your athletes bring a hot pot and adapter so that they can prepare pasta, hot cereal, soup, or chili in their room. Besides being more healthful, eating these foods is also much less expensive than eating out.

Another idea is to assign food items: Ask some athletes to bring cereal, ask some to bring juice, and ask others for bowls, cups, and utensils. You can also assign a snack coach or hydration coach whose job is to make sure that snacks and fluids are available before and after practice. If you are lucky enough to have parents who travel with the team, ask them to coordinate snacks and investigate eating venues in the places you travel to. Do as much planning as you can, because food is one of the few items you can control.

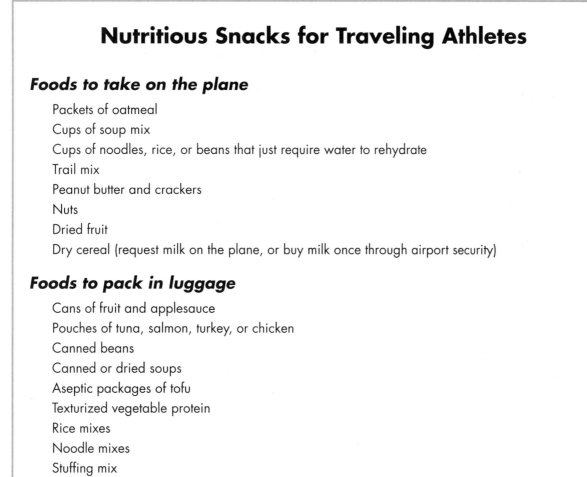

Nutritious Snacks for Traveling Athletes

Foods to take on the plane

Packets of oatmeal

Cups of soup mix

Cups of noodles, rice, or beans that just require water to rehydrate

Trail mix

Peanut butter and crackers

Nuts

Dried fruit

Dry cereal (request milk on the plane, or buy milk once through airport security)

Foods to pack in luggage

Cans of fruit and applesauce

Pouches of tuna, salmon, turkey, or chicken

Canned beans

Canned or dried soups

Aseptic packages of tofu

Texturized vegetable protein

Rice mixes

Noodle mixes

Stuffing mix

Sports drink powder

Juice concentrate

Nonfat dry milk powder

Microwave light popcorn

Have athletes pack measuring cups and spoons for mixing and simple cooking.

FIGURE 12.3 Snacks for travel.

If you travel by car or by bus, you can bring more items compared with when you're flying. Consider packing a cooler with milk, yogurt, lunch meats, condiments, and fresh fruits and vegetables.

Because time is always at a premium when you travel, use your food coach or food scout to survey the team about their meal preferences after games. If the team will eat at a family-style restaurant after a game, get a menu ahead of time, ask each athlete for their menu choice, and call the restaurant so they can be prepared. Your food coach can call the restaurant to give an estimated time of arrival so you don't have to wait a long time before the food appears.

Another option is to order the food to be delivered or picked up. This doesn't limit you to pizza, however. For example, you could order Chinese, Mexican, Ital-ian, or Thai food. This is a pleasant surprise for your athletes and puts some variety into the food choices.

Appendix A lists healthy choices available at some popular chain restaurants.

Figure 12.4 lists some healthy foods usually available at restaurants or hotels; if you call ahead, it's likely that they will have these foods available for you.

Create a nutrition plan for a typical road trip, using the food guidelines in this chapter. Select what types of food to bring in the vehicle, determine what restaurants are available on the road, and decide how to handle any anticipated logistic issues. (Preseason Activities)

Healthy Foods Available on the Road

Breakfast

Cereals—hot and cold

Low-fat milk, soy milk, yogurt

Breads

Eggs

Pancakes and waffles

Butter and margarine

Peanut butter

Honey and jam

Syrup

Fruit

Dinner

Soup—broth- or vegetable-based

Salad

Cooked vegetables

Grilled or baked meats

Pasta with meat sauce and nonmeat option

Rice or other grains

Bread

Dessert: pudding, sorbet, frozen yogurt, light ice cream

Fruit

Lunch

Breads for sandwiches

Meats such as turkey, ham, roast beef

Lettuce, tomato, pickles

Light cheese

Mayonnaise, mustard

Soup—broth- or vegetable-based

Pasta

Grilled chicken

Hamburger, turkey burger

Baked potatoes

Fruit

Beverages

Water

Juice

Tea

Coffee

Low-fat milk

Low-fat chocolate milk

FIGURE 12.4 Healthy foods usually available while traveling.

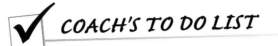

COACH'S TO DO LIST

- [ ] Help your athletes develop an eating schedule to optimize performance.
- [ ] Remind athletes to carry snacks to eat during the day so that they are not without food for long stretches of time.
- [ ] Work with the food service staff in your institution to optimize fueling your athletes.
- [ ] Assign an athlete to take part in the food committee.
- [ ] Make suggestions for a performance menu.
- [ ] Consider doing some food demonstrations for your athletes to give them ideas for nutritious meals and snacks that they can easily prepare.
- [ ] Develop a travel food plan by reminding your athletes to bring food with them and by making sure that you also bring appropriate snack items for your team.
- [ ] Assign a food coach or food scout to assist with overnight or tournament travel.
- [ ] Educate your athletes on performance-optimizing food choices they can make while on the road.

SUMMARY

- Developing and implementing a plan to feed athletes can optimize their health and sports performance.
- Athletes need to develop an eating schedule that supports their practice and class schedule.
- The food service staff is a valuable resource and ally to make sure that athletes receive foods that support a healthy immune system, expedite recovery from exercise, and achieve body composition goals.
- Athletes need to be able to provide feedback on foods being served to the team.
- Providing examples of foods that athletes can easily prepare can help them eat well on a regular basis.
- Traveling with appropriate snacks is a proactive approach to fueling athletes.
- A feeding plan is necessary for road events.

GAME PLAN QUESTIONS

1. Why is travel such a concern with regard to feeding athletes?

2. Why do you need to work with the food service staff?

3. How can you get parents involved with feeding the team?

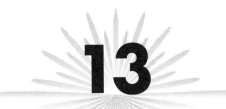

Budgeting Good Nutrition

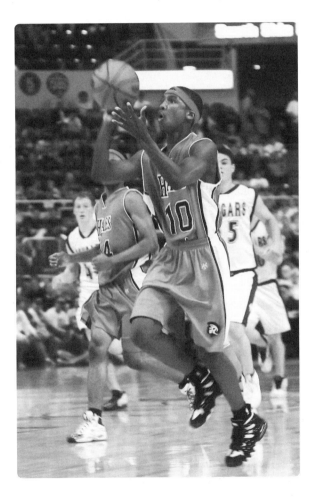

Dan is a university basketball player who is spending the summer between his freshman and sophomore year on campus to work and take classes. He is a scholarship athlete and receives a monthly stipend for food. Growing up, Dan never learned how to cook and ate most of his meals at fast food restaurants. He was thrilled that he had a stipend for food because he didn't always like the food choices at training table. However, he didn't budget well and after two weeks of eating out he ran out of money but wouldn't be getting another check for the rest of the month. The strength coach gave him extra shakes and bars, and some of his friends took him out for meals, but he ended up losing some weight that he really couldn't afford to lose.

The coach decided to have the sports dietitian meet with the players to teach them how to budget their money for food. They went to the grocery store, did some food preparation, and figured out how to eat out without breaking the bank. As a result, every athlete was able to have enough money to get through the summer and they gained some culinary skills along the way.

When you finish reading this chapter, you should be able to explain how to

- choose which foods to bring to competitions,
- get help from parents and booster clubs in providing food and drink,
- choose restaurants on the road that can supply healthy meals, and
- keep food costs down.

Working with professional athletes, I am always amazed by their food extravagances in terms of choices and quantity. However, in sports such as baseball, the major league players may dine on sushi or filet while the minor leaguers make do with peanut butter and jelly sandwiches. Most of you are not going to have a lobster budget, but this doesn't mean that your players can't eat well. A little creativity, parent participation, and collaboration with local food purveyors can help you to provide high-quality, tasty, and performance-enhancing meals.

This chapter is intended primarily for use by high school and club team coaches, given that for collegiate sports, the NCAA determines what and how much food teams can provide for their athletes.

Packing Food for Contests

It is always cheaper to travel with food rather than rely on eating out. Even snacks and drinks bought at a convenience store will be more expensive than food and beverages that you bring on the trip. Depending on the number of hours that you will travel, you can bring prepared sandwiches with you or have a team parent go the grocery store to buy the meat, cheese, and bread. Again, this is much cheaper than stopping at a sandwich shop to buy ready-made items.

Do a team inventory to see what items can be contributed before you spend money. For instance,

you may have parents who are willing to donate or lend coolers and thermoses. If you travel by bus you may have room to take a few folding tables or perhaps parents can bring tables, some chairs, tablecloths, and napkins so you can stop for a picnic instead of dining out.

You know how important it is for your athletes to be hydrated, but sports drinks and fitness water, as well as bottled water, are not inexpensive. To cut costs, buy gallons of water instead of the 20-ounce (600 ml) bottles or bring several gallon pitchers and some water filters and fill them with tap water at your sporting venue or in the hotel. Instead of bringing ready-to-drink sports beverages, buy the powder and mix the beverages yourself. You can also buy powdered mix for flavored water as well as juice concentrates and lemonade concentrate or powder. This will save a lot of money.

Foods with protein are also high priced. Lunchmeats are expensive, and if you have a large team, the costs can add up. So consider some alternatives that are cheaper. Peanut butter, tuna, chicken, and egg salad will go further than lunch meat. You can pack cold pasta, add some frozen vegetables and a few pouches of tuna or chicken breast, and toss with a vinaigrette to provide protein (tuna or chicken), carbohydrate (pasta and vegetables), and fat (vinaigrette).

Pack snacks instead of buying them. You pay a premium for snack-size bags of cookies or crackers or individual bags of trail mix. Instead, bring a large bowl, dump in cereal and dried fruit and nuts, and put a paper cup in the bowl so athletes can grab a cupful after practice or competition.

Perhaps a team parent would be willing to make low-fat muffins or peanut butter and jelly sandwiches. If you have a cooler, you can pack low-fat chocolate milk or yogurt, which will cost less than drinks and snacks at a convenience store.

Getting Help From Families and the Booster Club

Your school or club may impose an activity fee on athletes to cover travel, uniforms, and an end-of-the-season banquet. Bring up the subject of raising the fee to pay for food for practice and competition. This does not have to be an exorbitant amount, but if each player is assessed an additional $25 you will have money for beverages and snacks for the season.

Talk with your athletes and their parents and guardians about this. For some members of your team this extra fee would be a financial hardship, so perhaps a discreet scholarship fund could be established: Some families could contribute a little more to cover food costs for athletes who don't have the money.

If your team has a booster club, it can certainly assist with money and labor to make sure your athletes are fed and hydrated. There may be parents who love to cook, whereas others may be willing to help assemble the food, serve the food, or provide rides for your team. Everyone involved with the team should have a job.

When you have your preseason team meetings, ask the parents to fill out a questionnaire to indicate

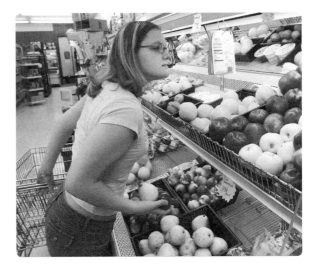

Shopping for and assembling grocery items is an inexpensive and healthy way to feed your athletes. It's also a great way to get parents involved.

how they would like to be involved. You may have a parent on your team who knows the owner of a local grocery store or a restaurant that may be willing to offer a deal on meals or food items. Another parent may be able to provide assistance through her business. If you don't ask, you are not going to know. Make the best use of your athletes' families; this is a great way for them to support their children and the team.

Brainstorm ideas on how to supply and prepare the necessary food. Consider resources such as parents, the booster club, local grocery stores, and restaurants. (Preseason Activities)

Example

John is a high school track coach in an inner-city neighborhood. Many of the kids on the team come from single-parent households and receive some type of food assistance. Although his team did well at meets, he was worried about tournaments and how these kids were going to be able to eat. He talked with the school about setting up a fund, he found local supermarkets that were willing to provide food, and some of the team parents contributed money to establish a travel fund. When the team traveled, all athletes were able to fuel well and play well regardless of their ability to pay.

In fact, John's program was so successful that other sports were able to take advantage, so the entire school sports program benefited.

Choosing Affordable (and Healthy) Chain Restaurants

Because you don't have unlimited time or financial resources to feed your athletes, cheap and fast may be the criteria you use. Unfortunately, fast food is not necessarily performance enhancing even though your athletes may love it. How can you find a happy medium? Consider buffets that have a one-price meal, but make sure that they offer a wide variety of acceptable items such as grilled or baked meats, pasta, potatoes, rice, fruits, and vegetables—not just wings and a huge dessert table. Help your overweight athletes make wise choices if you are at a buffet-type restaurant. Perhaps these athletes would be willing to forego some of the pasta or macaroni salad and have the ice cream instead. Show them all of the healthy low-calorie items and suggest that those foods take up the majority of the plate or bowl, so there is not as much room for the higher-calorie foods.

If your team tends to eat in the same places when you travel, or for a pregame meal, you may be able to negotiate a deal with the owner or manager. Keep in mind that protein is the most expensive item on the menu, so consider combination meals to keep the price down. Pasta with sauce, lasagna, ravioli, stir-fry dishes, and breakfast items are less costly than steak.

If your travel involves hotel dining, work out the cost and food details so you know what the final price will be. Streamline by offering only a few choices, and have your athletes decide ahead of time what they want to eat. This can save time and money.

The following types of restaurants will give you more options at a lower cost:

Italian

Asian

Buffet-style

Breakfast-type restaurants

Soup, salad, sandwich places

Diners

Beverages drive up the price of a meal, so when dining out, have athletes choose water. If they bring along powdered sports drinks, they can consume a drink with flavor without additional cost.

Another consideration is ordering family-style rather than individual entrees. If you have 20 athletes on your team and each orders a meal that costs US$15, you will pay US$300 not including your tax and tip. If you instead order five or six entrees for the table or large pans of a few entrees (some restaurants offer them for catering and carry-out customers) and a few salads, you will pay less money. And sharing food helps with team bonding.

Negotiating Food Budgets

If you are a collegiate coach, work with your food service or dining hall managers to develop a food budget that meets your needs and provides enough variety and tasty selections for your athletes. Take advantage of local vendors who are willing to supply snack items or beverages in exchange for recognition in the program book. Local farmers or dairy producers may be willing to provide produce and milk for postworkout snacks or may sell these items to you at reduced costs. Use one of your assistant coaches as the food broker to strike a deal.

A la carte items in a restaurant are pricey, so work with the restaurant to ensure that the final food choices are within the pre-established budget. Don't assume; check with the restaurant so you aren't surprised when the bill comes.

When traveling, if your schedule permits, take advantage of early-bird specials, which are offered by many restaurants. This may work if you have a night game or if your competition finishes in the early afternoon.

It may be cheaper to buy large items and then portion them yourself. For instance, a sub shop may charge more for two 6-inch subs than for one 12-inch sub. If so, order several 12-inch subs and have the shop cut them.

Don't forget to pack the snacks. Athletes are often hungry, and if they arrive at a restaurant starved, it will be more difficult to rein them in when they order from the menu. Provide them with something to eat right after practice or competition and even consider a mini-meal on the way to the restaurant, especially if you have to travel.

Before the season begins, sit down with your coaching staff and determine your food budget. Be sure to include snacks for both practices and competitions, along with meals while on the road. (Preseason Activities)

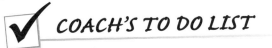

COACH'S TO DO LIST

- Don't be caught off guard when it comes to the food budget.
- Have your athletes, their parents, and the booster club pitch in to make sure that you have enough food and beverages for everyone.
- Encourage parents to get involved with meal planning for competition and preseason training camps.
- Have a budget discussion as part of your preseason meeting; consider rolling the food fee into the activity fee.
- Assign a food coach to negotiate costs with restaurants.
- Locate affordable restaurants for team travel and suggest that players supplement food while traveling by bringing breakfast and lunch items.
- Work with local grocery stores or farmers to provide food or beverages for your team without charge or at a minimal cost.
- Encourage parents and athletes to pack snacks or bring them from home for all-day competition to keep your athletes fueled and your food budget balanced.

SUMMARY

- Food can be a huge expense for a team.
- Packing food can cut down on expenses when traveling.
- Procuring coolers, thermoses, and paper products from parents can keep costs down.
- Researching lower-cost solutions for beverages, protein, and snacks will help to defray the food budget.
- Parental involvement and booster clubs can help offset food costs.
- Negotiating fees and items with restaurants can minimize expenses when traveling.
- Traveling with nonperishable food items for meals and snacks will lower eating out expenses.

GAME PLAN QUESTIONS

1. What types of food items should be part of your packing list?

2. How can you reduce food costs at restaurants?

3. How can team parents and booster clubs help with the food budget?

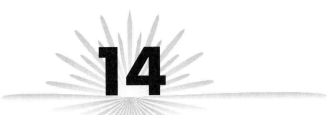

Implementing a Sport Nutrition Plan

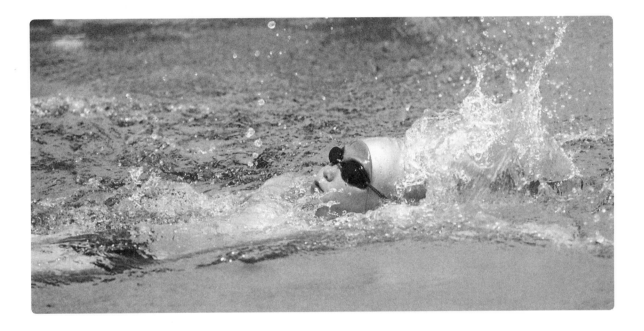

Mike is a high school swimmer with a promising future in the sport. He works hard, spending hours in the pool every day and maintaining a 4.0 GPA as well. However, his mom was concerned because he was very thin and every time he got a cold, he lost a few pounds. She brought Mike to see me and I devised a nutrition plan to help him put on a little weight. His times got better, and he stayed healthier as well.

Mike's mother asked if I would be willing to speak to his swim club. She said that the club couldn't pay me but that many of the parents asked for my number once they saw how well Mike had done. I did speak to the team and have since seen every one of the swimmers in my office.

When you finish reading this chapter, you should be able to explain how to

- create a sport nutrition game plan,
- get athletes and parents to buy into your sport nutrition game plan,
- present nutrition information in a positive way, and
- provide incentives for good nutrition.

Coaches need to spend a lot of time developing workouts, making game plans, and teaching athletes how to execute and fine-tune their technique. In addition, you need to educate athletes about fueling, hydration, injury prevention, weight management, life skills, alcohol and drug issues, and supplements. This is a full-time job often done on a part-time schedule.

To successfully accomplish the nutrition part of this job, you need to develop a **sport nutrition game plan** for your team. Here's an example of how one coach did it.

Creating a Sport Nutrition Game Plan

Coach Morrow, a high school girls' soccer coach, was very frustrated. He had many talented athletes on his team who played extremely well during the season but did poorly at postseason tournaments. The same issues kept coming up: As the season went on, players were weaker, were slower, and tired more quickly. In addition, he noticed that some of them had gotten thinner. What worried him most was that players who had been on top of their game early in the season were playing with less emotion, showing up later to practice, and not even trying.

He sat down with his team captains to get an idea of what was happening. They told him that some of the players were drinking, others were dieting, and a few had jobs in addition to practice and schoolwork and were overly tired.

Coach Morrow decided to develop a comprehensive sport nutrition plan for the following season. Soccer was a fall sport, so he decided to address some of these issues before the start of the season. He called a team meeting one week before the end of the school year. He asked each of his players to list goals that they wanted to work on over the summer. He also gave them a fueling and hydration game plan to follow over the summer (see figure 12.1 on page 177 for a sample plan).

One month before the start of the season, he contacted all of his athletes to ask how they were doing with their plan. He strongly encouraged those who had not done well to follow the plan or risk not playing at the start of the season.

One week before the start of the season, the coach sent a mailing to all of his players asking them to come prepared to every practice by doing the following:

- Drinking 20 ounces (600 ml) of fluid one hour before practice and eating something one hour before practice
- Bringing a water or sport bottle to practice
- Bringing a snack to eat after practice

He also talked with the school principal and athletic director to make sure that his team could be allowed to eat and drink something in their next-to-last period class.

He called a mandatory meeting for players and parents after the first team practice. At this meeting he presented the alcohol and substance abuse policy, which he had each student-athlete and parent sign. He also had each player complete an eating and health questionnaire and list any medications taken, including prescription and over-the-counter medications and supplements.

After reviewing the questionnaires, he was concerned with the number of players who stated they were very dissatisfied with their bodies. He arranged to have a sports dietitian and therapist talk about disordered eating so that his athletes would understand the performance-detracting effects. He invited parents to attend so they could learn what to watch for and how to best nourish their children. He also had the dietitian and therapist address players and parents separately so that both groups would feel comfortable asking questions.

Because the team had to play several schools that were three to four hours away, the coach worked with parents to establish a revolving food schedule for travel. He also reminded his athletes that he wanted them to eat and drink a little more at each meal two days before games. Parents volunteered to help by packing meals, searching out restaurants, or buying healthy snacks and drinks for the team to have on the bus as well as at tournaments.

Although this took extra time for Coach Morrow, the results were worth the effort. His team did extremely well: they won the state championship, and, best of all, the athletes felt well, played well, and stayed well throughout the season.

When you create your own sport nutrition game plan, use this checklist to guide you:

- ☐ Call a team meeting one week before the end of the season. Ask your players to list the nutrition goals they want to work on during the off-season.

- ☐ Provide an off-season fueling and hydration plan for your athletes.

- ☐ Contact your athletes one month before the start of the season to assess progress.

- ☐ Remind athletes that they may not start if they do not follow the plan.

- ☐ Send a hydration and fueling reminder to your team one week before the start of the season so that they come prepared for practice.

- ☐ Meet with your school principal and athletic director to request that your athletes be allowed to eat and drink in their next-to-last-period class.

- ☐ Call a mandatory athlete–parent team meeting after the first team practice.

- ☐ Review and have each athlete and parent sign the alcohol and substance abuse policy, supplement and medication form, and, if needed, weight contract.

- ☐ Get parents involved in supplying food and drinks.

- ☐ Have each athlete complete a nutrition questionnaire.

- ☐ Consider asking a sports dietitian and sport psychologist to address eating and body image issues with your athletes.

- ☐ Educate athletes about the effects of hydration and eating, as well as use of supplements or alcohol, on performance.

- ☐ Work with parents to develop a plan for eating on the road.

- ☐ Teach athletes how to make simple, nutritious meals.

> *Create a sport nutrition game plan. Describe that game plan with parents and athletes during the preseason meeting. (Start-Up Activities)*

Referring Athletes to a Sports Dietitian

You wouldn't send an athlete with a knee injury to an internist; you would send him to a sports medicine specialist. Likewise, when it comes to your athletes' nutritional management, you need a sports dietitian. A **sports dietitian** is a registered dietitian with an additional certification from the American Dietetic Association. He will possess the Certified Specialist in Sports Dietetics (CSSD) credential and will be identified as a Board-Certified Specialist in Sports Dietetics. A sports dietitian specializes in working with athletes on sport nutrition issues such as weight management, chronic diseases, eating disorders, and supplement education.

In some cases the fee for a sports dietitian may be covered by insurance, but often this is an out-of-pocket expense. If you have an athlete who might benefit from sitting down one-on-one

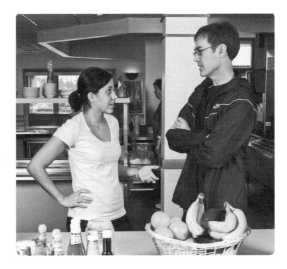

Your job as a coach is to help your athletes stay healthy and perform well. In some cases, that means referring an athlete to a qualified specialist such as a sports dietitian.

(continued)

Referring Athletes to a Sports Dietitian, *(continued)*

with a sports dietitian and the parents aren't sure they want to spend the money, suggest that they view the expense as being similar to the cost of athletic shoes or proper equipment and stress the performance-enhancing aspect of sport nutrition.

If your athletes or their parents express interest in meeting with a professional, remind them that they need to meet with someone who has expertise in both sport and nutrition. Personal trainers may give nutrition advice that is not necessarily accurate or appropriate for your athletes and may not know how to work with an athlete who has eating issues or health concerns. A registered dietitian has nutrition expertise but may not be familiar with the sport and may not be able to formulate a meal plan that fully addresses the athlete's concerns.

Talk to your booster club or the school administrator to see whether funds are available to have a sports dietitian talk to your team. You may be able to open up the presentation to other teams and share the cost or perhaps to include the entire school so that the fee is paid by the school district. At the college level, the NCAA offers speakers grants to cover the cost of health experts, including sports dietitians.

You may be able to negotiate a reduced fee with a sports dietitian for a team meeting and then offer his or her services to your individual athletes at a cost. Make sure that the parents attend the team meeting so that they can talk with the sports dietitian and schedule appointments for their student-athletes. Consider building the cost of having a sports dietitian address your athletes into the sport activity fee.

If you have an athlete with an underlying health issue such as diabetes, hypertension, eating disorder, or a weight concern, she should meet with a sports dietitian to develop a plan to stay healthy and able to participate fully in practices and competition. If the athlete cannot afford to meet with a dietitian, then the athlete's physician, school nurse, or athletic trainer should meet with her to discuss her particular health concern. Although you need to be aware of athletes' health issues, somebody else should be the primary health educator for the athletes. An athlete with an eating disorder will need to be cleared by a physician for sport participation and will need to work with a therapist, and ideally a dietitian, with expertise in eating disorders. Athletes with health issues are at increased risk of injury to themselves and potentially to teammates. In addition, if an athlete with diabetes whom you have allowed to compete becomes hypoglycemic, you may be held responsible for any complications that the athlete experiences. You cannot afford to take that chance. Explain this to the parents of athletes with special nutrition issues and reiterate that even if a visit to a professional is not covered by insurance, those issues need to be addressed to safeguard the athlete's health.

There are several ways that you can find a sports dietitian. Find out whether your local hospital has an outpatient nutrition department, and ask the chief dietitian whether a dietitian on staff can talk to your athletes. If you live near a university, find out whether it has a nutrition department and whether there is a faculty member who works with athletes. The university's department of athletics may have a sports dietitian on staff or available on a consulting basis. A sports medicine clinic, health club, spa, or Y in your area may use the services of a sports dietitian. You may be able to team up with other schools in your area to share the services of a sports dietitian to defray some of the cost.

You also can locate sports dietitians in the Yellow Pages. Look under "dietitian" instead of "nutritionist." Although many nutritionists are qualified and competent, some are not. The term *nutritionist* does not guarantee that the individual has completed coursework, has taken a registration exam, and is able to treat athletes who have medical issues. By contrast, a registered dietitian has completed the coursework in an accredited university nutrition and clinical dietetics program, has completed an internship, has passed a registration exam, and maintains continuing education status.

In addition, you can locate a sports dietitian through the American Dietetic Association or the Sports, Cardiovascular Disease, and Wellness Nutrition (SCAN) dietetic practice group of the American Dietetic Association.

The Web addresses for these organizations are as follows:

American Dietetic Association: www.eatright.org (select Find a Nutrition Professional)
SCAN: www.scandpg.org (select About Scan, then Search for a Dietitian)

Getting Athletes and Parents to Buy In

If you coach middle school and high school athletes, get parents involved. (If you are a college coach, you may need to involve your athletes' parents or guardians if athletes have health or substance abuse issues, but most likely you will not interact with parents on a regular basis.) To get both athletes and the parents on the same page, you need to be an enforcer. Insist on mandatory athlete and parent or guardian attendance at a preseason education session, and enforce consequences for absenteeism. For example, if the athlete or parent does not attend and does not make up the session, the athlete can't play. The athlete and his or her parents must realize that sport participation is a family affair. The athlete is on the team, but parents act as assistant coaches, teachers, and supporters; their role is invaluable.

At your mandatory team meeting, meet with the parents and athletes together and then with the parents separately. Emphasize that parents must support the alcohol and supplement policy. Inform them about your nutrition game plan. Ask them to let you know whether they are concerned about their child's health or weight or if they notice some change in their personality. Remind them that you will do the same. Tell parents that they must let you know about any medications, new health problems, or eating issues that may surface over the season or between seasons. Emphasize that parents should be good fans.

In your preseason meeting, make sure that every parent and athlete receives and signs off on the following forms:

Contract regarding alcohol and drug use (for athletes and, if desired, for parents too) (see figure 11.2 on page 170)

Supplement and medication form (see figure 7.2 on page 110)

Weight contract (see figure 5.8 on page 75)

Nutrition screening form (see appendix C on page 236).

Do not give these forms to your athletes ahead of time. Your athletes and parents must sign these in front of you or one of your staff. Each athlete can also turn in the preparticipation physical examination forms (see figure 14.1 for an example), completed by his or her physician, at this time.

Emphasize performance and fun, but also stress to your athletes and parents that you need to safeguard health. This is a great way to reinforce your message about making food a top priority. Make everyone aware that you have a zero-tolerance policy regarding coming to practice on empty. Put the responsibility on the athletes and parents and encourage parents to reinforce the fuel and hydration message to their children.

Involve all parents with the team in some way. If parents can't provide financial support, perhaps they can help with meal preparation, snack distribution, or transportation. Get parents involved in teaching athletes how to prepare simple meals. Perhaps you can have a team meeting at one of your athletes' homes and have everyone participate in meal preparation.

Make sure that your athletes recognize their parents at an event either at the end of the year or during the season. You could organize a weekend team brunch or weekday team dinner where the athletes prepare the food and get up to say a few words to honor their parents. Consider a weekly recognition or thank-you award printed in the school newsletter, or print the recognition on your letterhead and send it to the parent. This takes only a few minutes and means a lot to the recipient.

Plan a recognition event for parents during the season or at the end of the season to show your appreciation for their role on the sport nutrition team. (Season-Long Activities)

Presenting Nutrition Information

Present fueling and hydrating for optimal performance as positive messages. Consider posting signs around the training room and in the gym, weight room, and locker room. Here are some examples of positive messages:

- Come hydrated and ready to play.
- Fuel before you lift.
- Sit down to the plate, step up to the win.
- Eat to achieve.
- Right-size what goes into your body.
- Don't wait until it's too late—drink enough fluid, early and often.

Promote the message of "food first." Display posters of food. Make sure your athletes have access to healthy food items, such as fruit in the weight room. Allow your athletes to take fluid breaks and fueling breaks if necessary. End practice five minutes early

Preparticipation Physical Evaluation

This completed form must be kept on file by the school. This form is valid for 365 calendar days from the date of the evaluation as written on page 2.

Part 1. Student Information (to be completed by student or parent)

Student's Name: _____ Sex: _____ Age: _____ Date of Birth: _____ / _____ / _____

School: _____ Grade in School: _____ Sport(s): _____

Home Address: _____ Home Phone: (_____) _____

Name of Parent/Guardian: _____ E-mail: _____

Person to Contact in Case of Emergency: _____

Relationship to Student: _____ Home Phone: (_____) _____ Work Phone: (_____) _____ Cell Phone: (_____) _____

Personal/Family Physician: _____ City/State: _____ Office Phone: (_____) _____

Part 2. Medical History (to be completed by student or parent). Explain "yes" answers below. Circle questions you don't know answers to.

	Yes	No
1. Have you had a medical illness or injury since your last check up or sports physical?	___	___
2. Do you have an ongoing chronic illness?	___	___
3. Have you ever been hospitalized overnight?	___	___
4. Have you ever had surgery?	___	___
5. Are you currently taking any prescription or non-prescription (over-the-counter) medications or pills or using an inhaler?	___	___
6. Have you ever taken any supplements or vitamins to help you gain or lose weight or improve your performance?	___	___
7. Do you have any allergies (for example, to pollen, medicine, food or stinging insects)?	___	___
8. Have you ever had a rash or hives develop during or after exercise?	___	___
9. Have you ever passed out during or after exercise?	___	___
10. Have you ever been dizzy during or after exercise?	___	___
11. Have you ever had chest pain during or after exercise?	___	___
12. Do you get tired more quickly than your friends do during exercise?	___	___
13. Have you ever had racing of your heart or skipped heartbeats?	___	___
14. Have you had high blood pressure or high cholesterol?	___	___
15. Have you ever been told you have a heart murmur?	___	___
16. Has any family member or relative died of heart problems or sudden death before age 50?	___	___
17. Have you had a severe viral infection (for example, myocarditis or mononucleosis) within the last month?	___	___
18. Has a physician ever denied or restricted your participation in sports for any heart problems?	___	___
19. Do you have any current skin problems (for example, itching, rashes, acne, warts, fungus or blisters)?	___	___
20. Have you ever had a head injury or concussion?	___	___
21. Have you ever been knocked out, become unconscious or lost your memory?	___	___
22. Have you ever had a seizure?	___	___
23. Do you have frequent or severe headaches?	___	___
24. Have you ever had numbness or tingling in your arms, hands, legs or feet?	___	___
25. Have you ever had a stinger, burner or pinched nerve?	___	___

	Yes	No
26. Have you ever become ill from exercising in the heat?	___	___
27. Do you cough, wheeze or have trouble breathing during or after activity?	___	___
28. Do you have asthma?	___	___
29. Do you have seasonal allergies that require medical treatment?	___	___
30. Do you use any special protective or corrective equipment or devices that aren't usually used for your sport or position (for example, knee brace, special neck roll, foot orthotics, retainer on your teeth or hearing aid)?	___	___
31. Have you had any problems with your eyes or vision?	___	___
32. Do you wear glasses, contacts or protective eyewear?	___	___
33. Have you ever had a sprain, strain or swelling after injury?	___	___
34. Have you broken or fractured any bones or dislocated any joints?	___	___
35. Have you had any other problems with pain or swelling in muscles, tendons, bones or joints?	___	___

If yes, check appropriate blank and explain below:

___ Head	___ Elbow	___ Hip
___ Neck	___ Forearm	___ Thigh
___ Back	___ Wrist	___ Knee
___ Chest	___ Hand	___ Shin/Calf
___ Shoulder	___ Finger	___ Ankle
___ Upper Arm	___ Foot	

	Yes	No
36. Do you want to weigh more or less than you do now?	___	___
37. Do you lose weight regularly to meet weight requirements for your sport?	___	___
38. Do you feel stressed out?	___	___

39. Record the dates of your most recent immunizations (shots) for:
Tetanus: _____ Measles: _____
Hepatitus B: _____ Chickenpox: _____

FEMALES ONLY (optional)
40. When was your first menstrual period? _____
41. When was your most recent menstrual period? _____
42. How much time do you usually have from the start of one period to the start of another? _____
43. How many periods have you had in the last year? _____
44. What was the longest time between periods in the last year? _____

Explain "Yes" answers here: _____
_____
_____

We hereby state, to the best of our knowledge, that our answers to the above questions are complete and correct.

Signature of Student: _____ Date: ___ / ___ / ___   Signature of Parent/Guardian: _____ Date: ___ / ___ / ___

– 1 –

FIGURE 14.1 Sample preparticipation physical exam form.

Reprinted by permission of the Florida High School Athletic Association.

Preparticipation Physical Evaluation

This completed form must be kept on file by the school. This form is valid for 365 calendar days from the date of the evaluation as written on page 2.

Part 3. Physical Examination (to be completed by licensed physician, licensed osteopathic physician, licensed chiropractic physician, licensed physician assistant or certified advanced registered nurse practitioner).

Student's Name: _____ Date of Birth: ___/___/___

Height: _____ Weight: _____ % Body Fat (optional): _____ Pulse: _____ Blood Pressure: ___/___ (___/___ , ___/___)

Visual Acuity: Right 20/_____ Left 20/_____ Corrected: Yes No Pupils: Equal _____ Unequal _____

FINDINGS	NORMAL	ABNORMAL FINDINGS	INITIALS*
MEDICAL			
1. Appearance	_____	_____	_____
2. Eyes/Ears/Nose/Throat	_____	_____	_____
3. Lymph Nodes	_____	_____	_____
4. Heart	_____	_____	_____
5. Pulses	_____	_____	_____
6. Lungs	_____	_____	_____
7. Abdomen	_____	_____	_____
8. Genitalia (males only)	_____	_____	_____
9. Skin	_____	_____	_____
MUSCULOSKELETAL			
10. Neck	_____	_____	_____
11. Back	_____	_____	_____
12. Shoulder/Arm	_____	_____	_____
13. Elbow/Forearm	_____	_____	_____
14. Wrist/Hand	_____	_____	_____
15. Hip/Thigh	_____	_____	_____
16. Knee	_____	_____	_____
17. Leg/Ankle	_____	_____	_____
18. Foot	_____	_____	_____

* – station-based examination only

ASSESSMENT OF EXAMINING PHYSICIAN/PHYSICIAN ASSISTANT/NURSE PRACTITIONER

I hereby certify that each examination listed above was performed by myself or an individual under my direct supervision with the following conclusion(s):

_____ Cleared without limitation

_____ Not cleared for: _____ Reason: _____

_____ Cleared after completing evaluation/rehabilitation for: _____

_____ Referred to _____ For: _____

Recommendations: _____

Name of Physician/Physician Assistant/Nurse Practitioner (print): _____ Date: ___/___/___

Address: _____

Signature of Physician/Physician Assistant/Nurse Practitioner: _____

ASSESSMENT OF PHYSICIAN TO WHOM REFERRED (if applicable)

I hereby certify that the examination(s) for which referred was/were performed by myself or an individual under my direct supervision with the following conclusion(s):

_____ Cleared without limitation

_____ Not cleared for: _____ Reason: _____

_____ Cleared after completing evaluation/rehabilitation for: _____

Recommendations: _____

Name of Physician (print): _____ Date: ___/___/___

Address: _____

Signature of Physician: _____

Based on recommendations developed by the American Academy of Family Physicians, American Academy of Pediatrics, American Medical Society for Sports Medicine, American Orthopaedic Society for Sports Medicine and American Osteopathic Academy for Sports Medicine.

– 2 –

FIGURE 14.1 *(continued)*

so you can see your athletes refuel after practice. Have cups available so athletes can rehydrate after workouts or games.

There is no need for you to develop new sports nutrition information. There are some great resources with information you can download and use including the following:

Gatorade Sports Science Institute: www.gssiweb.org

National Athletic Trainers' Association: www.nata.org

National Collegiate Athletic Association: www.ncaa.org

 Post signs and posters reminding athletes to eat and drink for performance. Allow your athletes to decide which phrases or messages to use. (Season-Long Activities)

Providing Incentives for Good Nutrition

Your athletes are more likely to practice good eating and hydrating habits if you not only constantly reinforce the importance of doing so but also provide some motivation for them until these habits become routine. Praise those athletes who "do it right" in terms of hydrating and fueling. If you have an athlete on your team who has successfully altered body composition because he gained or lost weight, compliment him on a job well done. Emphasize to other teammates that this athlete was able to make changes to accomplish his goals without compromising performance. The purpose of this praise is not to tell teammates that there is one way the body should look but rather to recognize the effort that the athlete put forth to change his eating habits and food choices to optimize athletic performance and health.

If you are a middle school or high school coach, consider putting a few lines about your athletes in the school newsletter. Allow athletes who take care of their bodies to choose the meal when the team travels. Work with food service to get them to name an entree after a healthy, successful athlete and serve it in the school cafeteria. Allow those who have done well to be first in line for lunch. Set up a rewards program whereby your athletes can accumulate points for being nutrition stars and redeem these points for a meal or athletic gear.

If you are a collegiate coach, try different incentives. Highlight exceptional athletes on your athletic

Design an incentive program to encourage athletes to eat and drink properly. (Start-Up Activities)

department Web site. Perhaps allow athletes who have worked hard on improving their bodies to leave practice a little early or come a little later to conditioning. Consider a point system, whereby athletes accumulate points for meeting their goals for hydration, recovery, energy, or body composition. The athletes can then redeem these points for tickets to a university-sponsored event such as a concert, for meal or food points on their meal plan, or for a rest day. If you make nutrition fun, you'll make it more worthwhile for your athletes, and they'll be more likely to practice what you preach.

A Final Word

To make sure that your athletes are doing all they need to do to prepare for practice and competition, you need to have a performance plan in place. Take the time to develop a comprehensive nutrition plan to address hydration, pregame meals, pre- and postpractice eating strategies, travel eating, weight management, disordered eating, and supplement and alcohol use policies.

To be successful over a season, your athletes need to play hard, have enough energy, and finish strong. Take advantage of resources in your community or find written and online materials. Challenge your athletes to step up to the plate to become nutrition superstars. At the middle and high school levels, make their parents or guardians part of the team to provide support, labor, and assistance when needed. What you teach your athletes about fueling their bodies the right way and about behaviors and items that detract from performance will stay with them the rest of their lives, even when they no longer play team sports. As a mentor, educator, facilitator, and nurturer, you make a difference.

The following Web sites offer useful information and reproducible handouts.

General sport nutrition information

American Dietetic Association: www.eatright.org

SCAN: www.scandpg.org

American College of Sports Medicine: www.acsm.org

National Athletic Trainers' Association: www.nata.org

National Collegiate Athletic Association: www.ncaa.org

Gatorade Sports Science Institute: www.gssiweb.org

Dairy Management Institute: www.drink-milk.com

Australian Institute of Sport: www.ais.org.au/nutrition

National Federation of State High School Associations: www.nfhs.org

Weight issues

ADA: www.eatright.org

SCAN: www.scandpg.org

Weight Control Information Network: http://win.niddk.nih.gov

National Dairy Council: www.nationaldairycouncil.org

Supplements

SCAN: www.scandpg.org

NATA: www.nata.org

NCAA: www.ncaa.org

National Federation of State High School Associations: www.nfhs.org

Australian Institute of Sport: www.ais.org.au/nutrition

ATLAS and ATHENA: www.ohsu.edu

RESOURCES

Clark N. *Sports Nutrition Guidebook*. 4th ed. Champaign, IL: Human Kinetics; 2008.

Dunford M, ed. *Sports Nutrition: A Practice Manual for Professionals*. 4th ed. Chicago: American Dietetic Association; 2006.

Training and Conditioning Journal, Momentum Media Publishing, www.momentummedia.com

SUMMARY

- Create and implement a sport nutrition game plan that spells out not only what athletes should eat and drink but when.
- Expect athletes to follow your plan during the off-season and remind them that there will be consequences for noncompliance.
- Investigate local hospitals, fitness centers, or universities to find a sports dietitian. This person can be a valuable resource to your team or to individual athletes.
- Get athletes and parents to buy into your nutrition policy by holding mandatory team meetings.
- Before the start of the season, be sure you have a file on every athlete that includes a completed preparticipation examination form, drug and alcohol contract, supplement form, and weight contract.
- Get all parents involved with the team.
- Post positive messages in the training room, gym, weight room, and locker room that reinforce proper fueling and hydration for sport.
- Reward athletes who take care of their bodies through eating and hydrating appropriately.

KEY TERMS

sports dietitian   sport nutrition game plan

GAME PLAN QUESTIONS

1. What are the differences between a dietitian, a nutritionist, and a sports dietitian?

2. Where can you find reliable sport nutrition information?

3. What can you do to get your athletes and parents to buy into your sport nutrition plan?

APPENDIX A

Restaurant Dining Guidelines

Applebees

Weight Watchers meals
Teriyaki steak and chicken and shrimp
Tilapia
Chicken quesadilla
Baja chicken roll-up
Sizzling chicken
Low-fat veggie quesadilla

Au Bon Pain

Southwest vegetable soup
Mediterranean pepper soup
Charbroiled salmon filet salad
Fields and feta wrap
Smoked turkey wrap
Thai chicken salad
Tuna garden salad with light vinaigrette
Thai chicken sandwich
Arizona chicken salad

Limit These Items Because of Calories and Fat

Soup bread bowl
Cheese on sandwiches

Burger King

Hamburger
Grilled chicken sandwich
Side salad (Choose light dressings instead of the regular
    ones, which are higher in fat and calories)

Limit Because of Calories and Fat

Whopper

Cheesecake Factory

Weight management salads
Cajun jambalaya over rice
Jamaican black peppercorn shrimp
Miso salmon

Limit Because of Calories and Fat

Cheesecake (share with a friend!)

Chick-Fil-A

Grilled sandwiches
Wraps
Carrot and raisin salad
Fruit
Chicken soup
Side salads
Small Ice Dream

Limit Because of Calories and Fat

Fried chicken
Chicken strips

Chipotle

Black beans
Chicken or steak fajitas

Limit Because of Calories and Fat

Guacamole
Sour cream
Cheese
Chips

KFC

Original recipe wing and leg
Honey BBQ chicken sandwich
Baked beans
Corn
Mashed potatoes without gravy
Green beans

Limit Because of Calories and Fat

Extracrispy chicken breast
Biscuits
Gravy

McDonald's

Egg McMuffin
Scrambled egg burrito
Grilled chicken salad with light dressing
Grilled chicken sandwich with mustard or honey
    mustard

Grilled chicken wrap with lots of vegetables, light on the
  sauces
Medium fries
Small order of nuggets with BBQ sauce instead of ranch
California cobb salad with low-fat balsamic vinaigrette

Limit Because of Calories and Fat

Big Mac
Quarter Pounder
Large fries

Outback

Grilled shrimp on the BBQ
Filet
Sautéed mushrooms
Rib eye steak
Outback special steak

Limit Because of Calories and Fat

Bloomin Onion
Prime rib
Porterhouse steak

Panera

Smoked turkey breast sandwich
Smoked ham and Swiss cheese sandwich
Turkey fresco
Mediterranean veggie
Sierra turkey
Chicken salad on nine-grain bread
Asian sesame chicken salad
Grilled chicken Caesar salad
Moroccan tomato lentil soup
Gumbo
Santa Fe roasted corn soup
Mesa bean and vegetable soup
Chicken noodle soup
Savory vegetable bean soup
Garden vegetable soup
Vegetarian baked bean soup

Quiznos

Small turkey light
Small honey bourbon chicken

Subway

Chicken teriyaki or barbecued chicken sandwich
Wheat, honey oat, or deli-style roll or low-
  carbohydrate wraps
Soups: minestrone, roasted chicken noodle, Spanish
  style chicken with rice, tomato garden vegetable with
  rotini, vegetable beef

Limit Because of Calories and Fat

Tuna salad
Cheese
Potato chips
Regular salad dressings

Taco Bell

Soft chicken taco
Soft beef taco
Fresco-style ranchero chicken soft tacos
Fresco-style grilled steak soft tacos
Fresco-style bean burrito
Fresco-style chicken burrito supreme
Fiesta chicken burrito
Steak fiesta burrito

Limit Because of Calories and Fat

Chalupas
Chimichangas
Double Stuft anything!

Wendy's

Grilled burger, no cheese, with side salad
Ultimate chicken grill sandwich
Chili and one half of a potato
Crispy chicken sandwich without mayonnaise
Potato with chili, broccoli, low-fat sour cream, chives
Roasted turkey and basil pesto frescata
Low-fat chocolate milk instead of a frosty
Chicken Oriental or Mandarin chicken salad, use half of
  the dressing

Chinese

Choose more	*Choose Less*
Lemon chicken	General Tsao's
Hunan dishes	Sweet and sour
Szechuan dishes	Ribs
Moo Shu dishes	Egg rolls or spring
Steamed dumplings	rolls
Egg drop soup	Fried rice
Hot and sour soup	Lo Mein
Fortune cookies	

Italian

Choose more	*Choose less*
Chicken cacciatore	Alfredo
Pasta with marinara	Sausage and
or meat sauce	pepperoni
Lasagna	Stuffed shells
Bread (try to limit	Garlic or cheese bread
amount eaten)	

Japanese

Choose more	*Choose less*
Edamame	Tempura
Miso soup	Rolls with mayonnaise
Maki sushi	
Sashimi	
Teriyaki	
Sukiyaki	

Pizza

Limit to two slices and have a salad or soup with the pizza

Choose more

Hand-tossed cheese—half the cheese
Pizza Hut—thin and crispy cheese
Hand-tossed with vegetables
Papa John's original crust garden special
Thin and crispy or hand-tossed chicken supreme
Thin crust or hand-tossed with ham

Choose less

Pepperoni
Sausage
Extra cheese
Stuffed
Deep dish
Wings
Garlic bread
Cheese bread
Cheese sticks
Bread sticks

Bars

Watch

Wings—each wing is 100 to 150 calories, and no one eats just one.
Blue cheese or ranch dressing adds more calories.
Cheese poppers
Fried cheese sticks
Fried shrimp
Chips
Fries

APPENDIX B

Performance Eating Handouts

Performance Eating for Endurance Sports
(Cross Country, Distance Swimming, Distance Cycling, Triathlon)

Drink Enough Fluids

A loss of as little as 2 percent of body weight caused by dehydration can increase fatigue and impair performance! Athletes who drink enough fluid can practice or perform up to 33 percent longer than those who don't drink enough.

Consume at least 90 ounces (2.7 L) of fluid daily. That's 11 cups (8 oz, or 240 ml, per cup) for females, 15 cups for males.

All fluids except alcohol count: coffee, tea, milk, juice, water, soda, and sports drinks as well as fruits, vegetables, soups, gelatin, and fruit ices. If you need extra calories, choose beverages such as juice, milk, and sports drinks. Limit soda consumption around the time of exercise because carbonated beverages take longer to empty from the stomach. Alcohol is a diuretic, which will take fluid away from the body. It can delay recovery from exercise and from injury.

Drink whenever you're dehydrated. You know you are dehydrated if you experience any of the following:

Noticeable thirst	Nausea
Muscle cramps	Fatigue
Weakness	Burning in stomach
Impaired performance	Dry mouth
Headache	Dizziness or lightheadedness

During the Day
Drink

- 16 to 20 ounces (480-600 ml) of fluid within one hour of waking up,
- 20 ounces of fluid with every meal, and
- 16 to 20 ounces with every snack.

For Exercise
Start exercise with some fluid already in your stomach. Drink 20 ounces (600 ml) an hour before exercise—either water or sports drink—and if you haven't eaten before practice or conditioning, choose a sports drink instead of water for the carbohydrate content.

During exercise drink 14 to 40 ounces (415 ml to 1.2 L) of fluid per hour of exercise. (If you are a light sweater, drink 14 ounces of fluid per hour; if you are a heavy sweater, drink about 40 ounces of fluid per hour.)

From L. Bonci, 2009, *Sport Nutrition for Coaches* (Champaign, IL: Human Kinetics).

Calculate your hourly sweat rate so you know how much fluid you need to drink per hour:

1. Weigh yourself before and after exercise. Wear as little clothing as possible while weighing.

2. Subtract your postexercise weight from your pre-exercise weight and then convert it to ounces. For example, there are 16 ounces (500 g) in a pound, so if you lose 2 pounds during exercise, you have lost 32 ounces (2 × 16), or 1 kilogram.

3. Add the number of ounces or milliliters of fluid you consumed during practice.

4. Divide the sum of the amount of fluid lost plus amount of fluid consumed by the number of hours you exercised to get your hourly sweat rate.

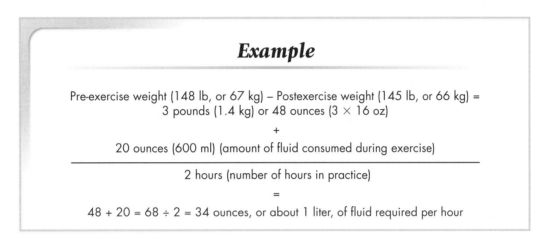

Example

Pre-exercise weight (148 lb, or 67 kg) – Postexercise weight (145 lb, or 66 kg) =
3 pounds (1.4 kg) or 48 ounces (3 × 16 oz)

+

20 ounces (600 ml) (amount of fluid consumed during exercise)

_____

2 hours (number of hours in practice)

=

48 + 20 = 68 ÷ 2 = 34 ounces, or about 1 liter, of fluid required per hour

When you consume fluid during exercise, remember these tips:

- Gulp, don't sip.
- Swallow fluids, don't spit.
- Drink, don't pour on your head.
- Do not overdrink (don't drink more than what your individual sweat rate calculation suggests).

During exercise, drinking sports drinks may be better than drinking water. You may need to experiment with a sports drink to find the one that works for you, but be careful with energy drinks. Drinks such as Red Bull, Amp, Lizard Fuel, Monster, and Rockstar are high in carbohydrate, which can delay the fluid from leaving your stomach so the fluid is not in your muscles. Also, the caffeine content of some of these beverages is high. The caffeine can make you feel nervous or jittery before events and can have a laxative effect.

After exercise, drink enough fluid to make up any loss in weight you have. Drink 24 ounces (700 ml) of fluid for every pound you lose during exercise.

Assess your hydration the next morning after exercise:

- Did your body weight return to baseline?
- Does your urine look more like lemonade than apple juice?
- Did your thirst subside?

If you answer no to any one of these questions, you need to drink more fluid.

Eat Small Meals Often

Eat within one hour of waking up. You need to eat breakfast or your body plays catch-up all day, which means you are tired during practice as well as in class or at work.

Try to eat small meals every four hours. Eat 17 to 22 calories per pound, or 37 to 48 kilo-calories per kilogram, of body weight if you are a female; 20 to 27 calories per pound, or 44 to 59 kilocalories per kilogram, of body weight if you are a male.

Eat Carbohydrate-Containing Foods for Energy

Two thirds of what's on your plate at each meal or snack should be carbohydrate-containing foods to fuel your muscles and brain during activity.

Good sources of carbohydrate include these:

Bread	Bagels	Pasta	Fruit	Vegetables
Barley	Potatoes	Corn	Pretzels	Tortillas
Juice	Crackers	Rice	Quinoa	

Try to limit these:

Pastries	Chips	Cookies	Pretzels	Fruit drinks
Soda	Ice cream	Crackers	Bagels	Juice
	French fries		Candy	

These foods contain carbohydrate but also have high amounts of fat and sugar, so eat them at nonexercise times of the day if you need extra calories.

Eat Protein for Muscle Growth and a Healthy Immune System

Although protein is not used as a fuel source for exercise, you need protein for muscle growth and repair and to support a healthy immune system. Your body needs both carbohydrate and protein to build new muscle. A third of what's on your plate at every meal and snack should be protein.

Minimum number of grams of protein a day:

.6 × body weight in pounds, or 1.3 grams × body weight in kilograms

Maximum number of grams of protein a day:

.9 × body weight in pounds, or 2 × body weight in kilograms

Include some protein as part of every meal and snack:

Eggs	Beef	Nuts	Yogurt	Reduced-fat cheeses
Chicken	Pork	Tofu	Low-fat milk	Fish and shellfish
Turkey	Jerky	Bean dip	Peanut butter	Baked beans

Try to limit these:

Bacon	Sausage	Pepperoni	Whole milk	Full-fat cheeses
Hot dogs	Fried meats			

Although these foods do contain protein, they are also high in fat and especially saturated fat, which is not healthy for the body.

Eat Fat as an Essential Fuel for Exercise

Fat is a fuel source for endurance exercise, so you need to include some fat as part of every meal and snack. Good sources of fat include these:

Nuts	Mayonnaise	Pesto	Olive oil	Safflower oil
Seeds	Nut butters	Olives	Canola oil	Sunflower oil
Guacamole	Avocados	Corn oil	Soybean oil	Soft margarines

From L. Bonci, 2009, *Sport Nutrition for Coaches* (Champaign, IL: Human Kinetics).

Try to limit these:

Creamy sauces	Cream cheese	Lard Butter	Sour cream Shortening	Stick margarines Creamy dressings

These foods are sources of fat but primarily of saturated or trans fats, which are not healthy for the body.

Limit the amount of fatty foods you eat before exercise, because they can upset your gut!

Add Salt If Necessary

Do you have salty sweat or salty residue on your skin or clothes after a workout or a tendency to develop muscle cramps? Then you may be a salty sweater. If so, you need to take in more salt. Here are some ways to add salt to your diet:

- Eat salty foods such as pickles and pretzels.
- Use salt, soy sauce, or Worcestershire sauce.
- Use sports drinks instead of water to provide sodium and help replace what is lost through sweating.
- Consider adding salt to a sports drink: Add 1/4 teaspoon of salt to 20 ounces (600 ml) of sports drink or 1/2 teaspoon of salt to 32 ounces (1 L) of sports drink.

Food Supplements

These are the best supplements to use for your sport:

- Sports drinks
- Sports bars that have more carbohydrate than protein
- Carbohydrate boosters such as gels, Clif shots, honey, honey wands, and sports beans
- High-carbohydrate sports drinks for use before or after exercise
- Sports drinks with protein for longer-duration exercise (more than two hours)

Eating, Drinking, and Exercise

Follow these guidelines when planning your daily routine.

One Hour Before Practice or Competition

Have a 20-ounce (600 ml) sports drink with a small amount of carbohydrate-containing food, such as a handful of pretzels or cereal or a granola bar.

During Practice or Competition

Take in 30 to 60 grams of carbohydrate per hour by consuming foods such as 32 ounces (1 L) of sports drink, one or two gels or honey packets, or four honey sticks. Drink enough fluid per hour based on your sweat rate.

After Practice or Competition

Drink enough to replace sweat losses. Eat or drink something with calories within 15 minutes of practice or play, such as the following:

- Two large handfuls of pretzels, crackers, or cereal
- Two large handfuls of trail mix
- Two high-carbohydrate sports bars
- A piece of fruit and a large handful of pretzels
- Two granola bars

If you are a salty sweater, choose pretzels, crackers, Chex mix, and sports drink after practice instead of sweet items.

From L. Bonci, 2009, *Sport Nutrition for Coaches* (Champaign, IL: Human Kinetics).

Sample Daily Menu

Breakfast

Men

- 1 1/2 cups (260 g) oatmeal with 1/4 cup nuts (35 g), 1/4 cup dried fruit or a large banana, and 8 ounces (240 ml) low-fat milk
- 12 ounces (360 ml) milk or 8 ounces (230) yogurt
- Two slices of toast or a bagel with peanut butter and jelly or a small amount of butter and jelly
- 8 ounces (240 ml) juice

Women

- 1/2 cup (120 g) oatmeal with 2 tbsp each nuts and dried fruit and 4 ounces (120 ml) low-fat milk
- 8 ounces (240 ml) skim milk or 6 ounces (170 g) low-fat yogurt
- A slice of toast with a teaspoon each of butter and jelly or 1 tbsp peanut butter and 1 tsp jelly
- 8 ounces (240 ml) water

Lunch

Men

- Sandwich on a roll or bagel: five slices of meat, two slices of cheese
- 1 to 2 tbsp of spread such as mayonnaise, salad dressing, pesto, or guacamole
- Piece of fruit
- Two large handfuls of crackers, pretzels, or baked chips and two granola bars or a low-fat muffin
- 12 ounces (360 ml) milk, juice, or lemonade and 12 ounces (360 ml) water

Women

- Sandwich on two slices of bread or a bagel: three slices of meat, one slice of cheese
- 1 tbsp of spread such as mayonnaise, salad dressing, pesto, or guacamole
- Small piece of fruit
- One handful of pretzels, crackers, or baked chips, or one granola or cereal bar
- 8 ounces (240 ml) milk, juice, or lemonade and 12 ounces (360 ml) water

Dinner

Men

- 8 ounces (225 g) lean meat, poultry, or fish
- 2 cups pasta, rice, or potatoes with some fat added
- A slice of bread or a roll with 1 to 2 teaspoons butter or margarine
- 2 cups vegetables, either cooked or in a salad with salad dressing
- 1 1/2 cups (200 g) reduced-fat ice cream, pudding, frozen yogurt, sherbet, or sorbet
- 12 ounces (360 ml) milk, juice, or lemonade and 8 ounces (240 ml) water

From L. Bonci, 2009, *Sport Nutrition for Coaches* (Champaign, IL: Human Kinetics).

Women

- 5 to 6 ounces (140-170 g) lean meat, poultry, or fish
- 1 cup pasta, rice, or potatoes, with some fat added
- 1 1/2 cups vegetables with some fat added
- 1 cup (130 g) low-fat ice cream, pudding, frozen yogurt, or sorbet
- 8 ounces (240 ml) milk, juice, or lemonade and 12 ounces (360 ml) water

Evening Snack

Men

- 2 cups (60 g) cereal (1 1/2 cups [45 g] flake-type cereal and 1/2 cup [15 g] granola) with 1 cup fruit and 8 ounces (240 ml) low-fat milk
- 20 ounces (600 ml) water

Women

- 1 cup (30 g) cereal (3/4 cup [22 g] flake-type and 1/4 cup [8 g] granola) with 1/2 cup fruit and 6 ounces (180 ml) low-fat milk
- 20 ounces (600 ml) water

From L. Bonci, 2009, *Sport Nutrition for Coaches* (Champaign, IL: Human Kinetics).

Performance Eating for Football

Drink Enough Fluids

A loss of as little as 2 percent of body weight caused by dehydration can increase fatigue and impair performance! Athletes who drink enough fluid can practice or perform up to 33 percent longer than those who don't drink enough.

Consume at least 125 ounces (4 L) of fluid daily. That's 15 cups (8 oz, or 240 ml, per cup).

All fluids except alcohol count: coffee, tea, milk, juice, water, soda, and sports drinks as well as fruits, vegetables, soups, gelatin, and fruit ices. If you need to put on mass, choose fluids with calories such as milk, juice, sports drinks, and lemonade. If you are trying to decrease body fat, stick with low-fat milk, lower sugar sports drinks, artificially sweetened beverages and of course water. Limit soda consumption around the time of exercise, because carbonated beverages take longer to empty from the stomach, delaying hydration. And remember that alcohol is a diuretic, which will take fluid away from the body. It can delay recovery from exercise and from injury. It also has a lot of calories and can increase your appetite.

Drink whenever you're dehydrated. You know you are dehydrated if you experience any of the following:

Noticeable thirst	Nausea
Muscle cramps	Fatigue
Weakness	Burning in stomach
Impaired performance	Dry mouth
Headache	Dizziness or lightheadedness

During the Day

Drink

- 16 to 20 ounces (480-600 ml) of fluid within one hour of waking up,
- 20 ounces of fluid with every meal, and
- 16 to 20 ounces with every snack.

For Exercise

Start with some fluid already in your stomach. Drink 20 ounces (600 ml) an hour before exercise—either water or sports drink—and if you haven't eaten before practice or conditioning, choose a sports drink instead of water for the carbohydrate content.

During exercise drink 20 to 40 ounces (600 ml to 1.2 L) of fluid per hour of exercise. (If you are a light sweater, drink 20 ounces of fluid per hour; if you are a heavy sweater, drink about 40 ounces of fluid per hour.)

Calculate your hourly sweat rate so you know how much fluid you need to drink per hour:

1. Weigh yourself before and after exercise. Wear as little clothing as possible while weighing.

2. Subtract your postexercise weight from your pre-exercise weight, then convert it to ounces (grams). For example, there are 16 ounces (500 g) in a pound, so if you lose 2 pounds during exercise, you have lost 32 ounces (2 × 16), or 1 kilogram.

3. Add the number of ounces or milliliters of fluid you consumed during practice.

4. Divide the sum of the amount of fluid lost plus amount consumed by the number of hours you exercised to get your hourly sweat rate.

From L. Bonci, 2009, *Sport Nutrition for Coaches* (Champaign, IL: Human Kinetics).

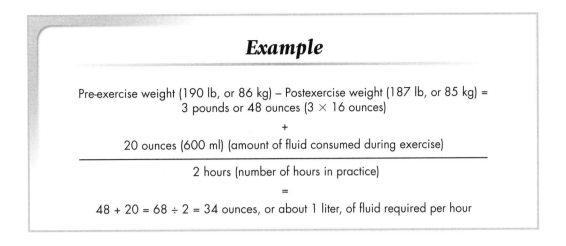

Example

Pre-exercise weight (190 lb, or 86 kg) − Postexercise weight (187 lb, or 85 kg) =
3 pounds or 48 ounces (3 × 16 ounces)

+

20 ounces (600 ml) (amount of fluid consumed during exercise)

_____

2 hours (number of hours in practice)

=

48 + 20 = 68 ÷ 2 = 34 ounces, or about 1 liter, of fluid required per hour

When you consume fluid during exercise, remember these tips:

- Gulp, don't sip.
- Swallow fluids, don't spit.
- Drink, don't pour on your head.
- Do not overdrink (don't drink more than what your individual sweat rate calculation suggests).

During exercise, drinking sports drinks may be better than drinking water. If you are concerned about the calories, pick a reduced-sugar sports drink to get the benefit of the sodium with fewer calories. Be careful with energy drinks. Red Bull, Amp, Lizard Fuel, Monster, and Rockstar are high in carbohydrate, which can delay the fluid from leaving your stomach so the fluid is not in your muscles. The caffeine content of some of these beverages is high, which can make you feel jittery and nervous. And they do not contain sodium, which is important for those of you who are salty sweaters.

After exercise, drink enough fluid to make up any loss in weight you have. Drink 24 ounces (700 ml) of fluid for every pound you lose during exercise.

Assess your hydration the next morning after exercise:

- Did your body weight return to baseline?
- Does your urine look more like lemonade than apple juice?
- Did your thirst subside?

If you answer no to any of these questions, you need to drink more fluid.

Eat More Frequently Throughout the Day

Eat within one hour of waking up. You need to eat breakfast or your body plays catch-up all day, which means you are tired during practice as well as in class or at work.

Try to eat something every four hours, but don't load up on snack foods. The goal is smaller meals every four hours. Eat 20 to 25 calories per pound (.45 kg) of body weight.

Eat Carbohydrate-Containing Foods for Energy

Football is a game of strength, speed, and stamina so you need to eat enough carbohydrate to fuel your muscles and brain during activity. Two thirds of what's on your plate at each meal or snack should be carbohydrate-containing foods.

Good sources of carbohydrate include these:

Bread	Bagels	Pasta	Fruit	Vegetables
Barley	Potatoes	Corn	Pretzels	Tortillas
Juice	Crackers	Rice	Quinoa	

From L. Bonci, 2009, *Sport Nutrition for Coaches* (Champaign, IL: Human Kinetics).

Try to limit these:

Pastries	Chips	Cookies	Pretzels	Fruit drinks
Soda	Ice cream	Crackers	Bagels	Juice
	French fries		Candy	

These foods contain carbohydrate but also have high amounts of fat and sugar.

Eat Protein for Muscle Growth and a Healthy Immune System

A third of what's on your plate at every meal and snack should be protein.

Your body needs both carbohydrate and protein to build new muscle. Don't eat protein to the exclusion of all else, because if you are eating too much protein you probably aren't eating enough carbohydrate.

Minimum number of grams of protein a day:

.6 × body weight in pounds, or 1.3 grams × body weight in kilograms

Maximum number of grams of protein a day:

.9 × body weight in pounds, or 2 × body weight in kilograms

Include some protein as part of every meal and snack:

Eggs	Beef	Nuts	Yogurt	Reduced-fat cheeses
Chicken	Pork	Tofu	Low-fat milk	Fish and shellfish
Turkey	Jerky	Bean dip	Peanut butter	Baked beans

Try to limit these:

Bacon	Sausage	Pepperoni	Whole milk	Full-fat cheeses
Hot dogs	Fried meats			

Although these foods do contain protein, they are also high in fat and especially saturated fat, which is not healthy for the body.

Eat Fat as an Essential Fuel for Exercise

Include some fat as part of every meal and snack
Good sources of fat include these:

Nuts	Mayonnaise	Pesto	Olive oil	Safflower oil
Seeds	Nut butters	Olives	Canola oil	Sunflower oil
Guacamole	Avocados	Corn oil	Soybean oil	Soft margarines

Try to limit these:

Creamy	Cream	Lard	Sour cream	Stick margarines
sauces	cheese	Butter	Shortening	Creamy dressings

These foods are sources of fat but primarily of saturated or trans fats, which are not healthy for the body.

Limit the amount of fatty foods you eat before exercise, because they can upset your gut!

From L. Bonci, 2009, *Sport Nutrition for Coaches* (Champaign, IL: Human Kinetics).

Add Salt If Necessary

Do you have salty sweat or salty residue on your skin or clothes after a workout or a tendency to develop muscle cramps? Then you may be a salty sweater. If so, you need to take in more salt. Here are some ways to add salt to your diet:

- Eat salty foods such as pickles and pretzels.
- Use salt, soy sauce, or Worcestershire sauce.
- Use sports drinks instead of water to provide sodium and help replace what is lost through sweating.
- Consider adding salt to a sports drink: Add 1/4 teaspoon of salt to 20 ounces (600 ml) of sports drink or 1/2 teaspoon of salt to 32 ounces (1 L) of sports drink.

Food Supplements

These are the best supplements to use for your sport:

- Sports drinks
- Low-sugar sports drinks
- Protein isolate
- Sports bars with at least 40 percent carbohydrate

Eating, Drinking, and Exercise

Follow these guidelines when planning your daily routine.

One Hour Before Practice or Competition

Drink 20 ounces (600 ml) of sports drink or 20 ounces of water along with a small amount of carbohydrate, such as a handful of pretzels or cereal or a granola bar. Include some protein such as 1/4 cup (35 g) nuts, a few pieces of jerky, or 8 ounces (230 g) low-fat yogurt.

If you don't want to eat anything solid, have 20 ounces (600 ml) of sports drink and a yogurt, or 12 ounces (360 ml) of low-fat chocolate milk and 8 ounces (240 ml) of water.

During Practice or Competition

Drink enough fluid per hour based on your sweat rate. Alternate between sports drinks and water.

After Practice or Competition

Drink enough to replace sweat losses. Eat or drink something with calories within 15 minutes of practice or play, such as the following:

- A peanut butter sandwich
- Two large handfuls of trail mix
- A high-carbohydrate sports bar (300-400 calories)
- A few pieces of jerky and a handful of pretzels

If you are a salty sweater, drink sports drinks and eat salty foods instead of sweet items.

From L. Bonci, 2009, *Sport Nutrition for Coaches* (Champaign, IL: Human Kinetics).

Sample Daily Menu

Breakfast

- Three eggs
- Two slices of whole-grain toast with butter or margarine
- A slice of ham
- 12 ounces (360 ml) low-fat milk or 8 ounces (230 g) yogurt
- 8 ounces (240 ml) juice + 12 ounces (360 ml) water

Lunch

- Sandwich on a hoagie roll: five slices of meat, two slices of cheese
- Piece of fruit
- Two handfuls of crackers, pretzels, or baked chips and two granola bars or a low-fat muffin
- 12 ounces (360 ml) water and 12 ounces (360 ml) milk, juice, or lemonade

Dinner

- 8 to 10 ounces (225-280 g) lean meat, poultry, or fish
- Two cups pasta, rice, or potatoes, with some fat added
- Two cups vegetables, either cooked or in a salad, with some fat added
- 2 cups (260 g) light ice cream, frozen yogurt, sherbet, sorbet, or pudding
- 12 ounces (360 ml) milk, juice, or lemonade and 8 ounces (240 ml) water

Evening Snack

- Sandwich on a whole-grain roll or bread: five slices of turkey breast, lettuce, tomato, mayonnaise
- Pickles
- A handful of baked chips or pretzels
- 20 ounces (600 ml) water

From L. Bonci, 2009, *Sport Nutrition for Coaches* (Champaign, IL: Human Kinetics).

Performance Eating for Intermittent, High-Intensity Sports
(Tennis, Volleyball, Track and Field, Crew, Swimming)

Drink Enough Fluids

A loss of as little as 2 percent of body weight caused by dehydration can increase fatigue and impair performance! Athletes who drink enough fluid can practice or perform up to 33 percent longer than those who don't drink enough.

Consume at least 90 ounces (2.7 L) of fluid daily. That's 11 cups (8 oz, or 240 ml, per cup) for females, 15 cups for males.

All fluids (except alcohol) count: coffee, tea, milk, juice, water, soda, and sports drinks as well as fruits, vegetables, soups, gelatin, and fruit ices. Alcohol is a diuretic, which will take fluid away from the body. It can delay recovery from exercise and from injury.

Drink whenever you're dehydrated. You know you are dehydrated if you experience any of the following:

Noticeable thirst	Nausea
Muscle cramps	Fatigue
Weakness	Burning in stomach
Impaired performance	Dry mouth
Headache	Dizziness or lightheadedness

During the Day

Drink

- 16 to 20 ounces (480-600 ml) of fluid within one hour of waking up,
- 20 ounces of fluid with every meal, and
- 16 to 20 ounces with every snack.

For Exercise

Start exercise with some fluid already in your stomach. Drink 20 ounces (600 ml) an hour before exercise—either water or sports drink—and if you haven't eaten before practice or conditioning, choose a sports drink instead of water for the carbohydrate content.

During exercise drink 14 to 40 ounces (415 ml to 1.2 L) of fluid per hour of exercise. (If you are a light sweater, drink 14 ounces of fluid per hour; if you are a heavy sweater, drink about 40 ounces of fluid per hour.)

Calculate your hourly sweat rate so you know how much fluid you need to drink per hour:

1. Weigh yourself before and after exercise. Wear as little clothing as possible while weighing.

2. Subtract your postexercise weight from your pre-exercise weight and then convert it to ounces. For example, there are 16 ounces (500 g) in a pound, so if you lose 2 pounds during exercise, you have lost 32 ounces (2×16), or 1 kilogram.

3. Add the number of ounces or milliliters of fluid you consumed during practice.

4. Divide the sum of the amount of fluid lost plus amount of fluid consumed by the number of hours you exercised to get your hourly sweat rate.

From L. Bonci, 2009, *Sport Nutrition for Coaches* (Champaign, IL: Human Kinetics).

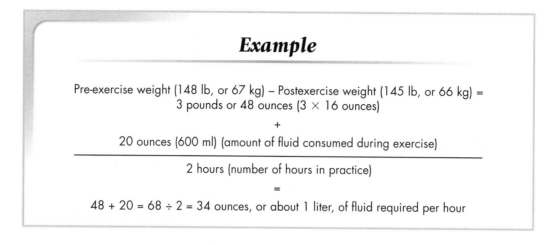

When you consume fluid during exercise, remember these tips:

- Gulp, don't sip.
- Swallow fluids, don't spit.
- Drink, don't pour on your head.
- Do not overdrink (don't drink more than what your individual sweat rate calculation suggests).

During exercise, drinking sports drinks may be better than drinking water. Be careful with energy drinks. Red Bull, Amp, Lizard Fuel, Monster, Rockstar are high in carbohydrate, which can delay the fluid from leaving your stomach so the fluid is not in your muscles. Also, the caffeine content of some of these beverages is high.

After exercise, drink enough fluid to make up any loss in weight you have. Drink 24 ounces (700 ml) of fluid for every pound you lose during exercise.

Assess your hydration the next morning after exercise:

- Did your body weight return to baseline?
- Does your urine look more like lemonade than apple juice?
- Did your thirst subside?

If you answer no to any of these questions, you need to drink more fluid.

Eat Small Meals Often

Eat within one hour of waking up. You need to eat breakfast or your body plays catch-up all day, which means you are tired during practice as well as in class or at work.

Try to eat small meals every four hours. Eat 15 to 20 calories per pound, or 33 to 44 kilo-calories per kilogram, of body weight if you are a female; 20 to 27 calories per pound, or 44 to 59 kilocalories per kilogram, of body weight if you are a male.

Eat Carbohydrate-Containing Foods for Energy

Carbohydrate is the primary fuel source for your sport, so make sure that two thirds of what's on your plate at each meal or snack contains carbohydrate to fuel your muscles and brain during activity.

Good sources of carbohydrate include these:

Bread	Bagels	Pasta	Fruit	Vegetables
Barley	Potatoes	Corn	Pretzels	Tortillas
Juice	Crackers	Rice	Quinoa	

From L. Bonci, 2009, *Sport Nutrition for Coaches* (Champaign, IL: Human Kinetics).

Try to limit these:

Pastries	Chips	Cookies	Pretzels	Fruit drinks
Soda	Ice cream	Crackers	Bagels	Juice
	French fries		Candy	

These foods contain carbohydrate but also contain high amounts of fat and sugar.

Eat Protein for Muscle Growth and a Healthy Immune System

A third of what's on your plate at every meal and snack should be protein. Your body needs both carbohydrate and protein to build new muscle. However, do not skimp on carbohydrate and load up on protein, because your performance will be impaired.

Minimum number of grams of protein a day:

$.6 \times$ body weight in pounds, or $1.3 \times$ body weight in kilograms

Maximum number of grams of protein a day:

$.9 \times$ body weight in pounds, or $2 \times$ body weight in kilograms

Include some protein as part of every meal and snack:

Eggs	Beef	Nuts	Yogurt	Reduced-fat cheeses
Chicken	Pork	Tofu	Low-fat milk	Fish and shellfish
	Jerky	Bean dip	Peanut butter	Baked beans

Try to limit these:

Bacon	Sausage	Pepperoni	Whole milk	Full-fat cheeses
Hot dogs	Fried meats			

Although these foods do contain protein, they are also high in fat and especially saturated fat, which is not healthy for the body.

Eat Fat as an Essential Part of Your Diet

Fat is not a major fuel source for high-intensity exercise but is still an essential part of your diet. Include some fat as part of every meal, but try to limit fat intake before practice and competition because it can upset your gut and delay carbohydrate from reaching your muscles.

Good sources of fat include these:

Nuts	Mayonnaise	Pesto	Olive oil	Safflower oil
Guacamole	Nut butters	Olives	Canola oil	Sunflower oil
Pesto	Avocados	Corn oil	Soybean oil	Soft margarines

Try to limit these:

Creamy	Cream	Lard	Sour cream	Stick margarines
sauces	cheese	Butter	Shortening	Creamy dressings

These foods are sources of fat but primarily of saturated or trans fats, which are not as healthy.

Before exercise, eat low-fat carbohydrate-containing foods such as bagels, cereal, and pretzels instead of muffins, granola, and chips.

Add Salt if Necessary

Do you have salty sweat or salty residue on your skin or clothes after a workout or a tendency to develop muscle cramps? Then you may be a salty sweater. If so, you need to take in more salt. Here are some ways to add salt to your diet:

- Eat salty foods such as pickles and pretzels.
- Use salt, soy sauce, or Worcestershire sauce.
- Use sports drinks instead of water to provide sodium and help replace what is lost through sweating.
- Consider adding salt to a sports drink: Add 1/4 teaspoon of salt to 20 ounces (600 ml) of sports drink or 1/2 teaspoon of salt to 32 ounces (1 L) of sports drink.

Food Supplements

These are best supplements to use for your sport:

- Sports drinks
- Sports bars that have more carbohydrate than protein
- Carbohydrate boosters such as sports gels, honey, honey sticks, and Clif Shots
- High-sodium foods and beverages if you are a salty sweater

Eating, Drinking, and Exercise

Follow these guidelines when planning your daily routine.

One Hour Before Practice or Competition

Drink 20 ounces (600 ml) of sports drink or 20 ounces of water along with a small amount of carbohydrate, such as a handful of pretzels or cereal or a low-fat granola bar. If you are a salty sweater, choose a sports drink and pretzels or low-fat crackers.

During Practice or Competition

Take in 30 grams of carbohydrate per hour by consuming foods such as 16 ounces (480 ml) of sports drink, a gel, a packet of honey, or two honey sticks. Drink enough fluid per hour based on your sweat rate.

After Practice or Play

Drink enough to replace sweat losses. Eat or drink something with calories within 15 minutes of practice or play, such as the following:

- Two handfuls of pretzels, crackers, or cereal
- Two handfuls of trail mix
- A high-carbohydrate sports bar
- A piece of fruit and a small handful of pretzels
- Two granola bars

If you are a salty sweater, eat something salty after exercise such as crackers, pretzels, or Chex mix with salted nuts. Choose a sports drink or tomato or vegetable juice instead of water.

From L. Bonci, 2009, *Sport Nutrition for Coaches* (Champaign, IL: Human Kinetics).

Sample Daily Menu

Breakfast

Men

- 1 cup (240 g) oatmeal with 1/4 cup nuts (35 g), 1/4 cup dried fruit or a large banana, and 8 ounces (240 ml) low-fat milk
- 12 ounces (360 ml) milk or 8 ounces (230 g) yogurt
- 8 ounces (240 ml) juice

Women

- 1/2 cup (120 g) oatmeal with 2 tbsp each nuts and dried fruit and 1/2 cup (120 ml) milk
- 8 ounces (240 ml) skim milk or 6 ounces (170 g) low-fat yogurt
- 8 ounces (240 ml) water

Lunch

Men

- Sandwich on a roll: five slices of meat, two slices of cheese
- Piece of fruit
- Two handfuls of crackers, pretzels, or baked chips and two granola bars or a muffin
- 12 ounces (360 ml) milk, juice, or lemonade and 12 ounces (360 ml) water

Women

- Sandwich on two slices of bread: three slices of meat, one slice of cheese
- Small piece of fruit
- One handful of pretzels, crackers, or baked chips, or a granola or cereal bar
- 8 ounces (240 ml) milk, juice, or lemonade and 12 ounces (360 ml) water

Dinner

Men

- 8 ounces (225 g) lean meat, poultry, or fish
- 2 cups of pasta, rice, or potatoes
- 2 cups of vegetables, either cooked or in a salad
- Fruit or 1 cup (130 g) low fat ice cream, pudding, frozen yogurt, sherbet, or sorbet
- 12 ounces (360 ml) milk, juice, or lemonade and 8 ounces (240 ml) water

Women

- 5 to 6 ounces (140-170 g) lean meat, poultry, or fish
- 1 cup of pasta, rice, or potatoes
- 1 1/2 cups vegetables
- Fruit or 1/2 cup (65 g) low-fat ice cream, pudding, frozen yogurt, or sorbet
- 8 ounces (240 ml) milk, juice, or lemonade and 12 ounces (360 ml) water

Evening Snack

Men

- 2 cups (60 g) cereal with 1 cup fruit and 8 ounces (240 ml) milk
- 20 ounces (600 ml) water

Women

- 1 cup (30 g) cereal with 1/2 cup of fruit and 6 ounces (180 ml) milk
- 20 ounces (600 ml) water

From L. Bonci, 2009, *Sport Nutrition for Coaches* (Champaign, IL: Human Kinetics).

Performance Eating for Weight- and Physique-Focused Sports
(Boxing, Diving, Gymnastics, Wrestling)

Drink Enough Fluids

Although you can lose weight quickly by limiting fluid intake, a loss of as little as 2 percent of body weight caused by dehydration can increase fatigue and impair performance!
There is never a reason to show up at practice or competition in a dehydrated state.

Consume at least 90 ounces (2.7 L) of fluid daily. That's 11 cups (8 oz, or 240 ml, per cup) for females, 15 cups for males.

All fluids except alcohol count: Coffee, tea, milk, juice, water, soda, and sports drinks as well as fruits, vegetables, soups, gelatin, and fruit ices. If you are trying to make weight, choose low-calorie fluids such as these:

Water
Low-sugar sports drinks
Artificially sweetened beverages
Vegetable juice
Unsweetened tea and coffee
Low-fat milk

All alcohol, even light or low-carbohydrate alcohol, acts as a diuretic, which will take fluid away from the body. Alcohol can delay recovery from exercise and from injury. It contains a lot of calories and can make you hungrier as well.

Drink whenever you're dehydrated. You know you are dehydrated if you experience any of the following:

Noticeable thirst	Nausea
Muscle cramps	Fatigue
Weakness	Burning in stomach
Impaired performance	Dry mouth
Headache	Dizziness or lightheadedness

During the Day

Drink

- 16 to 20 ounces (480-600 ml) of fluid within one hour of waking up,
- 20 ounces of low-calorie fluid with every meal, and
- 16 to 20 ounces of low-calorie fluid with every snack.

For Exercise

Start with some fluid already in your stomach. Drink 20 ounces (600 ml) an hour before exercise—either water or sports drink—and if you haven't eaten before practice or conditioning, choose a sports drink instead of water for the carbohydrate content.

During exercise drink 14 to 40 ounces (415 ml to 1.2 L) of fluid per hour of exercise. (If you are a light sweater, drink 14 ounces of fluid per hour; if you are a heavy sweater, drink about 40 ounces of fluid per hour.)

Calculate your hourly sweat rate so you know how much fluid you need to drink per hour:

1. Weigh yourself before and after exercise. Wear as little clothing as possible while weighing.

From L. Bonci, 2009, *Sport Nutrition for Coaches* (Champaign, IL: Human Kinetics).

2. Subtract your postexercise weight from your pre-exercise weight and then convert it to ounces. For example, there are 16 ounces (500 g) in a pound, so if you lose 2 pounds during exercise, you have lost 32 ounces (2 × 16), or 1 kilogram.

3. Add the number of ounces or milliliters of fluid you consumed during practice.

4. Divide the sum of the amount of fluid lost plus the amount of fluid consumed by the number of hours you exercised to get your hourly sweat rate.

When you consume fluid during exercise, remember these tips:

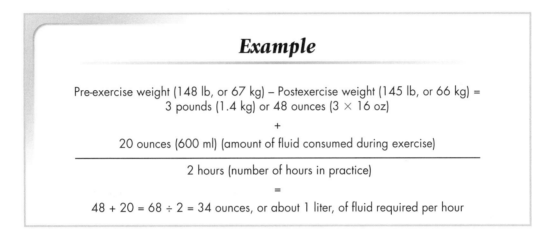

Example

Pre-exercise weight (148 lb, or 67 kg) – Postexercise weight (145 lb, or 66 kg) =
3 pounds (1.4 kg) or 48 ounces (3 × 16 oz)

+

20 ounces (600 ml) (amount of fluid consumed during exercise)

───

2 hours (number of hours in practice)

=

48 + 20 = 68 ÷ 2 = 34 ounces, or about 1 liter, of fluid required per hour

- Gulp, don't sip.
- Swallow fluids, don't spit.
- Do not overdrink (don't drink more than what your individual sweat rate calculation suggests).

During exercise, especially at all-day competitions, you may feel better drinking sports drinks than drinking water. But be careful with energy drinks. You may think that they help you perform better, but too much caffeine may make you jittery and nervous before competition. In addition, drinks such as Red Bull, Amp, Lizard Fuel, Monster, and Rockstar are high in carbohydrate, which can delay the fluid from leaving your stomach so the fluid is not in your muscles. They are also high in calories!

After exercise, drink enough fluid to make up any loss in weight you have. Drink 24 ounces (700 ml) of fluid for every pound you lose during exercise.

Assess your hydration status the next morning after exercise:

- Did your body weight return to baseline?
- Does your urine look more like lemonade than apple juice?
- Did your thirst subside?

If you answer no to any of these questions, you need to drink more fluid.

Eat Small Meals Often

Eat within one hour of waking up. You need to eat breakfast or your body plays catch-up all day, which means you are tired during practice as well as in class or at work.

If you are trying to make weight, you may want to skip meals, but this often results in overeating at the next meal or being too tired during the day. Instead, eat a small amount every four hours.

Eat 14 to 17 calories per pound, or 30 to 37 kilocalories per kilogram, of body weight if you are a female; 20 to 23 calories per pound, or 44 to 50 kilocalories per kilogram, of body weight if you are a male. Be selective about your food choices to get the most benefit with the fewest calories.

From L. Bonci, 2009, *Sport Nutrition for Coaches* (Champaign, IL: Human Kinetics).

Eat Carbohydrate-Containing Foods for Energy

Carbohydrate is an important fuel source for your muscles and brain during activity and should be part of every meal and snack. One third of what's on your plate should be a starchy food such as rice, pasta, or bread, and one third should be fruits and vegetables.

Good sources of carbohydrate include these:

Bread	Bagels	Pasta	Fruit	Vegetables
Barley	Potatoes	Corn	Pretzels	Tortillas
Pasta	Crackers	Rice	Quinoa	

If you are watching your weight, choose whole-grain foods such as whole-wheat bread, brown rice, oats, and corn and high-fiber items such as fruits and vegetables.

Try to limit these:

Pastries	Chips	Cookies	Pretzels	Fruit drinks
Soda	Ice cream	Crackers	Bagels	Juice
	French fries		Candy	

These foods contain carbohydrate but also contain high amounts of fat, sugar, and calories. Some are difficult to eat in small quantities, such as crackers, chips, cookies, and candy.

Eat Protein for Muscle Growth and a Healthy Immune System

Foods containing protein are important for muscle growth and repair. In addition, protein foods have a higher satiety value; they make you feel full longer so you don't get as hungry between meals. That's why it's important to have some protein at every meal and snack. Try to pick low-fat protein foods to control your calories.

Minimum number of grams of protein a day:

.6 × body weight in pounds, or 1.3 × body weight in kilograms

Maximum number of grams of protein a day:

.9 × body weight in pounds, or 2 × body weight in kilograms

Include some protein as part of every meal and snack:

Eggs	Beef	Nuts	Yogurt	Reduced-fat cheeses
Chicken	Pork	Tofu	Low-fat milk	Fish and shellfish
Turkey	Jerky	Bean dip	Peanut butter	Baked beans

If you are watching your weight, be careful with the amount of nuts or peanut butter you eat, and choose lean meats and low-fat dairy products.

Try to limit these:

Bacon	Sausage	Pepperoni	Whole milk	Full-fat cheeses
Hot dogs	Fried meats			

Although these foods do contain protein, they are also high in fat and especially saturated fat, which is not healthy for the body.

Eat Fat as an Essential Part of Your Diet

Fat is not a major fuel source for you during exercise but is still an essential part of your diet. Foods with fat can help you feel more satisfied longer so you will be less likely to overeat.

Include a small amount of fat in every meal, and don't be fooled by fat-free ice cream, cookies, and crackers. These foods still have a lot of calories, and they don't taste that great either!

Good sources of fat include these:

Nuts	Mayonnaise	Pesto	Olive oil	Safflower oil
Seeds	Nut butters	Olives	Canola oil	Sunflower oil
Guacamole	Avocados	Corn oil	Soybean oil	Soft margarines

Aim for about 1 tablespoon of oil, mayonnaise, soft margarine or pesto at a meal; 2 tablespoons of nut butter or salad dressing; 1/4 cup of guacamole, or 1/8 of an avocado.

Try to limit these:

Creamy	Cream	Lard	Sour cream	Stick margarines
sauces	cheese	Butter	Shortening	Creamy dressings

These foods are sources of fat but primarily of saturated or trans fats, which are not as healthy.

Food Supplements

These are the best supplements to use for your sport:

- Sports drinks (if needed during competition). Consider a low-sugar version to reduce the calories.
- A multivitamin mineral supplement if you are trying to lose weight.
- A low-calorie protein shake or bar (200 calories maximum). This can be a good snack because it is a limited portion.

Eating, Drinking, and Exercise

Follow these guidelines when planning your daily routine.

One Hour Before Practice or Competition

Have any of the following combinations: 20 ounces (600 ml) sports drink with 1/4 cup (35 g) nuts or a few strips of beef jerky; 8 ounces (230 g) fruit-flavored yogurt; 20 ounces (600 ml) water with a package of peanut butter crackers; or 1 cup (30 g) cereal with 4 ounces (120 ml) low-fat milk. If you are a salty sweater, choose a sports drink and pretzels or low-fat crackers.

During Practice or Competition

Drink enough fluid per hour based on your sweat rate.

After Practice or Play

Drink enough to replace sweat losses. Because practices can be long and meets and tournaments can last all day, eat something small or drink something with calories within 15 minutes of finishing, such as the following:

- One small handful of pretzels, crackers, or cereal
- One small handful of trail mix
- A 200-calorie sports bar
- A piece of fruit and a small handful of nuts

From L. Bonci, 2009, *Sport Nutrition for Coaches* (Champaign, IL: Human Kinetics).

Sample Daily Menu

Breakfast

Men

- Two eggs
- One slice whole-grain toast with 1 tsp margarine
- 8 ounces (240 ml) low-fat milk
- One piece of fruit

Women

- One packet of oatmeal made with skim milk
- Small banana
- One plain egg (cooked without oil)
- 8 ounces (240 ml) water

Lunch

Men

- Sandwich on two slices of whole-grain bread: four slices of meat, one slice of cheese
- One piece of fruit
- One handful of crackers, pretzels, or baked chips
- 12 ounces (360 ml) low-fat milk and 12 ounces (360 ml) water

Women

- Sandwich on a whole-grain wrap or small whole-grain pita: three slices of meat
- One small piece of fruit
- One small handful of pretzels, crackers, or baked chips, or a granola or cereal bar
- 8 ounces (240 ml) low-fat milk and 12 ounces (360 ml) water

Dinner

Men

- 8 ounces (225 g) lean meat, poultry, or fish
- 1 cups pasta, rice, or potatoes
- 2 cups vegetables, either cooked or in a salad
- 12 ounces (360 ml) low-fat milk and 8 ounces (240 ml) water

Women

- 5 to 6 ounces (140-170 g) lean meat, poultry, or fish
- 1/2 cup pasta, rice, or potatoes
- 1 1/2 cups vegetables
- 8 ounces (240 ml) low-fat milk and 12 ounces (360 ml) water

Evening Snack

Men

- 8 ounces (230 g) yogurt with 1/2 cup fruit
- 20 ounces (600 ml) water

Women

- 6 ounces (170 g) yogurt and a small piece of fruit or 1/2 cup fruit
- 20 ounces (600 ml) water

From L. Bonci, 2009, *Sport Nutrition for Coaches* (Champaign, IL: Human Kinetics).

Performance Eating for Precision Sports
(Baseball, Softball, Golf)

Drink Enough Fluids

Although you may not think you lose a lot of fluids, your games last a long time, which increases your risk of dehydration. A loss of as little as 2 percent of body weight caused by dehydration can increase fatigue and impair performance! Athletes who drink enough fluid can practice or perform up to 33 percent longer than those who don't drink enough.

Consume at least 90 ounces (2.7 L) of fluid daily. That's 11 cups (8 oz, or 240 ml, per cup) for females, 15 cups for males.

All fluids except alcohol count: coffee, tea, milk, juice, water, soda, and sports drinks as well as fruits, vegetables, soups, gelatin, and fruit ices. Alcohol is a diuretic, which will take fluid away from the body. It can delay recovery from exercise and from injury, and it can impair focus and reaction time as well.

Drink whenever you're dehydrated. You know you are dehydrated if you experience any of the following:

Noticeable thirst
Muscle cramps
Weakness
Impaired performance
Headache

Nausea
Fatigue
Burning in stomach
Dry mouth
Dizziness or lightheadedness

During the Day

Drink

- 16 to 20 ounces (480-600 ml) of fluid within one hour of waking up,
- 20 ounces of fluid with every meal, and
- 16 to 20 ounces with every snack.

For Exercise

Start exercise with some fluid already in your stomach. Drink 20 ounces (600 ml) an hour before exercise—either water or sports drink—and if you haven't eaten before practice or conditioning, choose a sports drink instead of water for the carbohydrate content.

During exercise drink 14-40 ounces (415 ml to 1.2 L) of fluid per hour of exercise. (If you are a light sweater, drink 14 ounces of fluid per hour; if you are a heavy sweater, drink about 40 ounces of fluid per hour.) Golfers, you need to bring fluid with you on the links. Try freezing water or sports drinks bottle so your liquids are cool and more palatable.

Calculate your hourly sweat rate so you know how much fluid you need to drink per hour:

1. Weigh yourself before and after exercise. Wear as little clothing as possible while weighing.

2. Subtract your postexercise weight from your pre-exercise weight, and then convert it to ounces. For example, there are 16 ounces (500 g) in a pound, so if you lose 2 pounds during exercise, you have lost 32 ounces (2 × 16), or 1 kilogram.

3. Add the number of ounces or milliliters of fluid you consumed during practice.

4. Divide the sum of the amount of fluid lost plus amount of fluid consumed by the number of hours you exercised to get your hourly sweat rate.

When you consume fluid during exercise, remember these tips:

From L. Bonci, 2009, *Sport Nutrition for Coaches* (Champaign, IL: Human Kinetics).

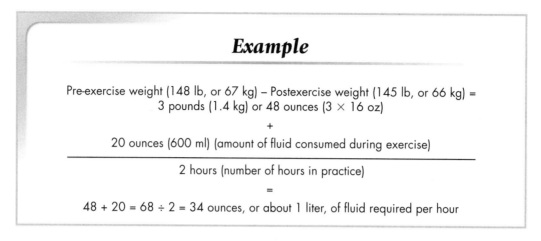

Example

Pre-exercise weight (148 lb, or 67 kg) – Postexercise weight (145 lb, or 66 kg) =
3 pounds (1.4 kg) or 48 ounces (3 × 16 oz)

+

20 ounces (600 ml) (amount of fluid consumed during exercise)

_____

2 hours (number of hours in practice)

=

48 + 20 = 68 ÷ 2 = 34 ounces, or about 1 liter, of fluid required per hour

- Gulp, don't sip.
- Swallow fluids, don't spit.
- Drink, don't pour on your head.
- Do not overdrink (don't drink more than what your individual sweat rate calculation suggests).

During exercise, drinking sports drinks may be better than drinking water. Be careful with energy drinks. You may think that you'll perform better with them, but too much caffeine may make you jittery and nervous before competition. In addition, drinks such as Red Bull, Amp, Lizard Fuel, Monster, and Rockstar are high in carbohydrate, which can delay the fluid from leaving your stomach so the fluid is not in your muscles.

After exercise, drink enough fluid to make up any loss in weight you have. Drink 24 ounces (700 ml) of fluid for every pound you lose during exercise.

Assess your hydration status the next morning after exercise:

- Did your body weight return to baseline?
- Does your urine look more like lemonade than apple juice?
- Did your thirst subside?

If you answer no to any of these questions, you need to drink more fluid.

Eat Small Meals Often

Eat within 1 hour of waking up. You need to eat breakfast or your body plays catch-up all day, which means you are tired during practice as well as in class or at work. Baseball or softball games may end late, which means you may eat late at night and not be hungry when you wake up. It may be a good idea to set your alarm so you can eat something light such as a handful of trail mix, a few peanut butter crackers, or a piece of fruit and a small handful of nuts and then go back to sleep for a few more hours. This way, you won't wake up starved and won't overeat at the next meal.

Try to eat small meals every four hours. Eat 14 to 17 calories per pound, or 30 to 37 kilocalories per kilogram, of body weight if you are a female; 20 to 23 calories per pound, or 44 to 50 kilocalories per kilogram, of body weight if you are a male.

Eat Carbohydrate-Containing Foods for Energy

Carbohydrate is an important fuel source for your muscles and brain during activity and should be part of every meal and snack. One third of what's on your plate should be a starchy food such as rice, pasta, or bread, and one third should be fruits and vegetables.

From L. Bonci, 2009, *Sport Nutrition for Coaches* (Champaign, IL: Human Kinetics).

Good sources of carbohydrate include these:

Bread	Bagels	Pasta	Fruit	Vegetables
Barley	Potatoes	Corn	Pretzels	Tortillas
Juice	Crackers	Rice	Quinoa	

If you are watching your weight, choose whole-grain foods such as whole-wheat bread, brown rice, oats, and corn and high-fiber items such as fruits and vegetables.

Try to limit these:

Pastries	Chips	Cookies	Pretzels	Fruit drinks
Soda	Ice cream	Crackers	Bagels	Juice
	French fries		Candy	

These foods contain carbohydrate but also contain high amounts of fat, sugar, and calories.

Eat Protein for Muscle Growth and a Healthy Immune System

For baseball, softball, and golf, you need to be strong to swing a bat or a club, so one third of what's on your plate at every meal and snack should be protein. Protein will not fuel you while you practice or play but along with carbohydrate will help you to build new muscle. Try to get more of your protein from food than from supplements, because many food sources of protein, such as low-fat chocolate milk, also provide valuable carbohydrate. However, if you do not believe that you get enough protein from food, consider adding a protein isolate, which is a pure protein powder without additives.

Minimum number of grams of protein a day:

.6 × body weight in pounds, or 1.3 × body weight in kilograms

Maximum number of grams of protein a day:

.9 × body weight in pounds, or 2 × body weight in kilograms

Include some protein as part of every meal and snack:

Eggs	Beef	Nuts	Yogurt	Reduced-fat cheeses
Chicken	Pork	Tofu	Low-fat milk	Fish and shellfish
Turkey	Jerky	Bean dip	Peanut butter	Baked beans

If you are watching your weight, be careful with the amount of nuts or peanut butter you eat, and choose lean meats and low-fat dairy products.

Try to limit these:

Bacon	Sausage	Pepperoni	Whole milk	Full-fat cheeses
Hot dogs	Fried meats			

Although these foods do contain protein, they are also high in fat and especially saturated fat, which is not healthy for the body.

Eat Fat as an Essential Fuel for Exercise

Fat is not a fuel source for high-intensity exercise but is still an essential part of your diet. Include a small amount of fat in every meal, but try to limit fat intake before practice and competition because it can upset your gut and delay carbohydrate from reaching your muscles.

Good sources of fat include these:

Nuts	Mayonnaise	Pesto	Olive oil	Safflower oil
Seeds	Nut butters	Olives	Canola oil	Sunflower oil
Guacamole	Avocados	Corn oil	Soybean oil	Soft margarines

Try to limit these:

Creamy sauces	Cream cheese	Lard Butter	Sour cream Shortening	Stick margarines Creamy dressings

These foods are sources of fat but primarily of saturated or trans fats, which are not as healthy.

Add Salt If Necessary

Have you ever noticed salty residue on your skin, clothes, visor, or cap after a workout, or do you tend to develop muscle cramps? Then you may be a salty sweater. If you are a salty sweater, you need to take in more salt. Here are some ways to add salt to your diet:

- Eat salty foods such as pickles and pretzels.
- Use salt, soy sauce, or Worcestershire sauce.
- Use sports drinks instead of water to provide sodium and help replace what is lost through sweating.
- Consider adding salt to a sports drink: Add 1/4 teaspoon of salt to 20 ounces (600 ml) of sports drink or 1/2 teaspoon of salt to 32 ounces (1 L) of sports drink.

Food Supplements

These are best supplements to use for your sport:

- Sports drinks
- Sports bars that have more carbohydrate than protein
- High-sodium foods and beverages if you are a salty sweater
- A protein isolate, such as whey protein or soy protein, if you are not getting enough protein through food

Eating, Drinking, and Exercise

Follow these guidelines when planning your daily routine.

One Hour Before Practice or Competition

Drink

- 20 ounces (600 ml) sports drink with a small handful of nuts or a few strips of beef jerky,
- 12 ounces (360 ml) low-fat chocolate milk or 8 ounces (230 g) fruit-flavored yogurt, or
- 20 ounces (600 ml) water with a handful of pretzels and nuts, or one half of a peanut butter sandwich, or a bowl of cereal.

If you are a salty sweater, choose a sports drink and pretzels or low-fat crackers.

During Practice or Competition

Drink enough fluid per hour based on your sweat rate.

After Practice or Play

Drink enough to replace sweat losses. Eat or drink something with calories within 15 minutes of practice or play, such as the following:

- One handful of pretzels, crackers, or cereal
- One handful of trail mix
- A 200-calorie sports bar
- One piece of fruit and a small handful of nuts
- One granola bar

If you are a salty sweater, eat something salty after exercise such as crackers, pretzels, or Chex mix with salted nuts. Choose a sports drink or tomato or vegetable juice instead of water.

From L. Bonci, 2009, *Sport Nutrition for Coaches* (Champaign, IL: Human Kinetics).

Sample Daily Menu

Breakfast

Men

- 1 cup (240 g) oatmeal with 1/4 cup nuts (35 g), 1/4 cup dried fruit or a large banana, and 8 ounces (240 ml) low-fat milk
- 12 ounces (360 ml) milk or 8 ounces (230 g) yogurt

Women

- 1/2 cup (120 g) oatmeal with 2 tbsp each nuts and dried fruit and 4 ounces (120 ml) low-fat milk
- 8 ounces (240 ml) skim milk or 6 ounces (170 g) low-fat yogurt
- 8 ounces (240 ml) water

Lunch

Men

- Sandwich on a roll: five slices of meat, two slices of cheese
- Piece of fruit
- One handful of crackers, pretzels, or baked chips
- 12 ounces (360 ml) low-fat milk and 12 ounces (360 ml) water

Women

- Sandwich on two slices of bread: three slices of meat, one slice of cheese
- Small piece of fruit
- One small handful of pretzels, crackers, or baked chips, or a granola or cereal bar
- 8 ounces (240 ml) low-fat milk and 12 ounces (360 ml) water

Dinner

Men

- 8 ounces (225 g) lean meat, poultry, or fish
- 2 cups pasta, rice, or potatoes
- 2 cups vegetables, either cooked or in a salad
- 12 ounces (360 ml) low-fat milk and 8 ounces (240 ml) water

Women

- 5 to 6 ounces (140-170 g) lean meat, poultry, or fish
- 1 cup pasta, rice, or potatoes
- 1 1/2 cups vegetables
- 8 ounces (240 ml) low-fat milk and 12 ounces (360 ml) water

Evening Snack

Men

- 1 1/2 cups (45 g) cereal with 1/2 cup fruit and 8 ounces (240 ml) milk
- 20 ounces (600 ml) water

Women

- Yogurt and a piece of fruit
- 20 ounces (600 ml) water

From L. Bonci, 2009, *Sport Nutrition for Coaches* (Champaign, IL: Human Kinetics).

Performance Eating for Stop-and-Go Sports
(Basketball, Lacrosse, Rugby, Field Hockey, Ice Hockey, Soccer)

Drink Enough Fluids

A loss of as little as 2 percent of body weight caused by dehydration can increase fatigue and impair performance! Athletes who drink enough fluid can practice or perform up to 33 percent longer than those who don't drink enough.

Consume at least 90 ounces (2.7 L) of fluid daily. That's 11 cups (8 oz, or 240 ml, per cup) for females, 15 cups for males.

All fluids except alcohol count: coffee, tea, milk, juice, water, soda, and sports drinks as well as fruits, vegetables, soups, gelatin, and fruit ices. Alcohol is a diuretic, which will take fluid away from the body. It can delay recovery from exercise and from injury.

Drink whenever you're dehydrated. You know you are dehydrated if you experience any of the following:

Noticeable thirst	Nausea
Muscle cramps	Fatigue
Weakness	Burning in stomach
Impaired performance	Dry mouth
Headache	Dizziness or lightheadedness

During the Day

Drink

- 16 to 20 ounces (480-600 ml) of fluid within one hour of waking up,
- 20 ounces of fluid with every meal, and
- 16 to 20 ounces with every snack.

For Exercise

Start exercise with some fluid already in your stomach. Drink 20 ounces (600 ml) an hour before exercise—either water or sports drink—and if you haven't eaten before practice or conditioning, choose a sports drink instead of water for the carbohydrate.

During exercise drink 14 to 40 ounces (415 ml to 1.2 L) of fluid per hour of exercise. (If you are a light sweater, drink 14 ounces of fluid per hour; if you are a heavy sweater, drink about 40 ounces of fluid per hour.)

Calculate your hourly sweat rate so you know how much fluid you need to drink per hour:

1. Weigh yourself before and after exercise. Wear as little clothing as possible while weighing.
2. Subtract your postexercise weight from your pre-exercise weight and then convert it to ounces. For example, there are 16 ounces (500 g) in a pound, so if you lose 2 pounds during exercise, you have lost 32 ounces (2 × 16), or 1 kilogram.
3. Add the number of ounces or milliliters of fluid you consumed during practice.
4. Divide the sum of the amount of fluid lost plus amount of fluid consumed by the number of hours you exercised to get your hourly sweat rate.

From L. Bonci, 2009, *Sport Nutrition for Coaches* (Champaign, IL: Human Kinetics).

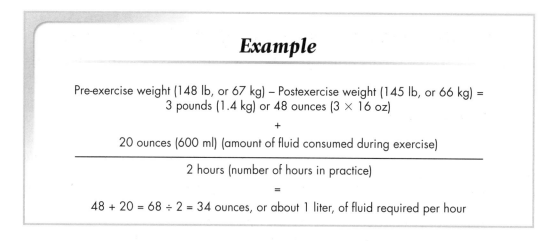

Example

Pre-exercise weight (148 lb, or 67 kg) – Postexercise weight (145 lb, or 66 kg) =
3 pounds (1.4 kg) or 48 ounces (3 × 16 oz)

+

20 ounces (600 ml) (amount of fluid consumed during exercise)

_____

2 hours (number of hours in practice)

=

48 + 20 = 68 ÷ 2 = 34 ounces, or about 1 liter, of fluid required per hour

When you consume fluid during exercise, remember these tips:

- Gulp, don't sip.
- Swallow fluids, don't spit.
- Drink, don't pour on your head.
- Do not overdrink (don't drink more than what your individual sweat rate calculation suggests).

During exercise, drinking sports drinks may be better than drinking water. Be careful with energy drinks. Drinks such as Red Bull, Amp, Lizard Fuel, Monster, and Rockstar are high in carbohydrate, which can delay the fluid from leaving your stomach so the fluid is not in your muscles. Also, the caffeine content of some of these beverages is high.

After exercise, drink enough fluid to make up any loss in weight you have. Drink 24 ounces (700 ml) of fluid for every pound you lose during exercise.

Assess your hydration status the next morning after exercise:

- Did your body weight return to baseline?
- Does your urine look more like lemonade than apple juice?
- Did your thirst subside?

If you answer no to any of these questions, you need to drink more fluid.

Eat Small Meals Often

Eat within one hour of waking up. You need to eat breakfast or your body plays catch-up all day, which means you are tired during practice as well as in class or at work.

Try to eat small meals every four hours. Eat 15 to 20 calories per pound, or 33 to 44 kilocalories per kilogram, of body weight if you are a female; 20 to 27 calories per pound, or 44 to 59 kilocalories per kilogram, of body weight if you are a male.

Eat Carbohydrate-Containing Foods for Energy

Two thirds of what's on your plate at each meal or snack should be carbohydrate-containing foods to fuel your muscles and brain during activity.

Good sources of carbohydrate include these:

Bread	Bagels	Pasta	Fruit	Vegetables
Barley	Potatoes	Corn	Pretzels	Tortillas
Pasta	Crackers	Rice	Quinoa	

Try to limit these:

Pastries	Chips	Cookies	Pretzels	Fruit drinks
Soda	Ice cream	Crackers	Bagels	Juice
	French fries		Candy	

These foods contain carbohydrate but also contain high amounts of fat and sugar.

Eat Protein for Muscle Growth and a Healthy Immune System

A third of what's on your plate at every meal and snack should be protein. Your body needs both carbohydrate and protein to build new muscle. If you eat too much protein, you are probably not eating enough carbohydrate.

Minimum number of grams of protein a day:

.6 × body weight in pounds, or 1.3 × body weight in kilograms

Maximum number of grams of protein a day:

.9 × body weight in pounds, or 2 × body weight in kilograms

Include some protein as part of every meal and snack:

Eggs	Beef	Nuts	Yogurt	Reduced-fat cheeses
Chicken	Pork	Tofu	Low-fat milk	Fish and shellfish
Turkey	Jerky	Bean dip	Peanut butter	Baked beans

Try to limit these:

Bacon	Sausage	Pepperoni	Whole milk	Full-fat cheeses
Hot dogs	Fried meats			

Although these foods do contain protein, they are also high in fat and especially saturated fat, which is not healthy for the body.

Eat Some Fat as an Essential Fuel for Exercise

Include some fat as part of every meal and snack. Good sources of fat include these:

Nuts	Mayonnaise	Pesto	Olive oil	Safflower oil
Seeds	Nut butters	Olives	Canola oil	Sunflower oil
Guacamole	Avocados	Corn oil	Soybean oil	Soft margarines

Try to limit these:

Creamy	Cream	Lard	Sour cream	Stick margarines
sauces	cheese	Butter	Shortening	Creamy dressings

These foods are sources of fat but primarily of saturated or trans fats, which are not as healthy.

Limit the amount of fatty foods you have before exercise, because they can upset your gut!

Add Salt If Necessary

Do you have salty sweat or salty residue on your skin or clothes after a workout or a tendency to develop muscle cramps? Then you may be a salty sweater. If you are a salty sweater, you need to take in more salt. Here are some ways to add salt to your diet:

- Eat salty foods such as pickles and pretzels.
- Use salt, soy sauce, or Worcestershire sauce.

- Use sports drinks instead of water to provide sodium and help replace what is lost through sweating.
- Consider adding salt to a sports drink: Add 1/4 teaspoon of salt to 20 ounces (600 ml) of sports drink or 1/2 teaspoon of salt to 32 ounces (1 L) of sports drink.

Food Supplements

These are best supplements to use for your sport:

- Sports drinks
- Sports bars that have more carbohydrate than protein

Eating, Drinking, and Exercise

Follow these guidelines when planning your daily routine.

One Hour Before Practice or Play

Have 20 ounces (600 ml) of sports drink or 20 ounces (600 ml) of water with a small amount of carbohydrate, such as a handful of pretzels or cereal or a granola bar.

During Practice or Play

Take in 30 grams of carbohydrate per hour by consuming foods such as 16 ounces (480 ml) of sports drink, a gel, a packet of honey, or two honey sticks. Drink enough fluid per hour based on your sweat rate.

After Practice or Play

Drink enough to replace sweat losses. Eat something or drink something with calories within 15 minutes of practice or play, such as the following:

- Two handfuls of pretzels, crackers, or cereal
- Two handfuls of trail mix
- A high-carbohydrate sports bar
- A piece of fruit and a small handful of pretzels
- Two granola bars

From L. Bonci, 2009, *Sport Nutrition for Coaches* (Champaign, IL: Human Kinetics).

Sample Daily Menu

Breakfast

Men

- 1 cup (240 g) oatmeal with 1/4 cup nuts (35 g), 1/4 cup dried fruit or a large banana, and 8 ounces (240 ml) low-fat milk
- 12 ounces (360 ml) milk or 8 ounces (230 g) yogurt
- 8 ounces (240 ml) juice

Women

- 1/2 cup (120 g) oatmeal with 2 tbsp each nuts and dried fruit and 1/2 cup (120 ml) milk
- 8 ounces (240 ml) skim milk or 6 ounces (170 g) low-fat yogurt
- 8 ounces (240 ml) water

Lunch

Men

- Sandwich on a roll: five slices of meat, two slices of cheese
- Piece of fruit
- Two handfuls of crackers, pretzels, or baked chips and two granola bars or a muffin
- 12 ounces (360 ml) milk, juice, or lemonade and 12 ounces (360 ml) water

Women

- Sandwich on two slices of bread: three slices of meat, one slice of cheese
- Small piece of fruit
- One handful of pretzels, crackers, or baked chips, or a granola or cereal bar
- 8 ounces (240 ml) milk, juice, or lemonade and 12 ounces (360 ml) water

Dinner

Men

- 8 ounces (225 g) lean meat, poultry, or fish
- 2 cups pasta, rice, or potatoes
- 2 cups vegetables, either cooked or in a salad
- Fruit or 1 cup (130 g) low-fat ice cream, pudding, frozen yogurt, sherbet, or sorbet
- 12 ounces (360 ml) milk, juice, or lemonade and 8 ounces (240 ml) water

Women

- 5 to 6 ounces (140-170 g) lean meat, poultry, or fish
- 1 cup pasta, rice, or potatoes
- 1 1/2 cups vegetables
- Fruit or 1/2 cup (65 g) low-fat ice cream, pudding, frozen yogurt, or sorbet
- 8 ounces (240 ml) milk, juice, or lemonade and 12 ounces (360 ml) water

Evening Snack

Men

- 2 cups (60 g) cereal with 1 cup fruit and 8 ounces (240 ml) milk
- 20 ounces (600 ml) water

Women

- 1 cup (30 g) cereal with 1/2 cup of fruit and 6 ounces (180 ml) milk
- 20 ounces (600 ml) water

From L. Bonci, 2009, *Sport Nutrition for Coaches* (Champaign, IL: Human Kinetics).

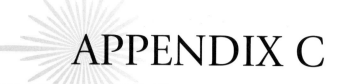

APPENDIX C

Nutrition Screening Form

1. Name:_____

2. Sport:_____

EATING HABITS

3. How would you describe your eating habits? **(Check one)**

    a. ___Good   b. ___Fair   c. ___Poor

4. How many times per day do you eat? _____

5. How many meals per week do you eat at restaurants and fast food places? _____

6. When you eat away from home, what kinds of foods do you choose?

    _____

    _____

    _____

7. If you eat at home, do you eat full meals? ___Yes ___No

    If yes, what types of foods? _____

    If no, what do you do for meals? _____

    _____

8. Who prepares meals at home? _____

9. Who does the shopping? _____

10. Are there foods that you exclude from your diet? **(Check all that apply)**

    If so, why?_____

    a. ___Red meat   b. ___Poultry (chicken, turkey)

    c. ___Fish   d. ___Dairy (milk, cheese)

    e. ___Vegetables   f. ___Fruit

    g. ___Fried food   h. ___Bread

    i. ___Grains (pasta, rice)   j. ___Fast food

    k. ___Sweets (candy, desserts)   l. ___Alcohol

    m. ___Fats and oils (mayonnaise, salad dressings, butter)

11. Have you made any changes to your eating in the past year?

If so, what type of changes? _____

_____

12. Have you tried to lose or gain weight in the past year? ___Yes ___No

If yes, what have you tried to do and how? _____

_____

13. How many glasses of fluid do you normally consume per day? _____

14. In a typical workout, about how many cups of water,
juice, sports drink, milk, soda, tea, or coffee do you drink *before* or *during* exercise? **(Check one)**

a. ___None   b. ___One or two cups

c. ___Three to five cups   d. ___More than five cups

15. Do you currently take any dietary supplements? ___Yes ___No

If yes, which ones? **(Check all that apply** and indicate brand, dose, and frequency of use.)

a.___Creatine   b. ___Protein shakes or powders

c.___Muscle-building supplements   d. ___Sports bars

   (Z-Mass, Meditropin)

e. ___Sports drinks   f. ___Amino acids

g. ___HMB   h. ___NO stimulator

i. ___Glutamine   j. ___Vitamins

k.___Herbs   l. ___Glucosamine or chondroitin

m. ___Pyruvate   n. ___Fat burners

o. ___Prohormones (Hgh, Andro, DHEA)   p. ___ Other_____

Weight History and Body Satisfaction Questions

16. Overall, how satisfied are you with the physical appearance of your body?

(Check one)

a. ___Very satisfied   b. ___Somewhat satisfied

c. ___Somewhat dissatisfied   d. ___Very dissatisfied

17. Do you have any personal goals for body composition? ___Yes ___No

If yes, which ones? **(Check all that apply)**

___Gain lean mass or gain weight

___Decrease body fat

___Lose weight

___Maintain current body composition

___None

18. Do you have weight or percent body fat goals?   ___Yes ___No

  If yes, what is the goal? _____

19. You believe that your body is

  ___fine as is.

  ___slightly overfat.

  ___overly fat.

  ___thin.

  ___too thin.

20. If you could change one thing about your body, what would it be and why?

  _____

21. What is your frame size?   ___small ___medium ___large

22. What is your current weight? _____lb

23. Are you satisfied with being at this weight?   ___Yes ___No

  If not, what would you like to weigh? _____ lb

  Why?_____

24. What was the most you weighed during the past year? _____lb

25. What was the least you weighed during the past year? _____lb

26. Does your weight fluctuate when your sport is in-season?   ___Yes___No

27. Has anyone ever recommended that you lose or gain weight for your sport? If so, which?

  _____

28. Do you avoid certain foods for reasons other than
allergies, intolerances, sensitivities, religious reasons, or dislike?   ___Yes___No

  If yes, why? _____

29. Do you eat at specific times of the day?   ___Yes ___No

30. If your eating times are disrupted, do you get upset or anxious?   ___Yes ___No

31. Do you now or have you ever restricted calories, carbohydrate, or fat?   ___Yes ___No

32. Do you now or have you ever restricted food intake to control your weight?   ___Yes ___No

  If yes, how did or do you restrict your foot intake? (**Check all that apply**)

  ___Cut down on the number of meals and snacks

  ___Eat less at meals

  ___Eliminate certain foods

  ___Other_____

33. Have you every tried to diet during your competitive season?

  ___Never ___Rarely ___Sometimes ___Often ___Always

From L. Bonci, 2009, *Sport Nutrition for Coaches* (Champaign, IL: Human Kinetics).

34. Do you or have you ever dieted in your off-season?

___Never ___Rarely ___Sometimes ___Often ___Always

35. Have you tried any of the following in the past year?

Commercial diets such as NutriSystem and Weight Watchers ___Yes ___No

Fad diets ___Yes ___No

Over-the-counter diet pills ___Yes ___No

Restriction of fluid intake ___Yes ___No

Restriction of carbohydrate intake ___Yes ___No

Restriction of fat intake ___Yes ___No

Restriction of calories ___Yes ___No

Diuretics or water pills ___Yes___No

Laxatives ___Yes ___No

Prescription diet pills __Yes ___No

Fat burners ___Yes ___No

Skipping meals ___Yes ___No

Self-induced vomiting ___Yes ___No

Exercise in addition to that required for sport ___Yes ___No

Nutritional counseling with a dietitian ___Yes ___No

36. What foods do you consider to be safe? **(Please list)**

_____

37. What foods do you consider to be trigger foods or foods you cannot control when you eat them?

_____

38. Do you ever feel guilty after eating?

___Never

___Sometimes

___Most of the time

___Always

39. How often do you think about food and what you eat?

___Never

___Rarely

___Sometimes

___All the time

40. How does exercise affect your appetite?

___I am hungry after exercise.

___I am not hungry after exercise.

___My appetite does not change.

41. Do you make an effort to modify your calorie intake when you don't exercise?

___I don't try to modify my intake.

___I try to eat less.

___I try to eat more.

42. How does exercise affect the amount of food you consume?

___I eat more.

___I eat the same amount.

___I eat less.

43. Do you ever feel that your eating is out of control?   ___Yes ___No

In what way?

___I eat too much.

___I am afraid to eat.

___I eat too little.

44. Do you think you have problems with eating?   ___Yes ___No

If yes, why? _____

_____

From L. Bonci, 2009, *Sport Nutrition for Coaches* (Champaign, IL: Human Kinetics).

APPENDIX D

Answers to Game Plan Questions

Chapter 1

1. Catabolism occurs during exercise because the body needs to break down nutrients to release energy to fuel the muscles. Anabolism can occur with strength training or resistance exercise because they both help build muscle.
2. Carbohydrate and fat.
3. For football, the energy systems used are anabolic and aerobic; for weightlifting, phosphagen and anaerobic.

Chapter 2

1. Carbohydrate is the preferred fuel source for the brain and nervous system as well as the primary fuel source of exercising muscles.
2. The main functions of protein are tissue growth and repair, bone health, and building and maintaining muscles.
3. The athlete will have lower levels of intramuscular triglycerides, which can result in earlier onset of fatigue during activity. Inadequate fat intake can also result in lowered testosterone levels and may adversely affect bone health.

Chapter 3

1. Work with principals, athletic directors, and teachers to establish fueling times in the hour before practice. Stress that your athletes need to eat and drink in the hour before practice for health as well as performance reasons.
2. They should consume at least 50 grams of carbohydrate within 15 minutes.
3. Stick with familiar foods, limit foods that can cause digestive distress, and think about the timing of intake.

Chapter 4

1. Before, during, and after exercise as well as whenever necessary to meet baseline needs.
2. Effects of dehydration include the following:

   Increased heart rate   Increased perceived effort of exertion

   Early-onset fatigue   Decreased ability to sustain attention.
3. They can calculate their sweat rate.
4. Do not drink water to the exclusion of all other fluids. Add salt to the diet in the form of salty condiments or salty foods.

Chapter 5

1. Athletes should consider their body composition, caloric intake, activity levels and caloric expenditure, and eating habits.

2. Calories are expended 24 hours a day. An athlete needs to know how many calories she spends for sport and all other activities so that she can determine how many calories she should eat to lose body fat.

3. Monitoring intake gives a better idea of not only what is consumed but when and how much. A food diary can also identify problem times of the day. Athletes who keep food diaries are more successful in achieving weight goals.

4. Identifying and modifying the rate of eating, manner of eating, volume of food consumed, and thoughts around mealtimes can help an athlete to develop healthy eating habits and to achieve and maintain weight goals.

5. Fad diets are low in calories so they do not provide enough energy for sport, and they are usually low in carbohydrate, protein, or fat, which can affect strength, speed, stamina, and recovery. In addition, these diets are very monotonous and cannot be followed for long periods of time, so the weight lost is usually regained.

Chapter 6

1. Resting metabolic rate, body composition, caloric intake, and energy expended through activity.

2. Lifting weights that are too light, not varying the exercise routine, consuming inadequate protein, and consuming inadequate calories.

3. The scale may not change quickly, but the athlete may notice changes in the size of biceps or pectoral muscles in response to lifting. These changes can be encouraging when the scale does not yield the desired number.

4. Many athletes who are trying to gain weight think that they eat a lot and all the time. A food diary can point out areas to improve upon. Keeping an activity log will help the athlete to see how many calories he expends in a day above and beyond the calories required for sport. This will help an athlete determine the calories needed to gain mass.

5. Supplements are not always effective, can be harmful or performance detracting, can be very costly, and may contain banned substances.

Chapter 7

1. Athletes are attracted to supplements for several reasons:

    Some athletes assume that a supplement provides the edge that food cannot.

    Supplements are easy to use.

    Athletes experience peer pressure to use supplements.

    Athletes think that supplements will provide a quick fix.

2. An athlete should look for one that provides 100 to 250 percent of the daily value for all the vitamins and minerals and that contains the United States Pharmacopeia (USP) symbol, which indicates that the supplement has been tested and reviewed by a U.S. regulatory agency.

3. A supplement policy should be established to keep your athletes safe, lessen your liability for any problems caused by a supplement, prevent overuse of supplements, and prevent use of banned substances.

4. The adverse effects of caffeine overuse include the following:

Rapid heartbeat	Jitters
Increased blood pressure	Anxiety
Insomnia	Inability to focus
Nervousness	Irritability

5. Problems with anabolic steroids include the following:

Growth stunting	Depression
Puffiness	Irritability
Acne	Mood swings
Weakened immune system	Suicidal thoughts

Chapter 8

1. Muscle cramps often occur because of muscle fatigue and overload, inadequate fluid consumption, inadequate sodium intake, and excessive sweat and sodium losses.

2. Main causes of digestive distress include the following:

Food-borne illness	Eating too much before exercise
Jostling during sport	Eating too soon before exercise
Eating unfamiliar foods	

3. Encourage athletes to fuel regularly during exercise, 30 to 60 grams of carbohydrate per hour. Have athletes practice with foods and fluids to determine what is tolerable.

Chapter 9

1. Encourage them to bring nonperishable foods along. Seek out buffets that have options for vegetarians.

2. If blood glucose levels are too high, the risk for dehydration and ketosis increases. If the levels are too low, the athlete may experience dizziness, fainting, and hypothermia.

3. The following foods should be available:

Dextrose or glucose tabs	Pretzels
Peanut butter crackers	Granola bars
Trail mix	Jerky

4. Give the athlete 15 grams of quickly absorbed carbohydrate, and test blood glucose. If the athlete is unconscious, put glucose gel between her cheek and gums and rub until dissolved. If blood glucose levels do not improve, a glucagon injection may be necessary.

5. Advise him to hydrate and fuel before sunrise and after sunset, wake up earlier to start fueling and hydrating, and break the fast as soon as he can.

Chapter 10

1. Athletes are at risk of developing eating disorders because they often have a desire to improve performance by dropping weight; an imbalance between calories consumed and calories expended, which decreases weight; and a fear of failure.

2. Health consequences of an eating disorder include the following:

   Anemia   Musculoskeletal injuries

   Amenorrhea   Gastrointestinal distress

3. An eating disorder can affect an athlete's performance in several ways:

   An athlete with an eating disorder is probably dehydrated.

   The athlete consumes inadequate calories to fuel the body for sport.

   The athlete has an increased risk of stress fractures.

   The athlete has delayed wound healing.

   The athlete may experience an increase in anxiety.

4. During a one-on-one meeting, remind the athlete that her place on the team or in the program will not be jeopardized. Reassure her that eating disorders are treatable.

5. Strategies to create a positive food environment include the following:

   Have a positive body image.

   Make good nutrition a priority for your athletes.

   Administer a preseason screening questionnaire.

   Ask athletes to complete a food log.

   Talk about nutrition in team meetings.

   Invite a sports dietitian to address the team.

Chapter 11

1. Alcohol must be discussed because it can impair performance, can adversely affect health, can have dangerous consequences, and can have legal consequences, especially in underage drinkers.

2. Performance consequences of alcohol consumption include the following:

   Delayed reaction time   Delayed recovery from injury

   Slower recovery   Hypothermia

   Poor concentration   Dehydration

3. Several strategies can be used:

   Ask athletes to complete a questionnaire that asks about alcohol use.

   Use the DISCUS tool kit.

   Dispel myths surrounding alcohol.

   Set a team policy.

   Have a mandatory meeting of athletes and parents in which you discuss alcohol policy.

Chapter 12

1. Traveling can affect athletes' food and beverage consumption in several ways:

   Altered sleep schedules   Changes in availability and accessibility

   Dehydration   of familiar foods

   Food safety issues   Skipped meals

2. Working with the food service staff is an effective way to develop creative and cost-effective solutions for feeding athletes and to ensure that athletes actually eat what is prepared.

3. Provide parents with a list of appropriate snacks for travel, ask them to provide snacks for practice and pregame meals, and appoint one to be the food scout.

Chapter 13

1. The packing list should include gallons of water, powdered sports drinks and lemonade mixes, peanut butter, packets of tuna and chicken, and trail mix.

2. To reduce food costs at restaurants, do not order a la carte, take advantage of early-bird special pricing, buy larger items and do your own portioning, and order family style.

3. There are many ways to get team parents and booster clubs to help with the food budget:

   Impose a food fee for each athlete.

   Consider establishing a food fund for athletes with financial hardships.

   Ask parents to help with the cooking or serving.

   Encourage every parent to find a way to contribute in some way.

Chapter 14

1. Dietitians, nutritionists, and sports dietitians have different credentials and areas of focus.

   • A *dietitian* is an expert in food and nutrition who works with patients on the nutritional management of health conditions.

   • A *nutritionist* may or may not be a dietitian and does not necessarily possess the clinical expertise in nutrition or food.

   • A *sports dietitian* is a registered dietitian with additional certification in sport nutrition and expertise in working with athletes.

2. Reliable sport nutrition information is available through various organizations:

ADA	American Dietetic Association
SCAN	Sports, Cardiovascular, and Wellness Nutrition
NATA	National Athletic Trainers' Association
ACSM	American College of Sports Medicine
NCAA	National Collegiate Athletic Association

3. You can persuade athletes and parents to buy in by taking the following actions:

   Make everyone accountable.

   Give parents a job on the team related to nutrition.

   Remind athletes of the consequences for not being fueled and hydrated.

   Reward athletes who take care of their bodies.

GLOSSARY

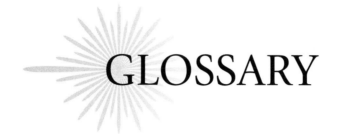

adenosine triphosphate (ATP)—A high-energy compound that is the cell's fuel source for muscle contraction, relaxation, and repair.

aerobic system—Energy system that fuels longer-duration activity and requires oxygen.

alcohol—An intoxicating fluid found in beer, wine, and liquor that can have adverse effects on the body and brain.

alcohol-related liver disease—Disease caused by alcohol consumption, resulting in cirrhosis or liver scarring.

amenorrhea—Absence of a menstrual period.

amino acids—Building blocks of protein.

anabolic steroids—Steroids are natural or synthetic substances that regulate body function. Anabolic steroids are compounds that mimic the effect of testosterone to promote tissue growth, especially increases in muscle mass; they are illegal, unless prescribed for a metabolic condition such as stunted growth. They can increase muscle mass and decrease body fat, but they can also have harmful physical and psychological side effects.

anabolism—The part of metabolism whereby something is synthesized or built, such as muscle mass.

anaerobic system—Energy system that provides fuel for bursts of activity and does not use oxygen.

anaphylaxis—A very severe allergic response where the throat swells in response to ingestion of the allergen.

anorexia—An eating disorder characterized by self-starvation resulting from an intense fear of becoming fat and body image distortion.

banned substance—Product that is not allowed in sporting organizations because it is harmful, may impair performance, or confers an unfair advantage.

binge eating disorder—An eating disorder characterized by periods of overconsumption of food.

blood glucose—Amount of glucose available in the blood. It is influenced by food consumed, physical activity levels, and insulin.

body composition—The ratio of fat mass (body fat) to lean or fat free mass (water, muscle, bone, organs) expressed as percent body fat to percent lean body mass.

bulimia—An eating disorder characterized by overconsumption of high-calorie foods (binge) followed by compensatory behavior to get rid of the calories (fasting, excessive exercise, laxative, diuretic or diet pill use, or vomiting) (purge).

caffeine—A stimulant found in coffee beans, tea leaves, and cocoa beans. In small amounts, caffeine can increase mental alertness and may improve performance, but it can be detrimental in large quantities.

carbohydrate—Macronutrient that is the primary source of energy for the body; includes sugars, starches, and dietary fibers.

carbohydrate loading—Increasing stored carbohydrate through an increase in intake (carbohydrate foods) and decrease in output (exercise) to delay fatigue during endurance exercise.

catabolism—The part of metabolism whereby something is broken down, such as the breakdown of protein to amino acids.

complete proteins—Proteins that contain all of the essential amino acids.

creatine—Creatine is synthesized in the liver, pancreas and kidneys from the amino acids glycine, arginine, and methionine commonly found in meat, poultry, and fish. The muscle converts creatine to phosphocreatine for ATP production for highly intense, short-term exercise. Creatine is a cell volumizer that causes the muscles to hold water and may also increase muscle mass.

creatine phosphate (CP)—Energy-rich compound that provides phosphate to form ATP.

daily energy expenditure—Calories burned through physical activity and all other activities such as personal hygiene and basic body functions.

dehydration—State in which the body is in negative fluid balance because it has lost too much fluid; it can adversely affect health and performance.

diabetes (types 1 and 2)—A disorder of glucose metabolism. Type 1 is characterized by the inability of the pancreas to produce insulin, the hormone that regulates blood glucose. In type 2, insulin is produced but in insufficient quantities. In both cases, blood glucose levels are higher than they should be, which can be harmful to the body.

Dietary Reference Intakes (DRIs)—Nutrition recommendations from the Institute of Medicine of the National Academies of the United States. The DRIs include average requirements and Recommended Dietary Allowances (RDAs; amounts considered adequate for healthy people) or Acceptable Intakes (AIs; amounts considered to pose no significant health risk).

disordered eating—Spectrum of abnormal or harmful eating behaviors undertaken for the purpose of altering body composition, as a coping mechanism, or as a means of exerting control.

diuretic—Substance that increases fluid loss through increased urination.

eating disorders not otherwise specified (EDNOS)—Clinical eating disorders that meet some but not all the criteria for anorexia or bulimia.

electrolyte—One of the three minerals—sodium, potassium, or chloride—that dissolve into charged particles or ions that are used by the cell to regulate the electric charge and flow of water molecules across cell membranes.

energy drinks—Beverages that contain caffeine and carbohydrate; they are often consumed with alcohol for "recreational" purposes.

essential amino acids—Amino acids (the building blocks of protein) that the body cannot make and must be supplied through food.

essential fatty acids—Fatty acids that the body requires but cannot make and must be supplied through food.

fat (lipids)—Macronutrient made of fatty acids; provides energy to the athlete during endurance exercise.

fat burners—Supplements marketed to help the body burn fat, such as ephedra and synephrine. Most of these are ineffective, and some can have stimulant effects that stress the heart.

fatty acids—Building blocks of fat. There are three types: saturated, monounsaturated, and polyunsaturated.

female athlete triad—The presence of undereating, low bone density, and amenorrhea that can occur across a spectrum of severity in female athletes.

food allergy—An autoimmune response in which the body is allergic to the protein in food, resulting in physical symptoms ranging from digestive distress to skin rashes or hives.

food intolerance—An inability to digest a particular food or food component.

glucose—Sugar found in the blood; also a component of carbohydrate.

gluten—The protein in wheat, rye, barley, and oats.

glycemic index—The effect that a carbohydrate-containing food has on blood glucose levels.

glycogen—Storage form of carbohydrate in the muscle and liver.

glycolysis—Breakdown of glycogen to yield glucose to fuel the body during exercise.

hitting the wall or bonking—Condition that occurs when glycogen use is greater than intake, resulting in fatigue.

hyperglycemia—High blood glucose levels.

hypoglycemia—Low blood glucose levels.

hyponatremia—State of low blood sodium levels that occurs in response to the following: excessive water intake, excessive sweat loss, excessive sodium loss, inadequate sodium intake, or some combination of these behaviors.

hypothermia—Low core body temperature.

incomplete proteins—Proteins that do not supply all of the essential amino acids.

ketosis—High concentration of ketone bodies (free fatty acids released from storage to be used as fuel) in the blood and body tissues.

lactate—Substance produced when there is insufficient carbohydrate available. High levels can cause fatigue during exercise.

lactate threshold—Point during exercise when muscle lactate levels rise above resting level resulting in early onset fatigue.

lactose—Milk sugar.

metabolic rate—Rate at which the body uses calories at rest.

metabolism—Chemical reactions in the body that result in energy production and utilization.

minerals—Inorganic compounds that are necessary to regulate body processes. They are divided into major and trace minerals.

monounsaturated fat—A fat with one double bond; may lower the risk of heart disease.

muscle-mass enhancers—Substances marketed to increase muscle mass. Most are ineffective at increasing muscle mass or strength.

orthorexia—Eating disorder characterized by an unhealthy obsession with healthy eating.

phosphagen system—Energy system that fuels muscles for highly intense, very short-term activities.

potassium—Mineral that is important to regulate fluid balance and assist in muscle contractions.

protein—Macronutrient composed of amino acids that is involved in cell functions and supports muscle growth and repair.

protein powders—Concentrated sources of protein derived from milk, egg, or soy protein. Some have vitamins, minerals, and herbs added.

reactive hypoglycemia—Low blood sugar that occurs about one to four hours after eating a carbohydrate-rich food; attributable to overproduction of insulin and a subsequent rapid decrease in blood glucose.

replete—Replace fuel sources after exercise.

salty sweater—Someone who loses a lot of salt in the sweat and may be at increased risk for muscle cramping.

saturated fat—A fat that is completely filled with hydrogen; may increase the risk of heart disease.

seasonal eating disorders—Restrictive eating behaviors used to make weight; seen in weight-class sports but only when the athletes are in their competitive season.

sodium—Mineral that speeds rehydration, replaces sweat loss, and improves fluid absorption.

sport nutrition game plan—A comprehensive education and action plan to address fueling, hydration, timing, supplements, weight, and substance abuse.

sports dietitian—A registered dietitian with additional credentialing and expertise in working with athletes.

supplements—Substances used in addition to food to alter body composition or improve performance. They can be vitamins, minerals, protein powders, gels, drinks, pills, or herbs.

trans fat—Polyunsaturated fat with hydrogen on opposite sides of the chain; may increase heart disease risk.

triglyceride—A fat that is composed of three fatty acids and glycerol (glyceride).

unsaturated fat—Fat with more than one double bond, such as omega-3 and omega-6 fats; lowers the risk of heart disease.

vegan—A person who consumes no animal products.

vegetarian—A person who excludes some animal products.

vitamins—Organic compounds necessary for growth and body processes. They are divided into fat- or water-soluble vitamins and are needed in very small amounts.

BIBLIOGRAPHY

ACSM Position Stand on Exercise and Fluid Replacement. *Med Sci Sports Exerc.* 2007;Vol 39 (2):377-390.

American Diabetes Association. Position Statement. Diabetes Mellitus and Exercise. Diabetes Care. 2002;25:S64

American Psychiatric Association. *Diagnostic and Statistical Manual of Mental Disorders.* 4th ed. Washington, DC: American Psychiatric Association; 1994.

Beals KA. *Disordered Eating Among Athletes. A Comprehensive Guide for Health Professionals.* Champaign, IL: Human Kinetics; 2004.

Bentley S. Exercise induced muscle cramp: proposed mechanisms and management. *Sports Med.* 1996;21:409-420.

Bergeron MF. Heat cramps: fluid and electrolyte challenges during tennis in the heat. *J Sci Med Sport.* 2003;6:19-27.

Byrne S, McLean N. Eating Disorders in athletes: A review of the literature. *J Sci Med Sport.* 2001;4:145-159.

Candow DG, Chilbeck PD, Burke DG, Davidson KS, Smith-Palmer T. Effect of glutamine supplementation combined with resistance training in young adults. *Eur J Appl Physiol.* 2001;86:142-149.

Casa D. Proper hydration for distance running: identifying individual fluid needs. A USA Track & Field advisory. *USA Track and Field.* April 2003.

Casa DJ, Armstrong LE, Hillman SK, et al. National Athletic Trainers' Association Position Statement: fluid replacement for athletes. *J Athl Train.* 2000;35:212-224.

Castillo EM, Comstock RD. Prevalence of use of performance enhancing substances among US adolescents. *Pediatr Clin North Am.* 2007;54:663-675.

Chao YM et al. *International Journal of Eating Disorders,* news release, Nov. 19, 2007.

Clark N. *Nancy Clark's Sports Nutrition Guidebook.* 4th ed. Champaign, IL: Human Kinetics; 2008.

Colberg S. *The Diabetic Athlete.* Champaign, IL: Human Kinetics; 2001.

Council on Scientific Affairs. American Medical Association. Caffeine labeling. *JAMA.* 1984. Aug 10; 252(6): 803-6.

Dorfman L. *The Vegetarian Sports Nutrition Guide.* New York: Wiley; 2000.

Food and Nutrition Board, Institute of Medicine, National Academies. *Dietary Reference Intakes (DRIs): Recommended Intakes for Individuals, Vitamins.* Washington, DC: National Academy of Sciences; 2004.

Froiland K, Koszewski W, Hingst J, Kopecly L. Nutritional supplement use among college athletes and their sources of information. *Int J Sports Nutr Exerc Metab.* 2004;14:104-120.

Grant BF, Dawson DA. Introduction to the National Epidemiologic Survey on Alcohol and Related Conditions. 2006. *Alcohol Research and Health.* Vol 79(2): 74-78.

Hallberg L, Rossander-Hulten L, Brune M, Gleerup A. Calcium and iron absorption: mechanism of action and nutritional importance. *Eur J Clin Nutr.* 1992, May;46(5): 317-27

Hartgens F, Kulpers H. Effects of androgenic-anabolic steroids in athletes. *Sports Med.* 2004;34:513-554.

Havala S. *The Vegetarian Food Guide and Nutrition Counter.* New York: Penguin; 1997.

Heaney RP, Recker RR, Hinders SM. Variability of calcium absorption. *Am J Clin Nutr.* 1988;47:262-4.

Institute of Medicine of the National Academies. *Dietary Reference Intakes: Water, Potassium, Sodium, Chloride, and Sulfate.* Washington, DC: National Academies Press; 2004.

Ivy JL, Goforth HW Jr, Dumon BM, McCauley TR, Parsons EC, Price TB. Early postexercise muscle glycogen recovery is enhanced with a carbohydrate-protein supplement. *J Appl Physiol.* 2002;93:839-846.

Johnston LD, O'Mlley PM, Bachman JG, Schulenberg JE. *Monitoring the future: national survey results on drug use, 1975-2007. Vol 1. Secondary School students.* NIH Pub No 08-6418-A. Bethesda, MD. National Institute on Drug Abuse. 2008. P. 26

Jonnalagadda SS, Rosenbloom CA, Skinner R. Dietary practices, attitudes, and physiological status of college freshman football players. *J Strength Cond Res.* 2001;15:507-513.

Jung AP, Bishop PA, Al-Nawwas A, Dale RB. Influence of hydration and electrolyte supplementation on incidence and time to onset of exercise-associated muscle cramps. *J Athl Train.* 2005;40:71-75.

Karp JR, Johnston JD, Tecklenburg S, Mickleborough TD, Fly AD, Stager JD. *Int J Sport Nutr Exerc Metab.* 2006;16:78-91.

Kleiner S, Kester K. *The Be Healthier, Feel Stronger Vegetarian Cookbook.* New York: Wiley; 1997.

Lambert MI, Hefer JA, Millar RP, et al. Failure of commercial amino acid supplements to increase serum growth hormone concentrations in male body-builders. *Int J Sport Nutr.* 1993;3:298-305.

Laos C, Metzl JD. Performance enhancing drug use in young athletes. *Adolesc Med Clin.* 2006;17:719-731.

Larson-Meyer DE. *Vegetarian Sports Nutrition.* Champaign, IL: Human Kinetics; 2007.

Levenhaugen DK, Carr C, Carlson MG, Maron DL, Borel MJ, Flakoll PJ. Postexercise protein intake enhances whole-body and leg protein accretion in humans. *Med Sci Sports Exerc.* 2002;34:828-837.

Levenson DI, Bockman RS. A review of calcium preparations. *N Engl J Med.* 1985;313:70-73.

Maravelias C, Dona A, Stefanidou M, Spilliopoulou C. *Toxicol Lett.* 2005;158:167-175.

Moses FM. The effect of exercise on the gastrointestinal tract. *Sports Med.* 1990;Mar 9(3):159-172.

Nawrot P, Jordan S, Eastwood J, Rotstein J, Hugenholtz A, Feeley M. Food Additives and Contaminants. 2003. Vol 20(1): 1-30.

National Athletic Trainers' Association (NATA). Position statement: fluid replacement for athletes. *J Athl Train.* 2000:35:212-224.

O'Dea JA. Consumption of nutritional supplements among adolescents: usage and perceived benefits. *Health Educ Res.* 2003;18:98-107.

Otis CL, Drinkwater B, Johnson M, Loucks A, Wilmore JH. American College of Sports Medicine position stand. The female athlete triad: Disordered eating, amenorrhea and osteoporosis. *Med Sci Sports Exerc.* 1997;29:i-ix.

Passe DH, Horn M, Murray R. Impact of beverage acceptability on fluid intake during exercise. *Appetite.* 2000;35:219-329.

Peters HP, DeVries WR, Vanberge-Henegouwen GP, Akkermans LM. Potential benefits and hazards of physical activity and exercise on the gastrointestinal tract. *Gut.* 2001;48:435-439.

Pope HG, Phillips KA, Olivardia R. *The Adonis Complex: The Secret Crisis of Male Body Obsession.* New York: Simon & Schuster; 2000.

Position of the American Dietetic Association, Dietitians of Canada, and the American College of Sports Medicine; Nutrition and Athletic Performance. *J Am Diet Assn.* 2000;100:1543-1556.

Rockwell, MS, Seldmand S. Body composition measurement: A tool of use, not abuse. *SCAN's PULSE* (Newsletter of the American Dietetic Association). 2002;21(3):9-11.

Rosen LW, McKeag DB, Hough DO, Curley V. Pathogenic weight control behavior in female athletes. *Phys Sportsmed.* 1988;14:79-95.

Schwellnus MP, Derman EW, Noakes TD. Aetiology of skeletal muscle "cramps" during exercise: a novel hypothesis. *J Sport Sci.* 1997;15:277-285.

Scofield DE, Unruh S. Dietary supplement use among adolescent athletes in central Nebraska and their sources of information. *J Strength Cond Res.* 2006;20:452-455.

Stover EA, Petrie HJ, Passe D, Horswill CS, Murray R, Wildman R. Urine specific gravity in exercisers prior to physical training. *Appl Physiol Nutr Metab.* 2006;31:320-327.

Stover EA, Zachwieja J, Stofan J, Murray R. Consistently high urine specific gravity in adolescent American football players and the impact of an acute drinking strategy. *Int J Sports Med.* 2006; Apr 27(4):330-5.

Sundgot-Borgen J, Torstviet MK. Prevalence of eating disorders in elite athletes is higher than the general population. *Clin J Sport Med.* 2004;14:25-32.

Thompson RA, Sherman RT. *Helping Athletes With Eating Disorders.* Champaign, IL: Human Kinetics; 1993.

U.S. Department of Health and Human Services and U.S. Department of Agriculture. *Dietary Guidelines for Americans, 2005.* 6th ed. Washington, DC: U.S. Government Printing Office; January 2005.

Varnier M, Leese GP, Thompson J, Rennie MJ. Stimulatory effect of glutamine on glycogen accumulation in human skeletal muscle. *Am J Physiol Endocrinol Metab.* 1995;269:E309-E315.

Willoughby DS. Effects of an alleged myostatin binding supplement and heavy resistance training on serum myostatin, muscle strength and mass, and body composition. *Int J Sports Nutr Exerc Metab.* 2004;14:461-472.

Yaspelkis BB, Ivy JL. The effect of carbohydrate-arginine supplement on postexercise carbohydrate metabolism. *Int J Sports Nutr.* 1999;9:241-250.

Zanker CL, Swaine IL, Castell LM, et al. Responses of plasma glutamine, free tryptophan and branched chain amino acids to prolonged exercise after a regime designed to reduce muscle glycogen. *Eur J Appl Physiol.* 1997;75:543-548.

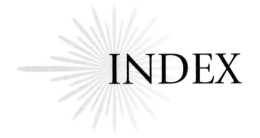

INDEX

Note: The italicized *f* and *t* following page numbers refer to figures and tables, respectively.

A

Acceptable Intakes (AIs) 102
activity logs 60*f*, 61*f*, 85*f*, 86*f*
adenosine triphosphate (ATP) 4-5
Adonis Complex, The (Pope) 148
aerobic system 5-6, 7*t*
air-displacement plethysmography 59
AIs 102
alcohol-related liver disease 167
alcohol use
       athlete contracts 169, 170*f*
       drug interactions 166
       educating athletes 164
       hydration and 49, 53
       hypoglycemia and 142, 143, 165
       long-term effects 166-167
       myths 168, 168*t*
       one-drink equivalents 169*f*
       short-term effects 165-166
       talking about 167-168
       team policies 169
       underage drinking 164
all-day events 42
amenorrhea 150-151*t*, 153
American Dietetic Association 158, 194
amino acids 21. *See also* protein
amino acid supplements 106, 125
anabolic steroids. *See* steroids
anabolism 4
anaerobic system 5, 7*t*
anaphylaxis 143
anorexia 149. *See also* disordered eating
answers to game plan questions 241-245
aristolochic acid 109
Arnolds 111
artificial sweeteners 16, 17*t*
Athletes Training and Learning to Avoid Steroids
    (ATLAS) 112
ATP 4-5

B

balance 10. *See also* food choices
banned substances 95, 95*t*, 96, 108, 109-113, 111*t*, 112*t*

beta-hydroxy-beta-methyl butyrate (HMB) 108
beverage choices. *See also* alcohol use; caffeine; hydration
       caloric intake and 71
       cutting cost of 186, 188
       dehydration and 48-49
       for hydration 49-50, 53, 124
BIA testing 58
binge eating disorder 149. *See also* disordered eating
bioelectrical impedance (BIA) testing 58, 83*t*
bitter orange 108
blank forms
       activity logs 61*f*, 86*f*
       blood glucose monitoring form 140*f*
       body changes chart 88*f*
       drug and alcohol agreement 170*f*
       food diaries 65*f*, 91*f*
       food frequency form 27*f*
       food pattern form 66-67*f*
       nutrition screening form 236-240
       supplement and medication form 110*f*
       weight contract 75*f*
blood glucose levels
       controlling 142-143
       monitoring 138, 139*f*, 140*f*
BMI 58, 83
BOD POD 59, 83*t*
body changes chart 88*f*
body composition
       assessment of 58-59, 83, 83*t*
       foods to meet goals 179
body fat, reducing. *See* weight loss
body image issues 156
body mass index (BMI) 58, 83
bonking 126
booster clubs 187
boron 108
budgets 186-188
bulimia 149. *See also* disordered eating

C

caffeine
       beverage content 107*t*
       combined with alcohol 166

caffeine *(continued)*
>hydration and 49, 53
>hypoglycemia and 143
>side effects 106-108
calcium 105, 124, 134
calories
>in carbohydrate 11
>expenditure calculation 59-62, 59*t*, 60*f*, 61*f*, 62*f*, 84-85, 84*t*, 85*f*, 86*f*
>in fat 17
>inadequate 155-156, 156*t*
>in protein 21
>for weight gain 89
carbohydrate
>calories per gram 11
>as energy source 5, 11-12
>during exercise 126, 141, 142*f*
>50-gram choices 43*t*
>food sources 13*t*, 92*t*
>for hypoglycemia 138, 141, 141*f*
>low-carb foods 12, 16, 125
>in meal plan example 14
>molecular structure 11, 11*f*
>pre-exercise 36
>recommended intake 12-13, 30-33
>simple vs. complex 11, 12*t*
>weight loss and 70
carbohydrate loading 37, 38
carbonated beverages 49, 124
catabolism 4
Certified Specialist in Sports Dietetics (CSSD) 193
Certo 125
chapparal 109
chromium 108
citrus aurantium 74, 108
comfrey 109
complementary proteins 131-132
complete proteins 22, 131-132
constipation 125
cooking lessons 180
creatine phosphate (CP) 4-5
creatine supplements 95*t*, 105-106, 125
CSSD 193

D
dehydration. *See also* hydration
>contributing factors 48-49
>disordered eating and 157
>effects 48
>GI distress and 122-124
>making weight and 72, 152
dehydroepiandrosterone (DHEA) 108
DEXA 58, 83*t*
DHEA 108
diabetes
>blood glucose control 142-143
>blood glucose monitoring 138, 139*f*, 140*f*
>exercise and 137-138
>fueling during exercise 141, 142*f*
>hydration and 141
>hypoglycemia in 137-142
>survival kit 141, 143
>types and characteristics 136-137
diarrhea 123, 125
Dietary Reference Intakes (DRIs) 102
Dieter's Tea 109, 125

dietitians 77, 158, 193-194
diets. *See* special diets; weight loss
DISCUS tool kit 167-168
disordered eating
>body image issues 156
>educating athletes 155-156
>in female athlete triad 152-155
>help for 157-158
>incidence rates 148
>nutrition screenings for 155
>parents and 158
>performance protocols 158, 159*f*, 160*f*
>risk factors 148-149
>signs of 150-151*t*, 152
>talking about 157
>types 149-152
diuretics 49, 53
DRIs 102
drug and alcohol policy agreement 169, 170*f*. *See also* alcohol use
drug-free environment 111-112
Drug Free Sport 112
dual-energy X-ray absorptiometry (DEXA) 58, 83*t*

E
eating disorders not otherwise specified (EDNOS) 149. *See also* disordered eating
eating habits and styles 67-69, 68*f*
eating schedules 177-178. *See also* timing of food intake
EDNOS 149. *See also* disordered eating
electrolytes 49-50, 113*t*, 121
energy availability 152
energy drinks 49, 106-108, 107*t*, 125, 166
energy expenditure 59-62, 59*t*, 60*f*, 61*f*, 62*f*, 84-85, 85*f*, 86*f*
energy production 4-6
energy systems 4-6, 7*t*
engineered foods 12, 25, 113*t*. *See also specific types*
Ephedra 74, 101*t*, 108
ephedrine 108
epinephrine 143
Epi-pen 143
epitonin 108
Epovar 109
essential amino acids 21. *See also* protein
essential fatty acids 17, 136
evening events 41
event day eating 39-42

F
fad diets 72, 73*t*
fast food 39-40, 68
fasts, religious 144
fat burner supplements 74, 108
fat-burning foods 70
fats (lipids)
>calories per gram 17
>as energy source 5
>food sources 20*t*, 92*t*
>functions 17
>inadequate 154
>in meal plan example 21
>molecular structure 17, 18*f*
>recommended intake 20, 30-33
>types 18, 19*t*
>weight loss and 71 (*See also* weight loss)
fat-soluble vitamins 102

fatty acids 17, 136
female athlete triad 152-155
fiber 11, 12t, 36, 123
fig bars 125
fish oil supplements 125
fluid intake. *See* hydration
food allergies 143
food-borne illness 122
food budgets 186-188
food choices
     assessment of 26f, 27f
     female athlete's guide 30-31
     food ratings for 29t
     for gaining weight 90, 92t
     goals for 28
     male athlete's guide 32-33
food diary
     nutrition screening 155
     weight gain 89, 90f, 91f
     weight loss 62-64, 64f, 65f
food frequency form 26f, 27f
food intake assessment. *See also* food choices; timing of
    food intake
     weight gain 89, 90f, 91f
     weight loss 62-69, 64f, 65f, 66-67f
food intolerances 143
food patterns 64-67, 66-67f
fructose 11, 43
fruit 43
fruit juice 49
fueling. *See* timing of food intake
FUEL protocol 159f, 160f
Furanone di-hydro 109

G
GAKIC 109
galactose 11
gamma butyrolactone (GBL) 109
gamma hydroxy butryone (GHB) 109
gamma-oryzanol 108
gastrointestinal distress 36, 122-125
GBL 109
gels 42, 113t
germander 109
GHB 109
ginger 101t, 125
glucagon injections 141
glucose 5-6, 11. *See also* blood glucose levels
glutamine 109
gluten sensitivity 143
glycemic index 13-16, 15t, 37, 38t
glycogen 5-6, 11, 126, 142
glycolysis 5
glycolytic system (anaerobic) 5, 7t
Good Gut Travel Kit 125
gym candy 111

H
herbal teas 125
hitting the wall 126
HMB 108
honey sticks 42, 113t
human growth hormone 108
hydration. *See also* dehydration
    beverage choices 49-50, 53, 71
    diabetics and 141

encouraging athletes 53
excessive 51
GI distress and 124
guidelines 50-52, 50t
sweat rate and 51-52
hydrostatic weighing 58-59, 83t
Hydroxycut 108
hyperglycemia 137, 138
hypoglycemia
    alcohol use and 165
    bonking and 126
    diabetes and 137, 138-142
    glycemic index and 37
hyponatremia 51, 124
hypothermia 137

I
immune system 178
incentives 198
incomplete proteins 22, 131-132
institutional food 178-180
iron 105, 124, 134-135

J
juice (slang term) 111

K
ketosis 137

L
lactate 5
lactate system (anaerobic) 5, 7t
lactate threshold 5
lactose 11, 11f, 143
liquid meals 36-37
liver disease, alcohol-related 167
low-carbohydrate foods 12, 16, 125

M
magnesium 124
ma huang 74, 108
maltose 11, 11f
medications 110f, 112-113, 166
meditropin 109
metabolic rate 59, 59t, 84, 84t
metabolism 4
microhydrin 109
midday events 41
minerals and mineral supplements
    as acceptable supplement 113t
    GI distress and 124
    muscle mass and 96
    types and requirements 103-105, 103t, 104t
    in vegetarian diets 133-134, 134-135t
moderation 10
monitoring body changes chart 88f
monounsaturated fat 18, 19t, 20
Mormon's tea 108
morning events 41
multivitamins. *See* vitamins and vitamin supplements
muscle cramps 120-122
muscle mass, increasing
    action plan 87-89
    beverage choices 49
    energy expenditure and 84-85, 84t, 85f, 86f
    food choices 90, 92t

muscle mass, increasing *(continued)*
    food intake assessment 89, 90*f*, 91*f*
    goals 88-89, 88*f*
    mistakes 96
    physical assessments 82-83, 83*t*
    requirements 82
    strategies 86-87, 92-94
    supplements 94-96, 95*t*, 108
    while losing body fat 69
muscle-mass enhancers 94-96, 95*t*, 108
myostatin blockers 95*t*, 108
MyPyramid Tracker 61, 62*f*, 85

N
Nancy Clark's Sports Nutrition Guidebook 180
nandrolone 96
natural vs. *safe* 113
net carbohydrate 16
nitric oxide stimulators 101*t*, 108
Nutrition Facts Panel 22, 22*f*, 89
nutrition screening form 236-240

O
off-season nutrition 176-177, 177*f*
omega-3 fatty acids 18, 136
orthorexia 149. *See also* disordered eating

P
parents 158, 187, 195
performance eating handouts
    endurance sports 204-209
    football 210-214
    high-intensity sports 215-219
    precision sports 225-230
    stop-and-go sports 231-235
    weight- and physique-focused sports 220-224
phosphagen system 4-5, 7*t*
physical assessments
    muscle mass increase 82-83, 83*t*
    preparticipation physical evaluation 196-197*f*
    weight loss 57-59
plant sitosterols 95*t*, 108
plums, dried 125
polyunsaturated fat 18, 19*t*, 20
Pope, Harrison 148
postexercise eating 42-43, 42*f*, 43*t*
potassium 121, 124
pre-event eating 38-40
pre-exercise eating 36-37, 124, 124*t*
preparticipation physical evaluation 196-197*f*
preseason meeting 155, 195
protein
    athlete type and 23*t*
    calories per gram 21
    complete vs. incomplete 22, 131-132
    cost comparison by source 114*t*
    as energy source 6
    excessive 96
    food budgets and 186, 188
    food sources 21-22, 23*t*, 92*t*, 114*t*, 133*t*
    functions 21
    getting enough 24-25
    inadequate 154
    in meal plan example 24
    molecular structure 21

    postexercise 43
    recommended intake 22-24, 23*t*, 30-33
    in vegetarian diets 131-133, 133*t*
    weight loss and 70
protein powders 25, 95*t*, 106, 113*t*, 125
prunes (dried plums) 125
pumpers 111
pyramid 111

R
Ramadan 144
RDAs 102
reactive hypoglycemia 142-143
recipes 40, 180
Recommended Dietary Allowances (RDAs) 102
recovery foods 179, 179*f*
Red Line 108
religious diets or fasts 144
restaurant dining guidelines 201-203
restaurants 39-40, 182, 182*f*, 188
Rest-Eze 109
resting metabolic rate (RMR) 59, 59*t*, 84, 84*t*
Ripped Fuel 108
RMR 59, 59*t*, 84, 84*t*
roid rage 111

S
SALT 52, 122
salty sweaters 52, 121
saturated fat 18, 18*f*, 19*t*, 20
scale weight 57-58, 69, 72
SCAN 194
schedules and eating 177-178
school cafeterias 178-180
seasonal eating disorders 152. *See also* disordered eating
shotgunning 111
sida cordifolia 108
skinfold calipers 58, 83*t*
Smoothie Recipe 40
snack coaches 40, 44
snacks, portable 40, 41, 181*f*, 186-187
sodium 50, 52, 120-122
sodium bicarbonate 125
special diets
    diabetic or hypoglycemic 136-143
    food allergies or intolerances 143
    religious diets or fasts 144
    vegetarian and vegan 130-136
Sports, Cardiovascular Disease, and Wellness Nutrition
    (SCAN) 194
sports bars 113*t*, 125
sports beans 113*t*
sports dietitians 193-194
sports drinks
    as acceptable supplement 113*t*
    cutting costs of 186
    diabetics and 141
    for hydration 49-50, 122
    for travel 125
sports nutrition game plan
    creating 192-193
    incentives 198
    information presentation 195
    parents in 195
stackers 111